Clinical Problem Solving in Periodontology & Implantology

Commissioning Editor: Alison Taylor
Development Editor: Carole McMurray
Project Manager: Caroline Jones
Designer/Design Direction: Miles Hitchin
Illustration Manager: Jennifer Rose

CLINICAL **PROBLEM SOLVING** IN PERIODONTOLOGY AND IMPLANTOLOGY

SERIES

FIRST EDITION

Clinical Problem Solving in Periodontology & Implantology

Edited by

Francis J. Hughes
Professor of Periodontology,
King's College London Dental Institute and Honorary Consultant in Restorative Dentistry,
Guy's & St. Thomas' NHS Trust,
London, UK

Kevin G. Seymour
Professor of Periodontology,
School of Dentistry,
The University of Manchester,
Manchester, UK

Wendy Turner
Senior Clinical Lecturer and Honorary Consultant in Restorative Dentistry,
Institute of Dentistry,
Barts and the London School of Medicine and Dentistry, QMUL

Shakeel Shahdad
Consultant in Restorative Dentistry,
Barts Health NHS Trust and Honorary Clinical Senior Lecturer
Institute of Dentistry,
Barts and the London School of Medicine and Dentistry,
London, UK

Francis Nohl
Consultant in Restorative Dentistry and Honorary Clinical Senior Lecturer,
University of Newcastle-upon-Tyne,
Newcastle, UK

CHURCHILL LIVINGSTONE

ELSEVIER

Edinburgh London New York Oxford Philadelphia St Louis Sydney Toronto 2013

CHURCHILL
LIVINGSTONE
ELSEVIER

ISBN 978-0-7020-3740-5
Reprinted 2012, 2013, 2014

British Library Cataloguing in Publication Data
A catalogue record for this book is available from the British Library

Library of Congress Cataloging in Publication Data
A catalog record for this book is available from the Library of Congress

Notices
Knowledge and best practice in this field are constantly changing. As new research and experience broaden our understanding, changes in research methods, professional practices, or medical treatment may become necessary.

Practitioners and researchers must always rely on their own experience and knowledge in evaluating and using any information, methods, compounds, or experiments described herein. In using such information or methods they should be mindful of their own safety and the safety of others, including parties for whom they have a professional responsibility.

With respect to any drug or pharmaceutical products identified, readers are advised to check the most current information provided (i) on procedures featured or (ii) by the manufacturer of each product to be administered, to verify the recommended dose or formula, the method and duration of administration, and contraindications. It is the responsibility of practitioners, relying on their own experience and knowledge of their patients, to make diagnoses, to determine dosages and the best treatment for each individual patient, and to take all appropriate safety precautions.

To the fullest extent of the law, neither the Publisher nor the authors, contributors, or editors, assume any liability for any injury and/or damage to persons or property as a matter of products liability, negligence or otherwise, or from any use or operation of any methods, products, instructions, or ideas contained in the material herein.

The publisher's policy is to use **paper manufactured from sustainable forests**

Printed in China

Last digit is the print number: 10 9 8 7 6 5 4 3

Contents

Preface

Students of periodontology typically have to master a range of specific diagnostic skills and clinical procedures and have to have a sound knowledge of the underlying disease processes, but in our experience they sometimes struggle particularly to master the clinical judgement required to make positive clinical decisions for diagnosis, treatment planning, and treatment execution. In this book, we describe the fundamentals of the practise of the subject and particularly illustrate the decision-making processes involved in the practise of periodontology in a clear and rational way.

The book is intended particularly for the undergraduate student, but we hope that it will also be useful for general dentists and postgraduate students embarking on further training in periodontology and implant dentistry. We have organized the book into three main sections: Periodontal Assessment and Diagnosis, Periodontal Treatment, and Introduction to Dental Implantology. We are particularly pleased to include Section 3 as a primer on the principles of the practice of dental implantology because this subject has rapidly become an important part of the specialty of periodontology, even though in many cases this subject has not traditionally been part of the undergraduate curriculum in periodontology. Authors FJH, WT, and KGS co-wrote Sections 1 and 2 of the book, FN wrote Chapters 16–18, and SS wrote Chapters 19–22.

We have adopted a problem-solving approach to coverage of the subject matter with the hope that this will have real clinical relevance that will be of continuing practical use for the reader. Therefore, the principles we wish to emphasise throughout the book are illustrated extensively with real clinical cases. In a few chapters, such as Chapter 4, we have strayed slightly from this approach in order to ensure appropriate coverage of the material we wish to emphasise. We have deliberately avoided the use of references in the text because we did not consider it to be appropriate for a book in this format, but we do provide a short list of selected further reading at the end of the book, which we hope will be useful and informative. The absence of references in the text does not, however, suggest that we reject the ideas of evidence-based practice—basing clinical decision making on the best available evidence. We also recognise that as further evidence becomes available, some of the ideas contained in the book will evolve or change markedly over time.

A case-orientated approach to description inevitably means that not all scenarios can be described in depth because all patients will have unique requirements, aspirations, expectations, and outcomes. Thus, we have also made extensive use of summary tables that we hope will underline the essential principles in solving specific problems. We are aware that students particularly like to use tables as easy ways of learning for the purpose of examinations, but we are confident that the reader will also recognise that although tables are very useful, they usually represent an oversimplification of problem-solving approaches to specific patient requirements.

The essential takeaway message from this is our wish that the clinical problem-solving process is based on positive decisions made by the clinician. For example, it is not unusual within our clinical practice to see patients who have been subjected to repeated unsuccessful nonsurgical treatment rounds for periodontitis without any active consideration of the reasons for this and what might be the appropriate management to rectify the situation. To paraphrase Albert Einstein, why would you expect to repeat the same procedure and expect a different outcome? If this book helps the clinician first to understand the principles of treatment and, most important, to make active decisions during treatment, then we will be very happy.

We are indebted to many people in writing this book. First, our sincere thanks to our patients who have unselfishly (and often enthusiastically) consented for us to publish their clinical records and photos here. Second, to our friends and colleagues who have generously allowed us to use some of their own clinical cases. These include Drs Eilis Lynch, Eleni Rizou, Paul Ryan, Sharan Sidhu, John Whitworth, and Emiliano Zanaboni. We are also grateful to Alison Taylor and Carole McMurray at Elsevier for encouraging and cajoling us from conception to completion of this project! Finally, we thank our partners and families for their support and encouragement and for tolerating the late nights working that inevitably seem to be involved in completing a project like this.

FJH
FN
KGS
SS
WT

Section 1

Periodontal assessment and diagnosis

Chapter 1

Periodontal assessment

Introduction

Periodontal diseases manifest themselves in the majority of the adult population. Therefore, it is mandatory that all patients presenting to a general practitioner, regardless of the first impressions made of their periodontal health, are screened to identify those at risk of periodontal disease who will need a more comprehensive assessment prior to making an appropriate diagnosis. A failure to assess the periodontal health of a patient in any routine dental examination is potentially a negligent omission.

An assessment of the clinical signs and symptoms along with the medical history generally form the basis for establishing the diagnosis and assessing the severity of periodontal disease. From the first visit, the clinician should make an overall appraisal of the patient, including taking a full history. This will subsequently need updating at every visit, and certain historical information is crucial for both the diagnosis and to form the background for developing the most appropriate treatment plan for the individual patient.

What factors in the dental history might indicate periodontal disease is present?

Often, patients are unaware that they have periodontal problems, which may cause significant symptoms only at a relatively late stage when teeth become loose or painful. It is common for patients to complain that their gums bleed, particularly on brushing or flossing; however, many patients accept this as being a normal occurrence and not an indicator that more significant disease is present. As disease progresses, particular concerns may be conveyed that teeth are becoming loose, gaps are opening up, and the teeth are becoming uneven or the gum is receding. This may make the patient particularly anxious about losing teeth or about their appearance.

The patient may also have pain, which can present in a variety of ways, from a dull pain after eating or on chewing to a more acute pain of short duration particularly after cold food or drinks.

A dental history should aim to address the following areas:

- How long has the patient been aware of the problem? Has the nature of the symptoms changed and does anything either relieve these symptoms or make them worse?
- Has the patient been a regular attendee, and has he or she received regular hygiene as part of this? In particular, if the patient has been having regular periodontal treatment, it is important to elicit if this has been comprehensive (i.e., subgingival debridement over several visits and if local anaesthesia was used), when it was last performed, and whether the patient felt any improvement as a result of the treatment. This may allow a more accurate picture to be formed of how the individual has responded to previous regimes when considering the possible treatment options.
- The patient's oral hygiene should be noted, including toothbrushing frequency and type of brush (powered or manual), if interdental brushes or floss are used daily, and type of toothpaste or any other oral hygiene aids (e.g., mouthwash type, interdental brushes, or water jet).
- If the patient had previous fixed or removable orthodontic treatment, the approximate dates of this should be noted. This might be of particular relevance if there are areas of gingival recession because certain tooth movement in the presence of thin bony and gingival architecture may need to be considered.
- If bleeding gums were one of the initial complaints, specific questions should be asked regarding if this is an occasional problem or whether it happens during each brushing, while eating, or even spontaneously.
- Is there a family history of periodontal problems? Specifically ask the patient whether he or she is aware of any immediate family members who have lost teeth through gum disease or have received regular periodontal treatment (rather than a routine scale and polish) at a young age (<40 years).

What is the relevance of a patient's medical history to his or her periodontal care?

Many aspects of a patient's medical history may be particularly relevant to his or her periodontal care. These are discussed further in subsequent chapters but may include the following:

- Medical problems can increase susceptibility to periodontal diseases (e.g., diabetes and HIV) and may, in whole or in part, explain the particular clinical presentation and disease severity.
- Medical problems can have periodontal and other oral manifestations (e.g., leukaemia and mucocutaneous disorders).
- Prescribed and nonprescribed medications can have oral and periodontal side effects (e.g., calcium channel blocker or phenytoin).

- Is periodontal infection a risk factor for systemic diseases or conditions that affect overall health? There is emerging scientific data on the association of periodontal disease with common systemic medical problems such as cardiovascular disease, stroke, diabetes, osteoporosis, and low-birth-weight infants. Future targeted anti-inflammatory therapies for patients with periodontal disease may modulate inflammation and, hence, lower risk for systemic conditions.
- Particular existing or previous medical conditions or medications may need specific precautions to be taken to avoid complications during or after treatment (e.g., antibiotic prophylaxis and patients on certain medications such as anticoagulants or bisphosphonates).
- Treating certain conditions may present additional risk to the dental team (e.g., communicable diseases) and may alter the way treatment is provided (e.g., not using ultrasonic instrumentation to avoid producing aerosol).

Why is it necessary to take a social history?

A social history should include details of habits such as tobacco use, including smokeless tobacco (see Table 1.1 for effects on periodontal health), and alcohol consumption. A smoking history should include not only whether patients are current smokers but also if they have smoked in the past, when they quit smoking, how many they smoked or are smoking now, and whether are they interested in quitting.

A social history may also give information about the patient's occupation that is both useful for interacting with the patient and may indicate specific dental issues (e.g., wind instrument player and importance of aesthetics in a job). It can also provide information about the patient's ability to attend appointments regularly and identify issues such as stress in a patient's life.

Table 1.1 Effects of smoking on periodontal health

Clinical findings	Less inflammation and bleeding on probing due to vasoconstriction within the gingivae that can mask the presence of periodontal disease Increased prevalence and severity of periodontitis with deeper probing depths and attachment loss related to amount and duration of smoking Two- or three-fold increase in vertical alveolar bone loss Increased rate of attachment loss Increased tooth loss
Microbiology	Tobacco smoke is selectively bactericidal and causes changes in the microflora Increased levels of periodontal pathogens in shallower and deeper periodontal pockets *F. nucleatum* ss *vincentii*, *P. intermedia*, *P. micros*, *P. nigrescens*, *B. forsythus*, *P. gingivalis*, *T. denticola*
Immunology	Reduced gingival crevicular fluid (GCF) Increases in TNF-α, MMP-8, and PGE_2 in GCF due to exposure of macrophages to nicotine Nicotine has depressive effect on the chemotaxis, phagocytosis, and migration of neutrophils in the gingival crevice—therefore a compromised immune function

Clinical periodontal examination

The examination should start with a general extra- and intraoral examination of the soft tissues, temporomandibular joint (TMJ), and lymph nodes to look at the mouth and surrounding tissues as a whole.

The periodontal tissue examination should be systematic, starting with an appraisal of gingival colour and contour, oral hygiene, and aesthetics. Oral hygiene and gingival inflammation can be measured in a number of ways using both full mouth scoring systems and partial scoring systems (Table 1.2), which act as a relatively objective way of scoring plaques present over time and reflect a patient's compliance with the oral hygiene instruction given. Objective measurements of plaque and bleeding are required to be able to measure and record changes in oral hygiene over time and are useful motivational tools as positive feedback for patients. The full mouth plaque and bleeding score is commonly used because it records the mesial, distal, buccal, and palatal/lingual surfaces of all the teeth present (Figure 1.1) in a dichotomous score (plaque present/absent). The graphical representation can act as a useful aid to the patient to illustrate and map out areas on which he or she needs to focus. Partial scoring systems often use Ramfjord teeth (Figure 1.2), which are considered to be a valid representation of full mouth scoring, particularly for epidemiological purposes. The main advantage of partial scoring indices is that they can be performed very rapidly; however, they fail to provide relevant site-specific information about plaque

Table 1.2 Examples of partial and full mouth plaque scoring indices

Full plaque recording system	Partial plaque scoring system
Plaque score (O'Leary)	Plaque index (Löe and Silness)
	Debris index (Grace and Smales)
	Turesky plaque index

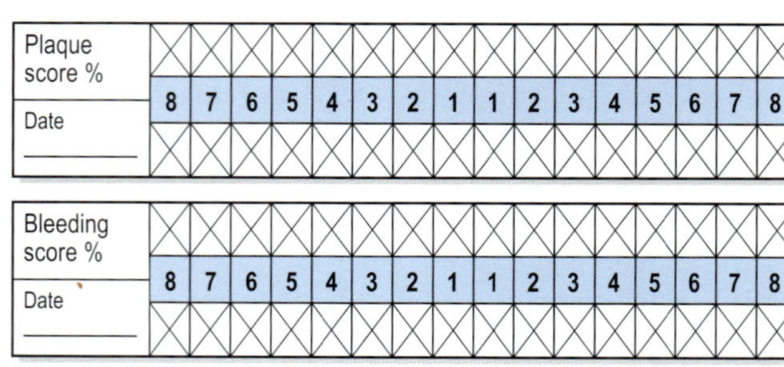

Fig 1.1 Plaque and bleeding scores.

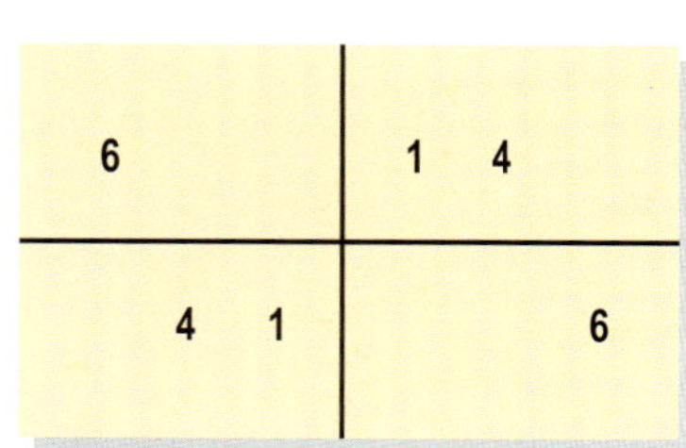

Fig 1.2 Ramfjord teeth are used as a representation of the full mouth for evaluation of plaque (FDI notation: 16, 21, 24, 36, 41, 44).

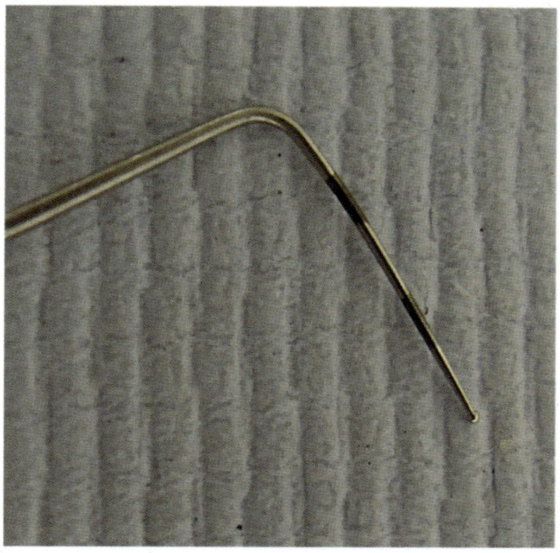

Fig 1.3 The WHO-C (clinical) probe. The key elements of this probe are a ball end with a 0.5-mm diameter, a black band at 3.5–5.5 mm, and a second black band at 8.5–11.5 mm.

and bleeding distribution. Plaque scoring is much more accurate if it is carried out after disclosing the patient.

What are the methods for screening for periodontal disease?

Periodontal screening for epidemiological study of the treatment needs of populations was developed and introduced in 1978 by the World Health Organization as the Community Periodontal Index of Treatment Needs (CPITN). Subsequent modification and development of CPITN for use as a periodontal screening method in general dental practice to identify "risk patients" has occurred. The Basic Periodontal Examination (BPE), developed in the United Kingdom and widely used throughout Europe, is an example of this and is very similar to the Community Periodontal Index and Periodontal Screening and Recording indices used worldwide. The BPE is a simple and rapid screening tool that is used to indicate the level of examination needed and to provide basic guidance on treatment need.

Employing a screening tool for periodontal disease is useful because with experience it can be carried out very rapidly (1 or 2 min) and therefore implemented for all patients. Because the majority of patients seen in a general practice setting may not have established periodontitis, a screening method allows the rapid identification of those with periodontal disease who will require more detailed periodontal assessment.

What do I need to carry out a BPE and how often should it be recorded?

A special probe called the WHO probe is required, and the key features are described in Figure 1.3. The BPE should be carried out on all new patients:

- For patients with codes 0, 1, or 2, the BPE should be recorded at least annually.
- For patients with BPE codes of 3 or 4, more detailed periodontal charting is required.

Table 1.3 BPE scoring codes

0	No pockets >3.5 mm, no calculus/overhangs, no bleeding after probing (black band completely visible)
1	No pockets >3.5 mm, no calculus/overhangs, but bleeding after probing (black band completely visible)
2	No pockets >3.5 mm, but supra- or subgingival calculus/overhangs (black band completely visible)
3	Probing depth 3.5–5.5 mm (black band partially visible, indicating pocket of 4 or 5 mm)
4	Probing depth >5.5 mm (black band entirely within the pocket, indicating pocket of 6 mm or more)
*	Furcation involvement

From The Basic Periodontal Examination. The British Society of Periodontology (2011). Download guidance document from www.bsperio.org.uk

BPE cannot be used to assess the response to periodontal therapy because it does not provide information about how sites within a sextant change after treatment. To assess the response to treatment, probing depths should be recorded at six sites per tooth pre- and post-treatment.

How do I record a BPE screening examination?

- The dentition is divided into six sextants: upper right (17 to 14), upper anterior (13 to 23), upper left (24 to 27), lower right (47 to 44), lower anterior (43 to 33), and lower left (33 to 37). NB third molars are not included for scoring.
- All teeth in each sextant are examined (with the exception of third molars) in adults.
- For a sextant to qualify for recording, it must contain at least two teeth. (If only one tooth is present in a sextant, the score for that tooth is included in the recording for the adjoining sextant.)
- The probe should be "walked around" the sulcus/pockets of each tooth in each sextant and the depth of insertion of the WHO probe read against the black band and the highest score recorded.
- Scores are recorded as 0, 1, 2, 3, 4, or * (Table 1.3).
- As soon as a code 4 is identified in a sextant, the clinician may then move directly to the next sextant, although it is better to continue to examine all sites in the sextant. This will help to gain a fuller understanding of the periodontal condition and will ensure that furcation involvements are not missed. If a code 4 is not detected, then all sites should be examined to ensure that the highest score in the sextant is recorded before moving to the next sextant.
- The scores are recorded in a grid, with the following being a typical example:

4	3	4*
3*	2	–

Is the BPE used for children and teenagers?

The BPE described previously was designed for adults, so a modified version is focused on fully erupted index teeth in children and teenagers, which are the first permanent molars—the maxillary right central incisor and the mandibular left central incisor.

How would I score a sextant where there are no probing depths greater than 5 mm but the furcation is detected?

Both the BPE code and the * should be recorded for each sextant where furcation involvement is found; for example, the score for this sextant would be 3*.

Can I probe around implants?

Peri-implantitis can create pockets around implants, so probing should include implants as part of the periodontal assessment. To prevent scratching of implant surfaces, a plastic periodontal probe can be used.

How do I interpret the BPE scores to reflect the treatment needs of an individual patient?

Interpreting the BPE score depends on many factors that are unique to each patient. The clinician should use his or her skill, knowledge, and judgement when interpreting BPE scores. General guidance is indicated in Table 1.4.

What are the limitations of the BPE?

The BPE-type screening is recognized worldwide and is a simple and rapid way of differentiating those patients who have periodontal health or gingivitis from those who have periodontitis. It is not a sufficiently detailed periodontal examination for patients who have significant periodontal disease because it does not give tooth- and site-specific information within a sextant or information on potential disease activity. In addition, it is not sufficiently discriminating to allow per- and postoperative comparisons of sites to evaluate treatment outcomes. Other limitations are illustrated in the following cases.

Table 1.4 Interpretation of BPE scores

Score	Interpretation
0	No indication for periodontal therapy
1	Oral hygiene instruction (OHI)
2	OHI, removal of plaque retentive factors (calculus, etc..)
3	OHI, root surface debridement
4	OHI, root surface debridement, assess the need for more complex treatment and referral to a specialist may be indicated
*	OHI, root surface debridement, assess the need for more complex treatment and referral to a specialist may be indicated

From British Society of Periodontology (2011).

Case 1

A 31-year-old patient presented as shown in Figure 1.4A complaining of intermittent bleeding of her gums, gum swelling, and difficulty in keeping her teeth clean. She had a noncontributory medical history and had been a reasonably regular dental attendee. On examination, there were visible plaque deposits on her teeth, and a full mouth plaque score was recorded as 72%.

Her BPE score was

3	3	3
2	3	2

Radiographs showed less than 10% crestal bone loss from the cement–enamel junction.

◇ ***Why are the BPE scores inconsistent with the minimal attachment loss experienced?***

The BPE scores of 3 show that the black band of the WHO probe is partly visible, indicating a pocket of 4 or 5 mm. True periodontal pockets result from the apical migration of the junctional epithelium following loss of connective tissue (alveolar bone and periodontal ligament). In this case, the increased probing depth is likely due to false pocketing (where there is no loss of connective tissue) due to inflammation resulting in swelling and fibrosis of the gingivae as a result of poor plaque control.

Case 2

A 55-year-old male returned for a routine recall appointment 6 months after receiving a course of periodontal therapy (Figure 1.4B).

On initial examination pre-periodontal therapy, the BPE scores were

4*	3	3*
4*	2	3*

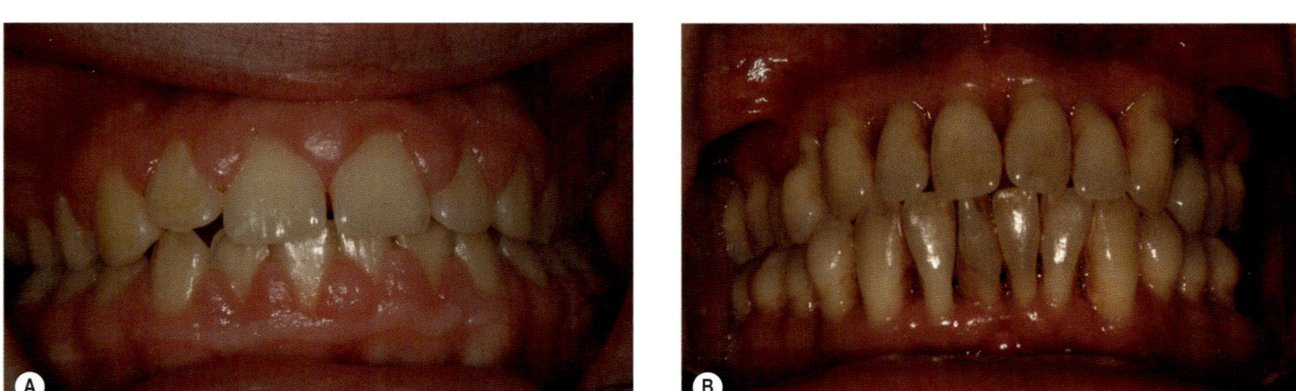

Fig 1.4 (A) Case 1; (B) Case 2.

On recall post-therapy, the BPE scores had not changed.

◇ ***Why did the BPE scores at recall not show any improvement?***

The BPE cannot be used to monitor disease due to the lack of detail within each sextant. This patient may well have had a good response to treatment on an individual site level, but this is not reflected in the global BPE score for each sextant. The * scores reflect that a tooth in that sextant has furcation involvement and is unlikely to change despite nonsurgical periodontal therapy. In this case, following the BPE scores of 3 and 4 at initial presentation, a full 6-point probing depth chart, bleeding on probing, and recession should have been recorded along with areas of furcation involvement and any tooth mobility.

Comprehensive periodontal assessment

As detailed previously, any patient with BPE scores of 3, 4, or * should have a full periodontal assessment carried out to record the following:

- Periodontal probing depths and gingival recession are recorded around six sites per tooth using a calibrated periodontal probe. The probe should be introduced to the base of the sulcus using a probing force of 20–25 g and walked around the tooth circumference. Periodontal probing is carried out at six sites around each tooth—mesiobuccal, mid-buccal, distobuccal, mesiolingual, mid-lingual, and distolingual—and recorded as a 6-point pocket chart. Various types of probes are available (Figure 1.5), and some are designed to standardize the pressure applied to improve consistency of measurements (Figure 1.6).
- Gingival recession is measured from the cement–enamel junction to the gingival margin and probing depth from the gingival margin to the base of the periodontal pocket. Gingival recession can be severe on some teeth, leading to exposure of root surfaces and furcations (Figure 1.7).
- Bleeding on probing is simultaneously recorded with the periodontal pocket charting and indicates inflammation is present within the periodontal pocket. The absence of bleeding on probing is a reliable indicator of periodontal stability in nonsmokers because non-inflamed sites rarely bleed.
- Suppuration (Figure 1.8) indicates the presence of pus within a periodontal pocket and can be determined clinically by placing a finger below the gingival margin and using pressure toward the crown of the tooth.
- Furcation involvement occurs when attachment loss has occurred between the roots of a multirooted tooth and can be examined using specially designed probes (e.g., Nabers probe; Figure 1.9).

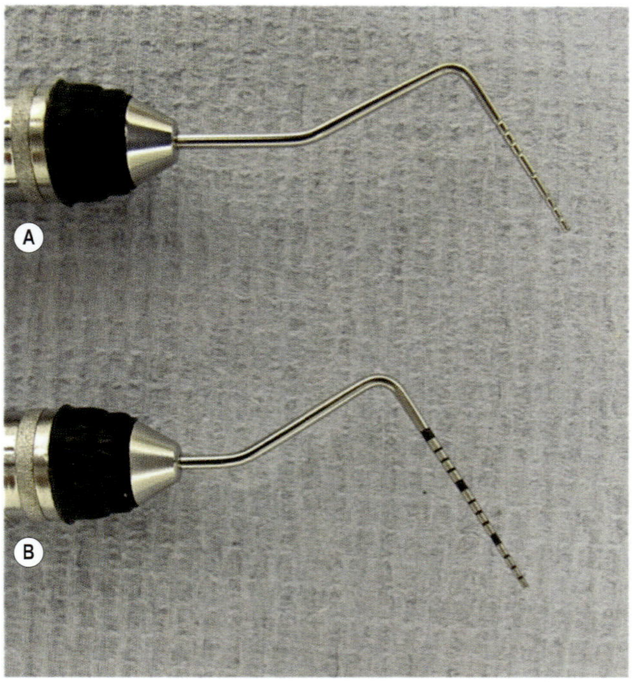

Fig 1.5 (A) Periodontal probe with Williams markings at 1, 2, 3, 5, 7, 8, 9, 10 and (B) UNC probe with 1, 2, 3, black band 4–5, 6, 7, 8, black band 9–10, 11, 12, 13, black band 14–15.

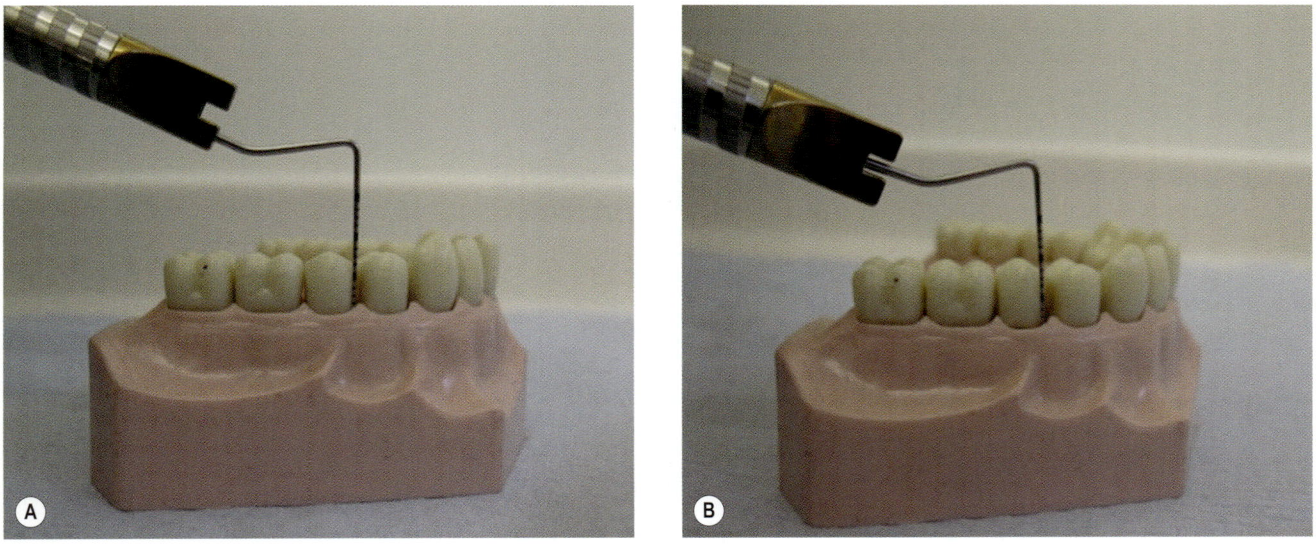

Fig 1.6 The Chapple constant force periodontal probe. (A) The probe is placed in the pocket and (B) the correct force is applied when the probe is aligned with the centre of the handle.

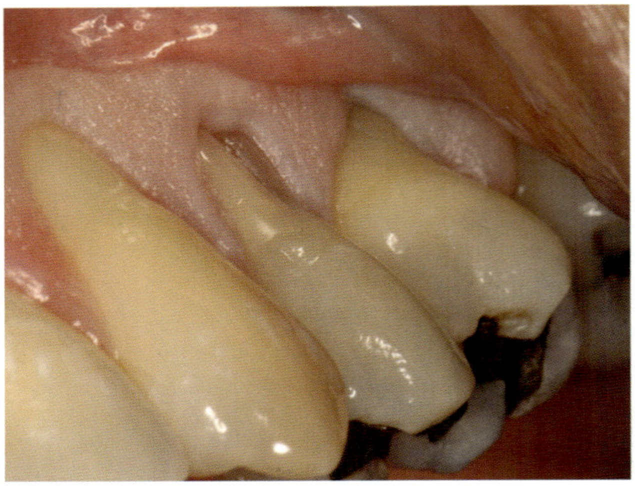

Fig 1.7 Severe gingival recession involving UL5 and UL6 and the furcation area in both teeth can be visualized.

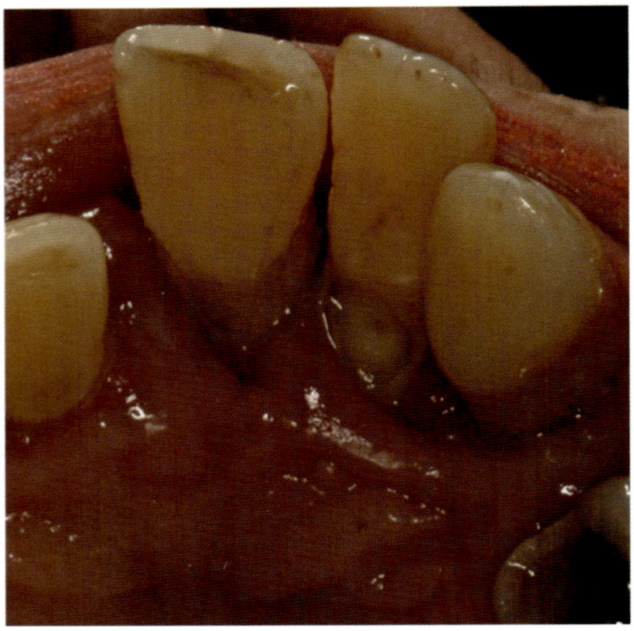

Fig 1.8 Suppuration from the periodontal pocket palatal to UL1.

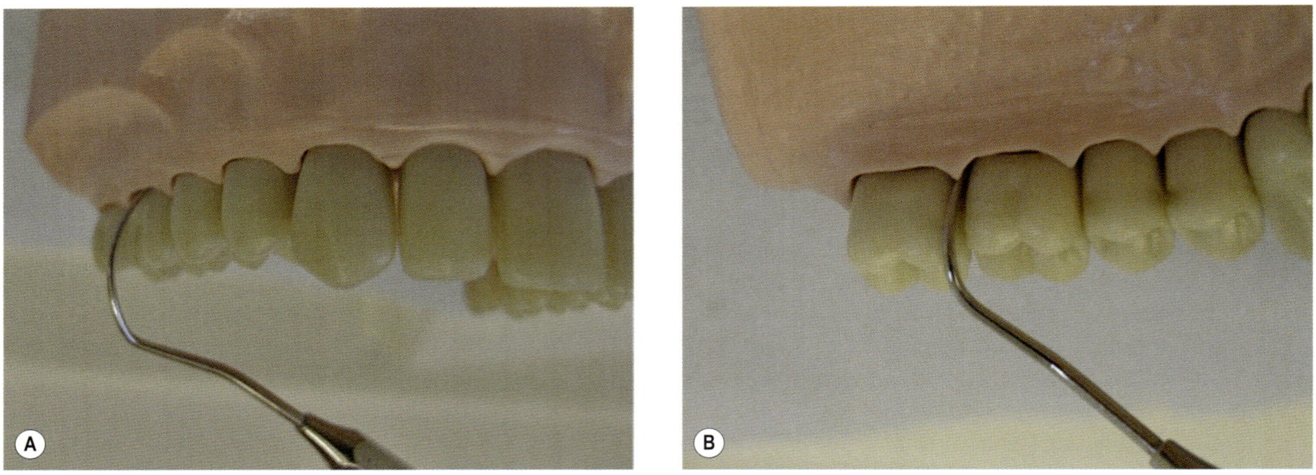

Fig 1.9 Using a Nabers probe to detect the buccal furcation (A) and the distal furcation (B).

- Assessment of functional occlusion and the presence of occlusal interferences and dysharmonies (also discussed in Chapter 15).
- Assessment of other local plaque retentive factors, including restoration margins, prostheses, root grooves, and other anatomical factors of the teeth.
- Assessment of the presence of co-morbidities.

Details of the scoring methods used for recording mobility, furcations, and recession are shown in Table 1.5.

Periodontal probing is a cornerstone of the assessment of the periodontal tissues and is the principal way that disease severity is assessed. Thus, it is important that the measurements taken are reasonably reproducible, and this can usually be greatly improved by general experience, although it is still inevitable that there will be small variations in some sites due to measurement error. In addition, a range of other factors may affect the pocket depth measurement; these are summarized in Table 1.6.

The assessment of tooth mobility requires consideration of the aetiology of the mobility. A full history of possible parafunctional habits, notably tooth grinding (bruxism) and habitual clenching, should be established and any history

Table 1.5 Common indices used in periodontal assessment

Mobility	Grade 1: Horizontal movement of up to 1 mm Grade 2: Horizontal movement >1 mm Grade 3: Severe mobility including movement in a vertical direction
Furcation involvement	Grade I: Furcation just detectable by probing Grade II: Probe can enter the furcation but cannot go all the way through Grade III: A through-and-through furcation (or the probe can touch the opposite root in upper molars)
Recession	Miller's classification: Class I: Marginal tissue recession, which does not extend to the mucogingival junction (MGJ). There is no periodontal loss (bone or soft tissue) in the interdental area Class II: Marginal tissue recession, which extends to or beyond the MGJ. There is no periodontal loss (bone or soft tissue) in the interdental area Class III: Marginal tissue recession, which extends to or beyond the MGJ. Bone or soft tissue loss in the interdental area is present, or there is a malpositioning of the teeth Class IV: Marginal tissue recession, which extends to or beyond the MGJ. The bone or soft tissue loss in the interdental area and/or malpositioning of teeth is so severe that root coverage cannot be anticipated

Table 1.6 Factors that may influence the accurate measurement of pocket depths

Factor	Comments
Operator variation	A small degree of variation (measurement error) is inevitable even when the same experienced operator is repeating measurements. The size of measurement error will increase when comparing measurements taken by two different operators
Probing force	The pocket depth will vary according to the force applied. Standardized forces should be of approximately 20–25 g (0.2–0.25 N of force); can be standardized by constant force probes such as electronic probes
Probe angulation and position	The probe should be angled along the contour of the root surface. Because the position of each site to be probed is not accurately defined, small variations in position can alter the pocket depth recorded. In clinical studies, accuracy can be improved by using custom-made stents that ensure the probe is used at the same angle and site on each occasion, but this is not feasible for clinical practice
The presence of subgingival calculus	The presence of subgingival calculus can make it more difficult to get the probe to the base of the pocket
Inflammation	The clinical probing depth does not necessarily correspond precisely to the anatomical (histologically defined) level of the epithelial attachment. In inflamed sites, the probe tends to travel beyond the true attachment level, and in uninflamed sites it tends to stop short of the true level of epithelial attachment

of TMJ-related symptoms considered. During examination, wear facets should be looked for, and an examination of occlusal dysharmonies should identify deviations on closure, premature contacts and displacements going into intercuspal position, followed by identification of interferences in lateral and protrusive movements.

What are clinical attachment loss and clinical attachment level?

The clinical attachment level represents the estimated position of the tooth-supporting structures that can be measured with the periodontal probe. Clinical attachment loss is the extent of periodontal support that has been lost around a tooth and is composed of two components: the periodontal pocket and gingival recession. The two components are added together at each of the points measured around a tooth to give the clinical attachment loss:

Probing depth (e.g., 5 mm) + gingival recession (e.g., 2 mm)
= clinical attachment loss (e.g., 7 mm)

Both of these terms are synonymously used and are abbreviated CAL.

Width of attached gingiva: How much is needed?

During assessment of a patient, it may be important to determine the width of attached gingiva, which is measured from the gingival margin to the mucogingival line and subtracting the pocket depth. In general, if the lip or cheek is stretched and this causes movement of the free gingival margin of the adjacent tooth, the width is considered insufficient. This is the case in Figure 1.10, in which stretching of the lower lip "pulls" on the free gingiva of the lower incisor, causing some blanching of the tissues. This type of mucogingival problem can be improved by mucogingival surgery to increase the width of attached gingiva, as discussed in Chapter 14. Generally 1- to 3-mm width of attached gingiva is considered consistent with periodontal health.

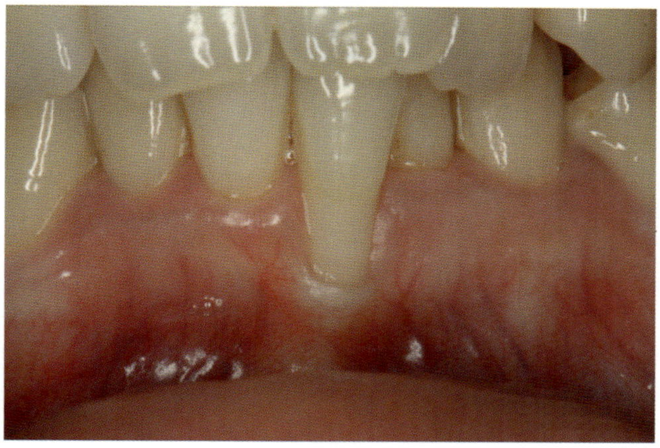

Fig 1.10 This lower left mandibular incisor shows a decreased width of attached gingiva on the labial aspect compared to the other lower incisors, which may not be compatible with gingival health.

The classification of localized recession defects is useful clinically because it gives an indication of the amount of root coverage that can be predictably achieved with mucogingival procedures . Miller class I and class II defects can predictably achieve up to 100% root coverage with the appropriate surgical technique.

When would I carry out a radiographic assessment?

The use of radiographs is widely accepted as being necessary in the full assessment of a patient with moderate to severe periodontal problems; however, they are an adjunct to clinical assessment, not a substitute for it. Bitewing radiographs will show the alveolar bone crest as long as the bone loss is not too severe, whereas periapical radiographs may be indicated in patients when bone loss is severe or a periodontal–endodontic lesion is suspected.

The main purpose is to assess the level of the alveolar crest and the pattern of bone resorption. However, it must be recognized that radiographs often underestimate the amount of alveolar bone loss. Bone levels are a good estimate of overall attachment loss that has occurred, and thus results from clinical and radiographic examinations should be compared. These may seen inconsistent when the probing depths noted are mainly the result of false pockets (bone loss is less than that expected from probing depth charts). In contrast, the bone loss is worse than the probing depths where the attachment loss is manifested as recession or where there has been healing and resolution after treatment.

The bone level in periodontal health is usually 2 or 3 mm apical to the cementoenamel junction (CEJ), and bone loss is normally determined according to the amount of root remaining in bone compared with the level of the CEJ and expressed as a percentage. On bitewing radiographs, the bone loss can also be expressed as millimetres of bone loss.

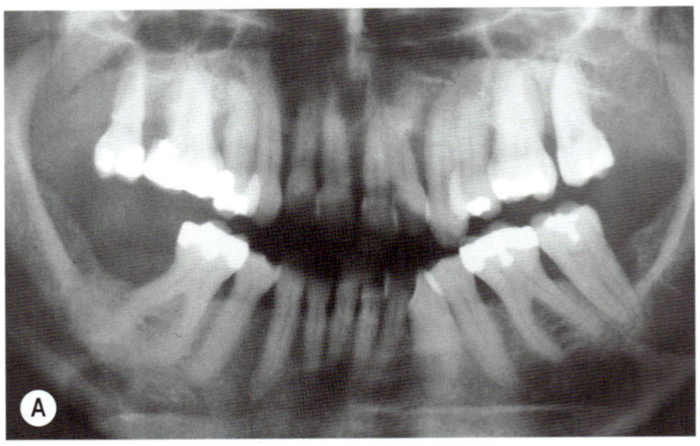

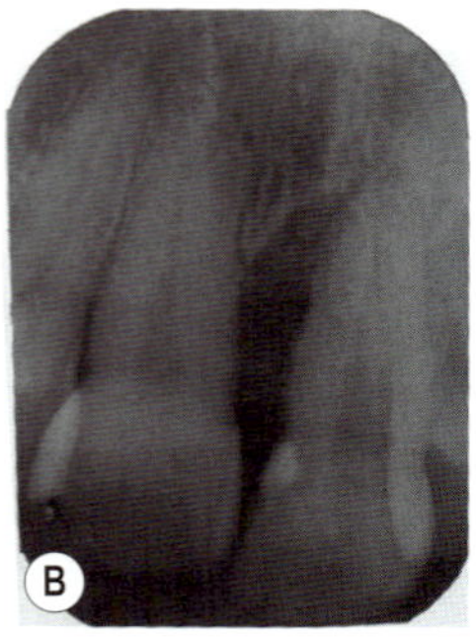

Fig 1.11 A panoramic radiograph demonstrating generalized horizontal bone loss supplemented with a periapical of the UL1 showing vertical bone loss almost to the apex.

Healthy bone levels can often be recognized by the presence of a lamina dura at the crestal bone.

In addition, radiographs are useful in assessing the presence of other co-morbidities, such as caries and endodontic involvements.

What are the appropriate radiographs to take?

- Horizontal bitewings show crestal bone and are indicated if attachment loss is less than 5 mm. They also give detail of overhanging restorations or interproximal caries that may act as local plaque traps.
- Vertical bitewings (where the film is turned 90° from the conventional horizontal bitewing) are more informative than horizontal bitewings in showing the bone levels in moderate to severe periodontitis around several teeth.
- Periapicals are indicated when severe periodontitis is present and may be useful for evaluating sites where vertical bony defects are suspected clinically; however, the detection of two- and three-walled vertical bony defects can still be a challenge to image. It will also allow an assessment of the root morphology, furcation involvement, root shape, and periodontal–endodontic status.
- Panoramic radiographs allow visualization of all teeth on one film. However, there is often lack of detail, particularly in the anterior region due to the shadow of the cervical spine. Because this makes interpreting the images challenging in this region, supplementation with periapical radiographs may be needed in certain cases (Figure 1.11).
- Cone beam computed tomography imaging may offer new perspectives on periodontal diagnosis and treatment planning, particularly for clearer three-dimensional visualization of vertical bony defects.

Is there a difference between horizontal and vertical bone loss?

- If the level of the bone is essentially equal interdentally, it is called horizontal bone loss (Figure 1.12) and measured as the percentage of bone lost (e.g., 20% of the original bone height is lost).
- Vertical/angular bone loss occurs when one tooth has lost more bone than the tooth next to it and is suggested when the bone crest is more apical to the CEJ adjacent to one tooth than to the other (Figure 1.12).
- Bone loss around an individual tooth can also be a combination of a horizontal component and a vertical component and is still expressed as the total amount of bone lost from the CEJ.

Assessment of co-morbidities

A key factor in considering the diagnosis, assessment of prognosis, and planning appropriate treatment is the assessment of co-morbidities—that is, other diseases and conditions that may also be present. Most commonly, these include the identification of caries and particularly endodontic lesions.

Most particularly impacting on prognosis is the identification of perio/endo lesions. A perio/endo lesion is where a periodontal pocket communicates directly with an endodontic lesion. These may occur where

- a periodontal pocket extends to cause loss of vitality of a tooth, most commonly if a pocket extends to the apex of the tooth but also if a furcation involvement results in loss of vitality due to the presence of lateral canals in the furcation, or if extension of a pocket to lateral canals occurring down the root surface of the tooth results in loss of vitality;
- a primary endodontic lesion results in drainage through the periodontal ligament, causing a periodontal pocket, or where there is a lateral perforation of the tooth that results in a pocket communicating to the defect; and
- there are coincident periodontal and periapical lesions that coalesce to form a combined perio/endo lesion.

Diagnosis of perio/endo lesions is particularly important because they have a major negative impact on the prognosis of a tooth. Distinguishing between possible primary aetiologies is important because those that arise primarily from the extension of a periodontal pocket have a particularly poor prognosis, whereas those that arise primarily from an endodontic lesion may respond well to

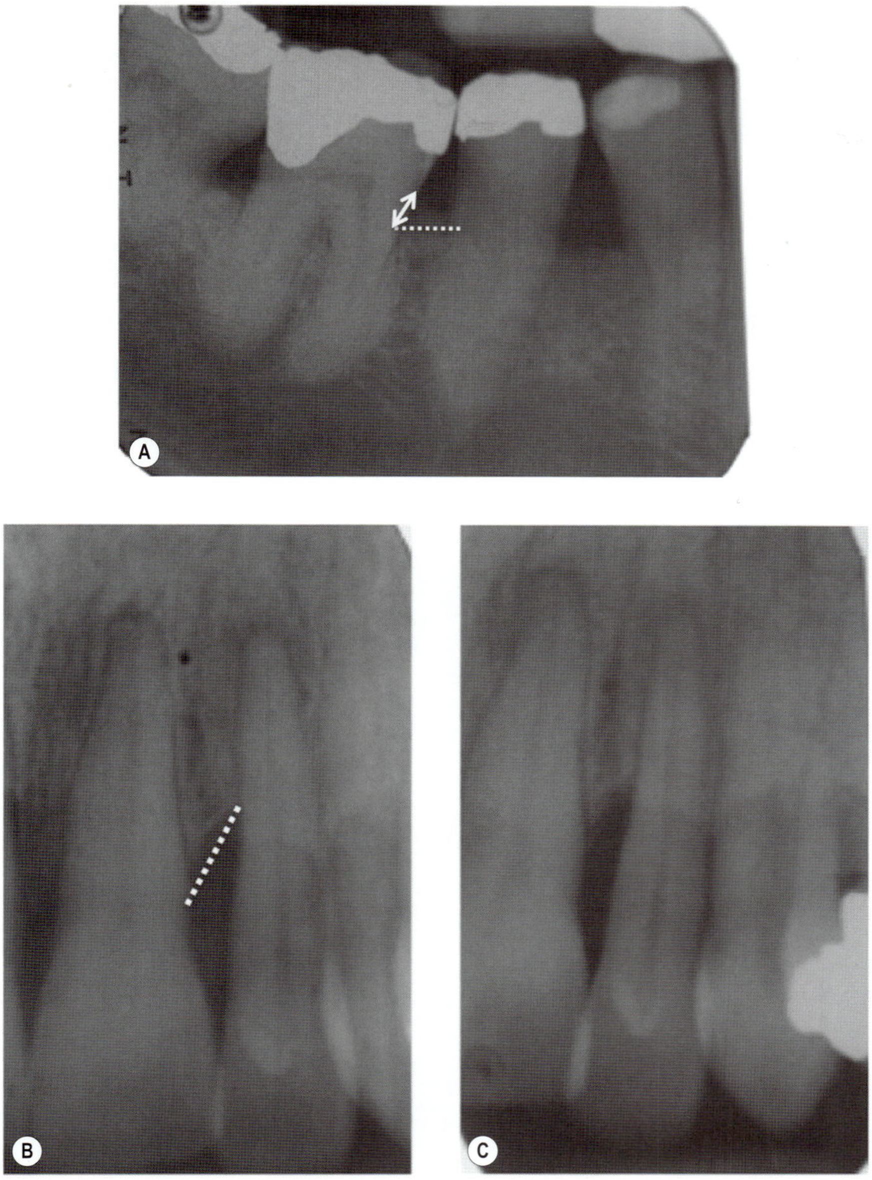

Fig 1.12 (A) Horizontal bone loss occurs when the level of the bone is below the CEJ (arrow) but equal interdentally (white dashed line), whereas in vertical bone loss, bone crest is more apical to the CEJ adjacent to one tooth than to the other (white dashed line in B).

endodontic treatment only, particularly if they are not long-standing.

Diagnosis of a perio/endo lesion is clinically difficult because the only consistent change is the loss of vitality of the tooth. Even here, where a multirooted tooth has a perio/endo lesion affecting one root, a vitality test may give a false-positive reading due to vitality remaining in the other roots. Radiographic evidence of continuous bone loss from a periodontal pocket to a radiolucent apex of the tooth is most commonly seen (Figure 1.13). However, occasionally, the diagnosis is more difficult. Deciding if a lesion is primarily endodontic or primarily periodontal can be judged only by the clinical findings in each case; if there is extensive periodontal disease elsewhere, then it is likely that the lesion is primarily caused by periodontitis, whereas if there is minimal periodontitis elsewhere and there is a plausible reason to suppose the tooth may have lost vitality, then the judgement may suggest a primarily endodontic lesion (Figure 1.14).

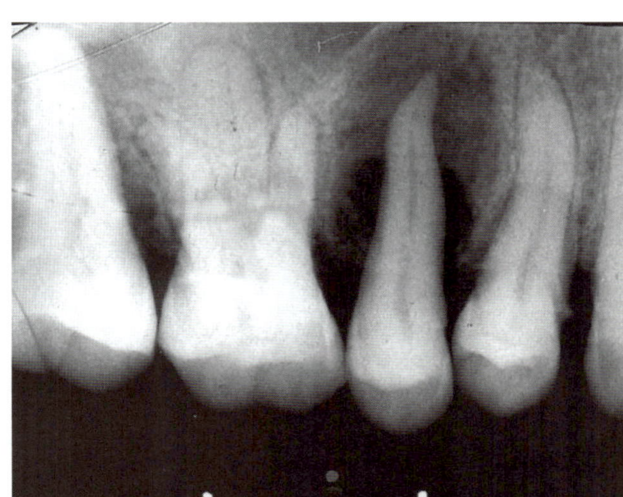

Fig 1.13 Radiographic appearance of perio/endo lesion on UR5 resulting from periodontal pocket extending to the apex of the tooth.

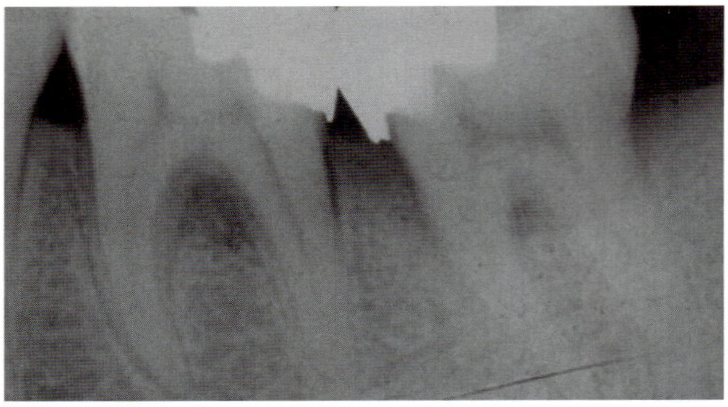

Fig 1.14 A rather innocuous-looking furcation lesion on LR6 turns out to be a perio/endo lesion, and the tooth has become nonvital (although at this stage there are no apical changes). Despite the presence of localized bone loss on the LR7 mesially associated with the overhanging restoration, there is no sign of periodontitis elsewhere, and the lesion on LR6 is diagnosed as being of primarily endodontic origin associated most likely with the deep DO restoration. Providing periodontal treatment for this furcation lesion will result in failure because the original diagnosis is actually an endodontic lesion resulting in a perio/endo lesion.

Conclusions

This chapter aimed to bring together the reasoning to support the routine use of screening of patients for periodontal disease and key elements of the history and clinical examination to arrive at an appropriate diagnosis and treatment plan for a patient. It is critical to correlate all the relevant indices and scores obtained from the examination to provide a meaningful and informative explanation to the patient regarding his or her periodontal disease. The clinical examination of the periodontal tissues described here provides the very important tooth-by-tooth assessment of the extent of periodontal disease in a patient. This information needs to be considered together with an assessment of patient-level aetiological and risk factors to allow a comprehensive diagnosis to inform treatment planning decisions.

Chapter 2

Classification of periodontal diseases

Introduction

The term "periodontal diseases" is usually used to describe the range of inflammatory conditions that affect the supporting tissues of the teeth, which are initiated by the accumulation of dental plaque. Potentially confusingly, in some instances, the term is alternately used to describe any condition affecting the periodontal tissues, which is not necessarily due to plaque accumulation and might be caused by any disease process. Here, and throughout this book, we use the conventional understanding for the term periodontal diseases to signify plaque-induced diseases. Other diseases that can affect the periodontal tissues are discussed further in Chapter 5. The use of the plural "periodontal diseases" signifies that these conditions can manifest themselves in a number of distinct ways that are clinically different and may have important influences in terms of management, future progression, and prognosis.

A classification system's basic attributes are to provide a structure to study the aetiology, pathological processes, and treatment of a specific disease or diseases and should also be flexible enough to permit the introduction of new diagnoses into the system as needed. The use of such a classification system for periodontal diseases is a convenient filing system for a broad spectrum of diseases and has developed as understanding about aetiology of periodontal diseases has increased during the past 20 years.

Diagnosis implies that a disease can be understood based on some of its key features and using this information will inform our overall treatment approach. However, reaching a diagnosis is often an inexact science because even when using a classification system, there is considerable overlap between categories and a "best fit" diagnosis (or differential diagnosis) is often reached after combining the aetiological factors elucidated during the patients' medical, dental, and social histories with the clinical oral examination findings. Reaching a working diagnosis is crucial (Table 2.1) because this "diagnostic label" will determine the subsequent initial treatment sequence.

A classification system may, in principle, be based mainly on the distinct clinical features of the conditions or, alternatively, may be based mainly on their different aetiologies. It can be argued that a classification system based on aetiology might be most useful in informing treatment planning decisions. However, periodontal diseases, like many other common chronic diseases, have a complex aetiology in which a range of different locally acting and systemically acting factors can combine to cause the disease, and thus it is difficult to use an aetiology-based system of classification. Furthermore, the same aetiological conditions may combine in different patients to cause clinically distinct disease entities.

What are the current possible periodontal diagnoses?

Plaque-related periodontal diseases are by far the most common of all conditions that can affect the periodontal tissues. Data from the 2009 United Kingdom Adult Dental Health Survey show that two-thirds of those examined had visible dental plaque on their teeth and other oral structures (e.g., dentures). In addition, 45% of people examined had pocket depths of ≥4 mm, and 9% of people examined had probing depths of ≥6 mm. Studies suggest that the overall prevalence of moderate to severe periodontitis in most populations throughout the world is approximately 15–20%. However, as noted previously, they are not the only possible conditions with such a presentation.

The classification for periodontal diseases and conditions is shown in Table 2.2. This classification is based on a consensus reached at the World Workshop in Periodontology in 1999 and supersedes other previous attempts to classify the periodontal diseases. The classification divides the conditions as follows:

- Gingival diseases—those that are confined to the superficial gingival tissues
- Periodontal diseases—inflammatory conditions that involve the deeper periodontal tissues and that have resulted in loss of alveolar bone, associated periodontal ligament, and apical migration of the junctional epithelium
- Developmental or acquired defects—gingival recession and other mucogingival problems (discussed in Chapter 14)

This classification, like all classifications, has prompted debate and disagreement, and no doubt as our knowledge of the aetiology and pathogenesis of periodontal diseases changes, new classification systems will be proposed. In addition, there is one obvious inconsistency: within the category "gingival diseases," there is a specific section on gingival lesions that are not due to plaque, whereas in the "periodontal diseases" section there is no equivalent attempt at classifying non-plaque-induced conditions that can affect the deeper periodontal tissues.

The cases presented in this chapter focus mainly on, and illustrate, the diagnosis of the following common plaque-related periodontal diseases:

- Gingival diseases
- Chronic periodontitis
- Aggressive periodontitis

Table 2.1 Importance of a diagnosis

What is the cause of the disease or condition? Is it plaque initiated?
What are the treatment options? What will happen if the condition is not treated?
Is referral to a more experienced or specialist clinician appropriate?
What is the expected response to the treatment proposed?
What is the prognosis?

Table 2.2 Classification of periodontal diseases and conditions

Gingival diseases
Dental plaque-induced gingival diseases
Gingivitis associated with dental plaque only
Gingival diseases modified by systemic factors
Gingival diseases modified by medications
Gingival diseases modified by malnutrition
Non-plaque-induced gingival lesions
Gingival diseases of viral origin
Gingival diseases of fungal origin
Gingival lesions of genetic origin
Gingival manifestations of systemic conditions
Traumatic lesions (factitious and iatrogenic)
Foreign body reactions
Not otherwise specified (NOS)
Periodontal diseases
Chronic periodontitis
Localized
Generalized
Aggressive periodontitis
Localized
Generalized
Periodontitis as a manifestation of systemic diseases
Associated with hematological disorders
Associated with genetic disorders
Not otherwise specified (NOS)
Necrotizing periodontal diseases
Necrotizing ulcerative gingivitis (NUG)
Necrotizing ulcerative periodontitis (NUP)
Abscesses of the periodontium
Gingival abscess
Periodontal abscess
Pericoronal abscess
Perio/endo lesions
Developmental or acquired deformities

Adapted from Armitage (1999).

How do I reach a periodontal diagnosis? Basic checklist

1. Is it a plaque-related periodontal disease or another disease affecting the periodontal tissues?
2. What is the severity of the periodontal problem? Is it limited to the gingival tissues or is there associated attachment loss?
3. Is the periodontal problem localized to a few teeth or a generalized condition?
4. Are there significant risk factors and systemic factors that might have impacted on the progression or susceptibility of the presenting periodontal problems?
5. Are there any additional conditions (co-morbidities) also present?

Gingival diseases

Plaque-related gingival disease is almost ubiquitous in all populations, and this inflammatory reaction is a response to the microbial challenge presented to the gingival tissues. It can be modified by the presence of plaque-retentive factors, particularly dental restorations, dental caries, or abnormal tooth anatomy. It is usually painless and is reversible if meticulous oral hygiene is maintained. The clinical features are red, swollen gingivae often associated with accumulation of plaque and calculus deposits and the commonly reported symptom of bleeding when brushing. Gingival diseases are confined to the gingival tissues, and gingivitis may be regarded as a normal immune-related reaction aimed to prevent periodontal destruction. Although plaque-related periodontal disease is always initiated by gingivitis, the progression into periodontitis is not the rule.

Case 1

A 61-year-old man presented complaining that his "lower teeth were worn down." In addition, he had experienced bleeding on brushing for some time. Crowns had been placed on the upper anterior teeth more than 10 years previously because these teeth had chipped, and he found it difficult to clean in between them. On examination, ceramometal crowns were present on upper canine to canine, which had bulky margins. The gingivae were red and bled rapidly on gentle probing; however, no probing depths of >3 mm were found. Chronic gingivitis was diagnosed because there was no loss of periodontal attachment. The patient was shown where plaque was accumulating, and oral hygiene instruction was given. On review after 2 weeks, the gingival inflammation and the patient's symptoms showed signs of resolution (Figure 2.1). This case illustrates that despite long-standing gingival inflammation, no progressive attachment loss was observed, with resolution possible after good home care from the patient.

Case 2

A 47-year-old woman was concerned about her generalized gingival swelling that had been slowly getting worse for 2 years, and spaces were now opening up between her teeth. Medical history revealed that she had been prescribed a calcium channel blocking drug, nifedipine, 2½ years previously to control her hypertension.

The clinical presentation was predominantly interproximal, lobular, gingival overgrowth covering one-third to one-half of the clinical crowns particularly in the anterior teeth (Figure 2.2). A diagnosis of drug-induced gingival disease was made.

Although it has been shown that a side effect of this calcium channel blocker-induced overgrowth occurs by an accumulation of extracellular matrix and disruption of collagen synthesis in gingival tissues, it is exacerbated by gingival inflammation and poor oral hygiene.

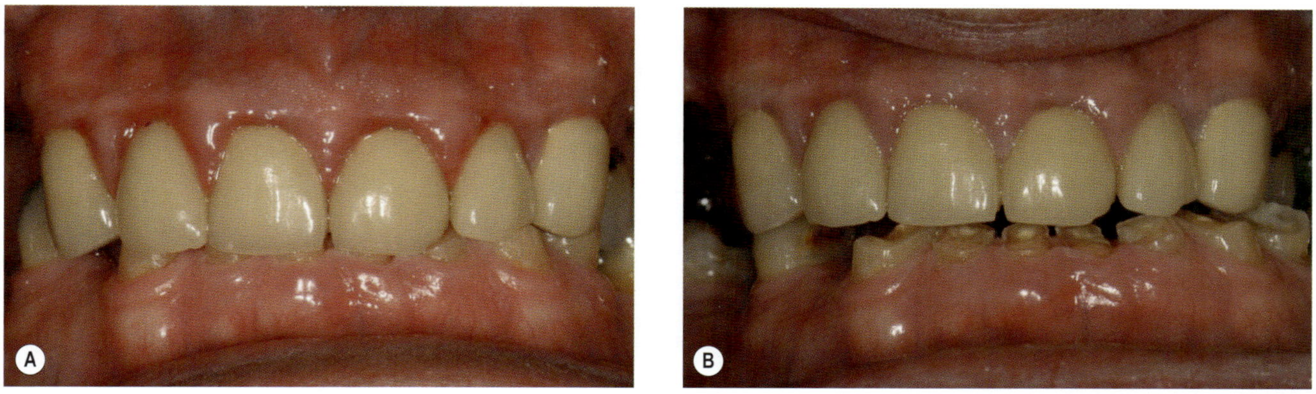

Fig 2.1 Case 1: (A) Presentation of well-established gingivitis and (B) signs of resolution occurring 2 weeks after giving oral hygiene instruction.

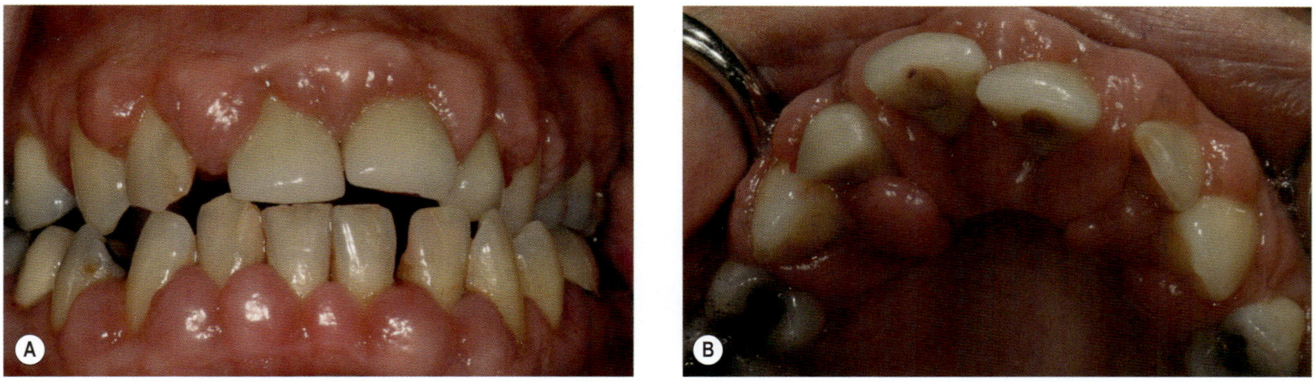

Fig 2.2 Case 2 on presentation: Drug-induced gingival overgrowth associated with nifedipine therapy.

Periodontal diseases

Chronic periodontitis

As previously noted, chronic periodontitis is extremely common, affecting the majority of adults during their lifetime. In some cases, the gingivae superficially appear healthy, making diagnosis only possible after periodontal screening and assessment. The aetiology of chronic periodontitis is multifactorial, and the rate of progression varies widely among individuals and is influenced by the individual host response.

Chronic periodontitis is generally slowly progressing, with some intermittent bursts of more rapid progression. Prevalence increases with age; however, this is not thought to be due to an increased susceptibility with age but, rather, a cumulative lifetime disease experience. In most cases, there is minimal tooth loss, and the level of disease is generally correlated with oral hygiene.

Chronic periodontitis can be further categorized into mild, moderate, or severe, reflecting the general amount of clinical attachment loss (CAL) at time of presentation. Mild chronic periodontitis is present when 1 or 2 mm of CAL is recorded, moderate when 3 or 4 mm CAL is recorded, and severe chronic when ≥5 mm is recorded. Some clinicians use the terms slight for mild or advanced when severe disease is present, but these are interchangeable terms and reflect the same levels of CAL. It must be remembered, however, that probing pocket depths, although extremely valuable, in isolation do not give the entire picture because the gingival margin might be above the cement–enamel junction if false pockets due to gingival swelling or enlargement are present or below if there is gingival recession, leading to a misrepresentation of the true level of clinical attachment.

Table 2.3 Features of aggressive periodontitis

Noncontributory medical history
Familial aggregation
Rapid attachment loss
Destruction not consistent with amount of plaque
Localized (first molar/incisor) and generalized (involving at least three other teeth)
Phagocyte abnormalities
Hyperresponsive macrophages
High proportions of *A. actinomycetemcomitans* and, in some Far Eastern populations, *P. gingivalis*

When a full probing depth assessment has been carried out, together with radiographical examination if indicated, the disease is further subdivided into localized or generalized disease. Localized disease occurs when up to 30% of teeth are affected, whereas in generalized disease, 30% or more of the teeth present are affected. A sensible approach is to give a general diagnosis that is reflective of the overall clinical picture, such as generalized moderate chronic periodontitis.

Aggressive periodontitis

Aggressive periodontitis is characterized by severe, rapidly progressing periodontitis. The features of the condition are considered to be sufficiently different from chronic periodontitis to justify classification as a distinct clinical entity. The features of aggressive periodontitis were described by the World Workshop in Periodontology and are listed in Table 2.3. These features include both clinical and laboratory findings. However, there is little evidence that laboratory testing of neutrophil and macrophage function, or microbiological testing, is actually of diagnostic value. Thus, a diagnosis of aggressive periodontitis is usually made by the demonstration of rapid periodontal breakdown in an otherwise healthy individual, together with the highly subjective judgement that the amount of plaque is not consistent with the amount of destruction present. Therefore, the diagnosis is usually made in a young patient with severe attachment loss (and thus where periodontal breakdown has demonstrably occurred rapidly) in the presence of reasonable plaque control.

As in chronic periodontitis, the disease can be subdivided into localized disease with first molar/incisor and no more than two other permanent teeth being affected or generalized disease when the pattern shows more teeth affected. Localized aggressive periodontitis has a very distinct pattern of disease presentation and may affect patients from early adolescence.

Case 3

A 56-year-old woman presented with mobility of her lower anterior teeth and a history of losing several teeth during the past 10 years. She had been a fairly regular lifelong dental attender; however, since moving 3 years ago, she had had only one visit when a tooth became loose. She has occasionally had a "scaling" by her dentist but cannot recall having any prolonged gum treatment. She had a noncontributory medical history and had previously smoked 10–15 cigarettes a day for 20 years. Oral hygiene was poor, with generalized supra- and subgingival plaque and calculus deposits (Figure 2.3).

The following BPE score was recorded.

4	4	4*
4*	4	3

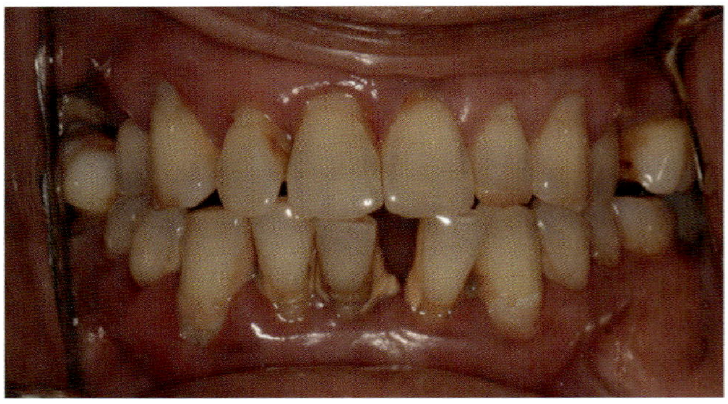

Fig 2.3 Case 3 on presentation.

A full periodontal assessment showed probing depth range of 4–6 mm; LL2 and LR1 were grade 2 mobile, and LR2 was grade 1 mobile. Radiographs show generalized horizontal bone loss of 40–50%, with loss of up to 70% associated with the lower incisors.

Is this plaque-related periodontitis?

The clinical findings show the classical signs of periodontitis. Her oral hygiene is poor, and there are visible plaque and calculus deposits. Thus, it is likely that the aetiology is plaque related, although the periodontal destruction has been exacerbated by long-term smoking. The patient was diagnosed with generalized moderate chronic periodontitis. Although the lower incisors have severe bone loss, an overall diagnosis of generalized moderate chronic periodontitis is more reflective of the clinical picture.

Although she has relatively severe probing depths, this woman would benefit from a course of initial nonsurgical periodontal therapy to improve her oral hygiene, followed by supra- and subgingival debridement. If left untreated, it would be expected that attachment loss would increase slowly over time, resulting in the loss of several teeth. The LL2 and LR1 are of a questionable prognosis, and early extraction could be considered as part of the treatment plan. On reassessment, if despite maintenance of good oral hygiene significant probing depths ≥5 mm remain, a specialist referral could be sought for advice on further management.

Case 4

A 60-year-old woman presented expressing great anxiety about the appearance of her upper teeth, which had been slowly drifting for a number of years. A number of teeth in both arches had been extracted due to dental pain and because they became loose. She was a nonsmoker, had a noncontributory medical history, and, as in Case 2, oral hygiene was poor, with generalized supra- and subgingival plaque and calculus deposits. The patient did admit to being under severe stress for several years because her husband had been ill and she had been caring for him. On clinical examination, she had lost the majority of her lower teeth and could not wear her partial denture due to supra-eruption of the UL2, leaving a very disrupted occlusion and lack of restorable space. The gingivae were red and swollen, with generalized loss of the interdental papillae (Figure 2.4).

The following BPE score was recorded:

4	4	-
X	3	X

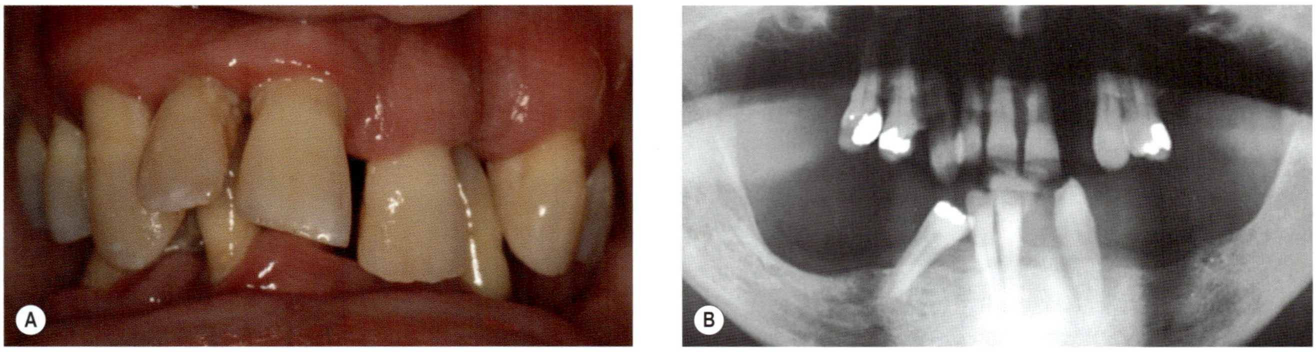

Fig 2.4 Clinical and radiographic presentation of Case 4.

A full periodontal assessment showed probing depth range of 4– 8mm, with significant mobility of the majority of the remaining teeth. Radiographs show horizontal bone loss of 40–50%, with loss of up to 90% associated with the upper and lower incisors.

◈ ***Is this plaque-related periodontitis?***

As in the previous case, the clinical findings are typical of periodontitis. Her oral hygiene is poor, and plaque and calculus deposits are visible, supporting the aetiology being plaque related. However, the stress she experienced in the past few years may have exacerbated periodontal destruction. The findings are consistent with a diagnosis of generalized severe chronic periodontitis (even though there are few remaining teeth, they are almost all affected), and the overall prognosis of the remaining teeth is poor. Treatment of this case may benefit from early strategic extractions because they may not be useful teeth for support of a removable partial denture, and it would also improve aesthetics.

Case 5

A 28-year-old woman was very concerned about the spaces opening up between her front teeth and worried that she was going to lose her teeth. She recalled that her mother had experienced some periodontal problems but was unsure if this had led to tooth loss. Her medical history was clear, and she was a nonsmoker.

On examination, her oral hygiene was good, although some localized plaque and calculus deposits were visible (Figure 2.5). Spacing was evident between UL1 and UL2, and there was some swelling on the gingiva of UL1 and localized gingival recession.

The following BPE score was recorded:

4*	4	4*
4	4	4*

Probing depths in all sextants were 5–10 mm. A panoramic radiograph showed generalized bone loss of 50%, with areas of up to 80%, and the pattern of bone loss was irregular (see Figure 2.5).

◈ ***Is this plaque-related periodontitis?***

Although there is relatively good plaque control in this patient, the clinical features of generalized bone loss, pocket formation, and drifting are clearly those of periodontitis. As in Cases 2 and 3, this form of periodontitis is plaque related, and the periodontal destruction is a result of the host response to the bacterial challenge. This woman presented with reasonably good oral hygiene but severe attachment loss that was inconsistent with the amount of plaque present. In addition, there is a suggestion from the history of a potential familial tendency. In this case, because the periodontal destruction is not localized to the first molars and incisors, a diagnosis of generalized aggressive periodontitis was made.

Case 6

A 13-year-old girl was referred to a periodontist by her general dentist following a chance finding of periodontal pocketing affecting some teeth.

The patient had not had any symptoms, and there was no history of gingival bleeding on brushing. There was no known family history of periodontal disease, although the patient has two older sisters. The gingivae appeared uninflamed, and plaque control was good. However, on examination, pocketing was noted at the lower incisors and the first molars, and radiographically there were early signs of vertical bone loss on the mesial surfaces of the first molars and up to 50% bone loss on the lower incisor teeth. The upper incisors were unaffected (Figure 2.6).

The clinical presentation is typical of early localized aggressive periodontitis because of the characteristic distribution of disease (incisors and first molars) and the very early presentation of attachment loss. Although there was no positive family history in this case, self-reported family history is unreliable and certainly not a very useful diagnostic criterion, particularly when the history is negative. However, as a precaution, screening of the patient's older sisters was organized in this case. Localized aggressive periodontitis also shows a strong racial predilection and may be up to 10 times more common in black Afro-Caribbean racial groups (as with the patient here) compared with those of white northern European racial origin.

Localized aggressive periodontitis may start in the second decade of life, but it is common for it to present later. In this case, the prompt vigilance of the general dentist enabled the very early diagnosis of what is often a very destructive condition, and prompt appropriate intervention should prevent the progression to a much more destructive process.

Often, if left untreated, the condition may result in early tooth loss and progress to involve other teeth, thus

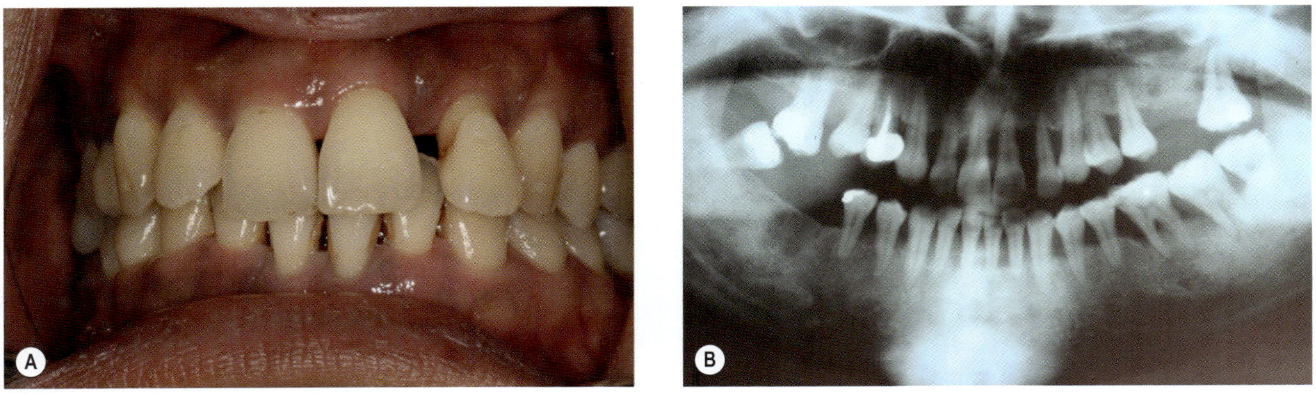

Fig 2.5 Clinical and radiographic features of Case 5 on presentation. The gingivae look largely uninflamed, but radiographically, severe generalized bone loss is evident. There has been drifting of the upper left anterior teeth.

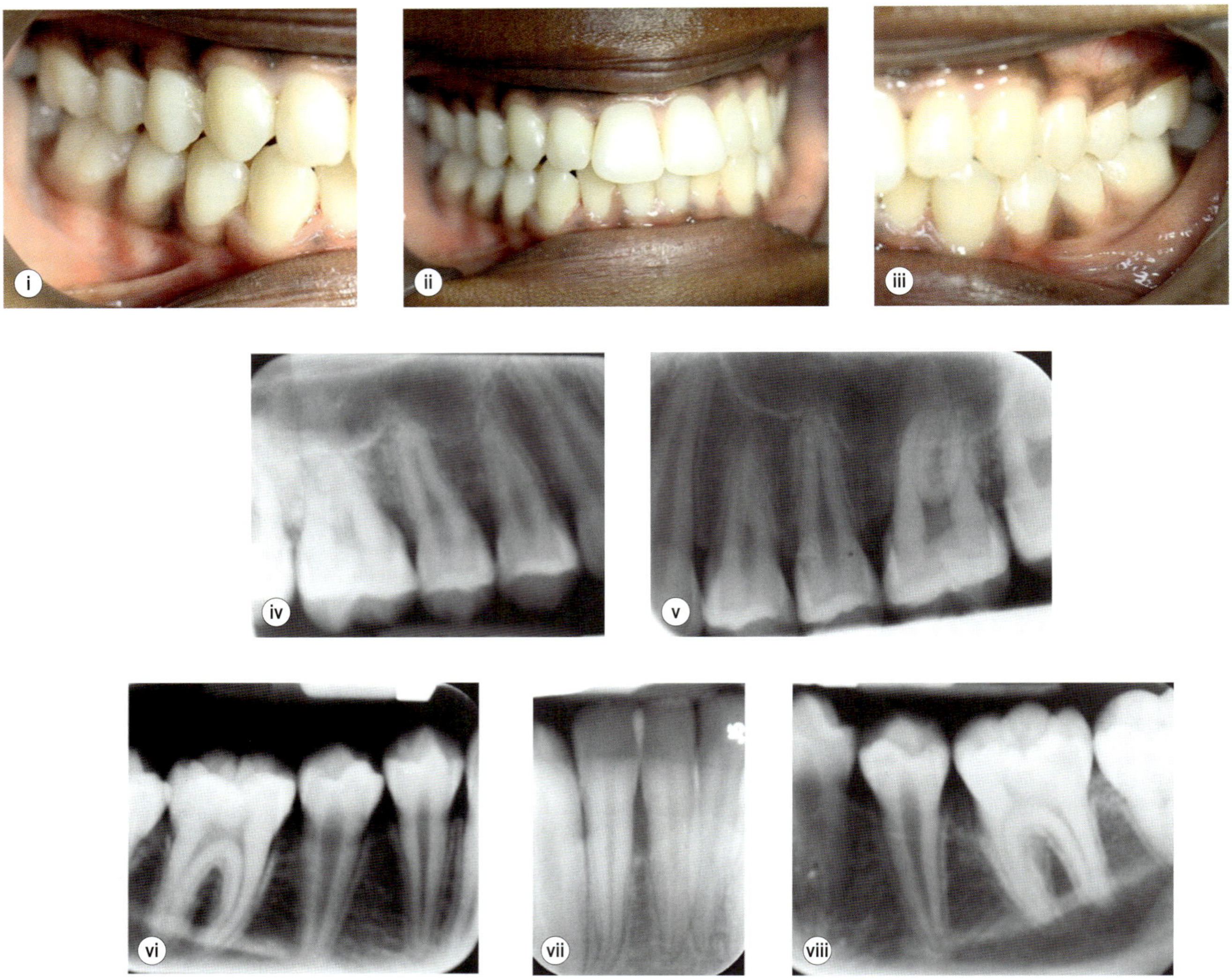

Fig 2.6 Clinical and radiographic presentation of Case 6 at age 13 years. The plaque control is good, and the gingivae appear uninflamed, illustrating the importance of proper periodontal screening of all patients, even where their gingival health is apparently good. The radiographs show up to 50% bone loss affecting the lower incisor teeth and early bone loss at the mesial sites of the first molars.

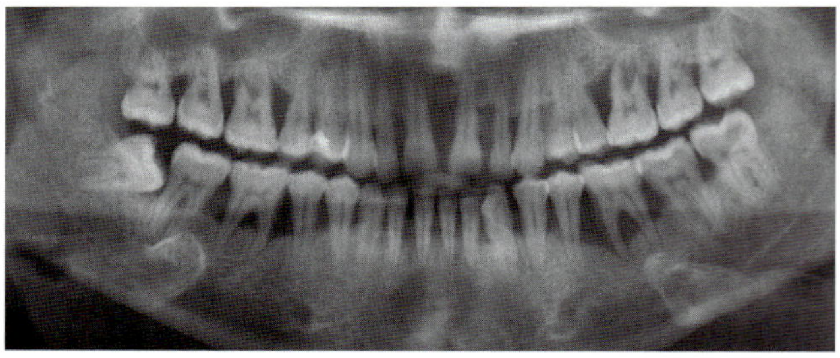

Fig 2.7 Radiographic presentation of a 24-year-old man who was originally from Trinidad. There is severe bone loss, which particularly affects the first molars and incisors but has also spread to affect many other teeth. The appearance and clinical features are suggestive of an initial diagnosis of localized aggressive periodontitis that had now progressed to a generalized aggressive form of the disease.

becoming generalized aggressive disease (Figure 2.7). Unfortunately, it is common for the condition to be recognized only following the severe destruction seen in Figure 2.7, probably because of the relative lack of clinical signs of inflammation of the condition until at a very late stage of the disease process.

◇ *Comparing chronic and aggressive periodontitis: A diagnostic dilemma?*

Chronic and aggressive periodontitis share many similarities, and it can be difficult to be confident in the initial diagnosis between generalized severe chronic periodontitis and generalized aggressive periodontitis. A comparison of some of the features of chronic and aggressive periodontitis is shown in Table 2.4.

The clinical features of all types of chronic periodontitis are essentially similar, with clinical signs of redness and swelling depicting an inflammatory response that is associated with accumulation of plaque and calculus deposits. Other common risk factors, such as smoking and systemic health, may increase the rate of progression of chronic periodontitis.

In contrast, there are some distinct differences between localized aggressive periodontitis and generalized aggressive periodontitis. Often in cases of localized aggressive periodontitis, there is very mild inflammation and minimal plaque deposits, although this is not exclusively the case. The main difference is the number of teeth affected and the pattern of periodontal destruction.

Table 2.4 Clinical features of chronic and aggressive periodontitis

Chronic periodontitis	Aggressive periodontitis
Very common; most prevalent in adults, and increasing prevalence with age	Uncommon; usually affecting persons younger than age 30 years but may be older at time of diagnosis
Amount of destruction consistent with the presence of local factors	Plaque deposits inconsistent with amount of destruction
Subgingival calculus a frequent finding	Often few calculus deposits
Slow to moderate rate of progression, but may have periods of rapid progression	Rapid rate of progression, often episodic
Associated with a variable microbial pattern	A variable microbial pattern; often associated with *A. actinomycetemcomitans*, particularly in localized form
Can be associated with local predisposing factors (e.g., tooth-related or iatrogenic factors)	
May be associated with systemic diseases (e.g., diabetes mellitus) and other risk factors, such as cigarette smoking and emotional stress	No underlying medical condition
Mainly generalized distribution but may be localized	May be generalized or localized; localized form has distinctive molar/incisor presentation and involves no more than two additional teeth

Although age is not a diagnostic criterion for aggressive periodontitis, in practice it is useful because severe periodontitis in a young patient is often the most reliable evidence of rapid periodontal breakdown over time. Perhaps the most important question to ask is whether it makes any difference if a patient is diagnosed as having aggressive periodontitis or severe chronic periodontitis. The main issue that might arise clinically is that of potential use of adjunctive antimicrobials for the management of aggressive periodontitis, which is discussed in Chapter 13. For the periodontal researcher, the distinction may also be important, particularly when searching for factors that are important determinants of susceptibility to disease.

Conclusions

Periodontal diseases are a group of chronic inflammatory conditions of the gingival and periodontal tissues caused by the presence of dental plaque. The current classification of periodontal diseases describes a wide range of different clinical phenotypes based on their presentation and aetiologies.

A number of previous classifications have been described in the historic literature, which are of significance mainly so that the reader can understand how a previous disease type might relate to the disease type in the existing classification. In particular, the term "adult periodontitis" has been used previously to describe chronic periodontitis, and a range of different terms have been used previously that equate approximately to aggressive periodontitis, including "early onset periodontitis," "juvenile periodontitis," and "rapidly progressive periodontitis." Despite possible limitations in the existing classification, it is important that clinicians use the same terms so they can all talk about the same thing. Thus, these older terms should be regarded as obsolete.

Chapter 3

Periodontal diagnosis

Systemic factors

It is well-recognized that taking a full medical history from a patient is an important part of diagnosis and assessment. Taking a medical history requires a systematic approach to obtaining information about the patient's past medical history. This can be carried out using a standard pro forma. If preferred, the patient can be asked to complete the pro forma him- or herself, and this can be checked by the clinician. The relevance of the medical history in periodontal diagnosis and treatment is mainly due to the following:

- The medical history may affect the management of the patient in some way.
- The medical history may affect the susceptibility, presentation, and progression of periodontal disease.
- The medical history may identify a condition that can directly manifest itself in the periodontal tissues.

Conditions that may affect periodontal management

Conditions that may affect the management of the patient include those that might adversely affect the ability to successfully carry out treatment, including surgical procedures. The major examples of such conditions include bleeding disorders and other blood dyscrasias where there is an obvious risk of uncontrolled bleeding following any type of periodontal treatment. In addition, any patient who is severely immunocompromised may be at increased risk of infection postoperatively.

It has long been suggested that patients with valvular heart disease, prosthetic cardiac valves, and those with a previous history of infective endocarditis may be at risk of infective endocarditis following the bacteraemia that is inevitably caused by any periodontal procedure, including both nonsurgical and surgical instrumentation. This has resulted in the suggestion that these patients should be provided with antibiotic prophylaxis prior to carrying out any invasive procedure. However, current guidelines for the United Kingdom have failed to find sufficient evidence that dental procedures are a cause of infective endocarditis or that the routine use of antibiotic prophylaxis regimes is helpful. As such, antibiotic prophylaxis prior to invasive dental procedures is not currently recommended.

Bisphosphonates are anti-bone resorptive drugs that are widely used for the management of osteoporosis, but they are also used in less common conditions such as neoplastic bone disease (e.g., the presence of bony secondary metastases from carcinomas). These drugs include alendronate, zoledronate, and pamidronate. Most patients take these drugs orally, but some patients, particularly those with neoplastic bone disease, may be given intravenous bisphosphonates. It is now recognized that bisphosphonate therapy results in the risk of the very serious complication of osteonecrosis of the jaw, which may occur, for example, following tooth extractions. This is particularly the case for those who are being treated with intravenous bisphosphonate therapy. Therefore, although people taking oral bisphosphonates can be managed normally, in those with a history of intravenous bisphosphonate therapy, tooth extractions are best avoided if possible, and where necessary, it may be appropriate to refer to a specialist centre for management.

Medical conditions may also affect periodontal management in many other ways. For example, they may have an important influence on a patient's ability to regularly attend periodontal treatment, may impair manual dexterity and the ability to carry out oral hygiene procedures (e.g., in those with severe rheumatoid arthritis), and in some cases may also influence goals and expectations of periodontal treatment outcomes. In addition, knowledge of a patient's past medical history may be invaluable during dental treatment if a medical emergency should arise.

Many medical conditions can occasionally manifest themselves in the gingival or periodontal tissues. The ability to distinguish between periodontal disease and the periodontal manifestations of another disease is discussed in Chapter 5.

Systemic aetiological factors in periodontal disease

From the epidemiology of periodontal disease, it is clear that susceptibility to periodontal disease varies considerably among patients, independent of the level of plaque control. Systemic factors have often been called secondary modifying factors of disease because in the presence of plaque, they may modify the host response, resulting in increased susceptibility to destructive disease or altered inflammatory response to the plaque. In general, these systemic factors can be categorized as those that predominantly affect the presentation of gingival inflammation and those that affect disease progression and susceptibility to periodontitis. Some of these conditions, such as type 2 diabetes mellitus, are extremely common, whereas there are a number of very rare, typically genetically inherited conditions that may also have profound effects on the presentation of periodontal disease.

Systemic factors predominantly affecting the gingival tissues

Pregnancy

It is well-recognized that the gingivae may show increased bleeding during pregnancy. Pregnancy gingivitis is an

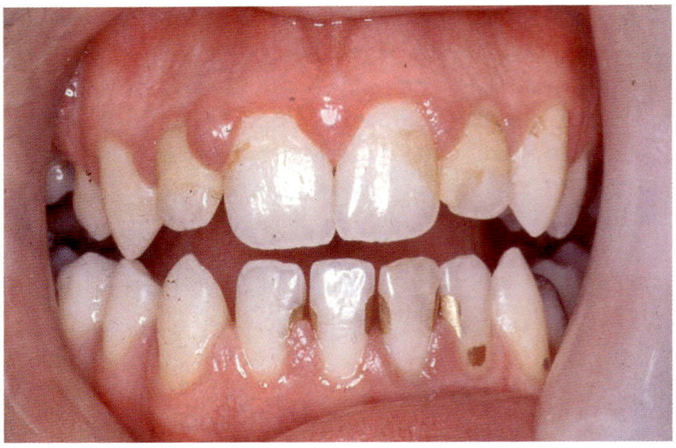

Fig 3.1 Swollen and inflamed gingivae, most marked here in the upper incisor regions, in pregnancy gingivitis. (Corsodyl staining of composite restorations in lower incisors is also evident.)

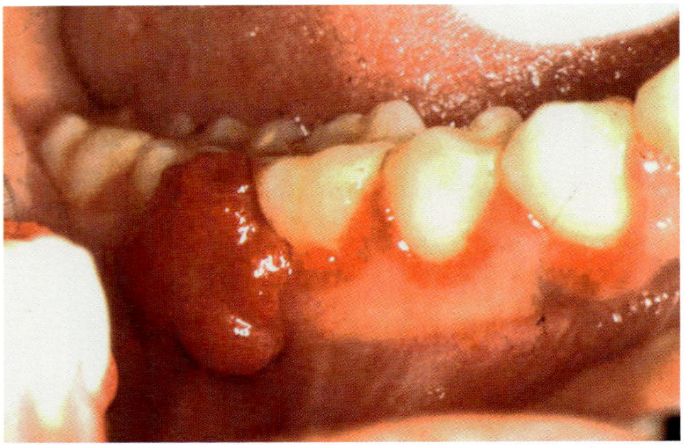

Fig 3.2 Pregnancy epulis arising from buccal interdental papilla between LR6 and LR7. Note the size of the lesion, which extends to the occlusal table, as seen by the indentation of the upper molar cusp that is visible. Note also profuse pregnancy gingivitis affecting the other teeth.

increase in gingivitis seen during pregnancy, which is thought to be due largely to the increased vascular blood flow associated with elevated progesterone levels. Pregnancy gingivitis in its mild form may simply be manifest as profuse gingival bleeding on minor trauma such as tooth brushing and even when eating. More typically, the gingivae show increased swelling, redness, and are extremely haemorrhagic (Figure 3.1). Pregnancy gingivitis may manifest at any time during pregnancy, but in the absence of adequate management it will persist throughout the term of the pregnancy. As with all conditions, prevention is better than cure, and it is essential that patients understand the importance of maintenance of a high standard of plaque control measures during pregnancy. Once pregnancy gingivitis is established, it is still managed by normal plaque control measures, but achieving full resolution can be quite a challenge and may occasionally benefit from the use of adjunctive local antimicrobial agents such as chlorhexidine mouthwash or gel.

Occasionally, the inflammation may be sufficiently severe as to result in the formation of a localized pyogenic granuloma known as a pregnancy epulis. The pregnancy epulis is a localized inflammatory swelling that is extremely haemorrhagic and can often become quite large—for example, growing sufficiently to interfere with the occlusion (Figure 3.2). Management of a large pregnancy epulis is a particular challenge because surgical removal during pregnancy results in considerable bleeding and is best avoided until after the pregnancy term is complete, if possible. Occasionally, these lesions can alternatively be managed by cryosurgery or laser surgery, but these techniques are not readily available in all centres. Again, the emphasis is on primary plaque control as the initial management tool. Following the birth of the infant, the pregnancy epulis will often become considerably more fibrous in a relatively short period of time, which may make it much more amenable to subsequent surgical removal.

Other hormonal factors

Less marked increased gingival bleeding, similar to pregnancy gingivitis, may be seen in patients taking the contraceptive pill and in girls at puberty, and occasionally patients report marked variations in gingival bleeding during their menstrual cycle. Again, the emphasis is on establishment and maintenance of good plaque control measures together with professional cleaning and careful oral hygiene instruction.

There is little evidence that pregnancy gingivitis or other hormonally related gingival inflammation results directly in increased periodontal breakdown. However, the establishment of poor periodontal health, such as may occur during pregnancy, may well be associated with risk of future periodontitis. Once it has become established, gingival inflammation is much more difficult to resolve than if there has been maintenance of good gingival health from the outset.

Drug-induced gingival enlargement

Drug-induced gingival enlargement, also known as drug-induced gingival overgrowth, is caused by three distinct classes of drugs:

- Phenytoin
- Ciclosporin
- Calcium channel blocker drugs

The general feature of drug-induced gingival enlargement is a variable degree of enlargement of the gingivae, particularly focused at the dental papillae, which is associated with the dose of the drug and the level of plaque and inflammation present. The mechanisms of action of these drugs to cause gingival enlargement are not fully understood, and it is not clear whether the same mechanisms account for the gingival response in each class of drug.

Phenytoin-induced gingival enlargement

Phenytoin is an anticonvulsant drug used mainly for the treatment of epilepsy. Many patients with epilepsy take phenytoin, but it is not usually the first drug of choice for epilepsy management. Although there are sporadic cases of gingival enlargement reported with the use of other anticonvulsant drugs, notably lamotrigine, these cases appear to be very rare and the gingival enlargement is mainly a specific side effect of phenytoin. The clinical features of phenytoin-induced gingival enlargement are principally

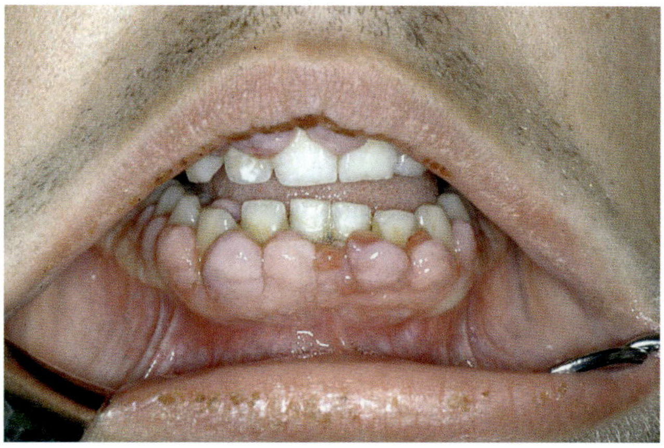

Fig 3.3 Marked, predominantly fibrous, gingival enlargement in a patient taking phenytoin.

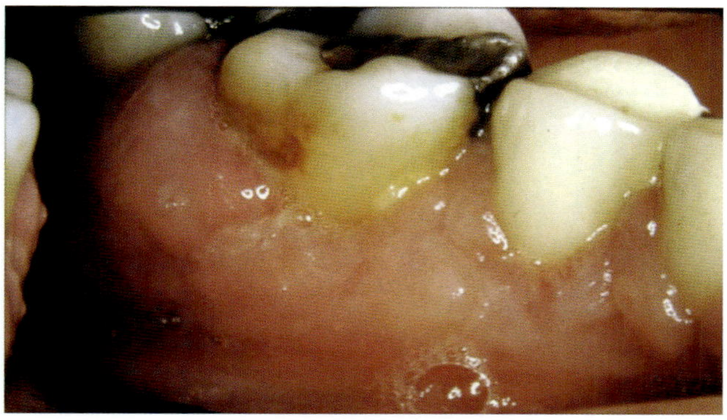

Fig 3.4 Gingival enlargement in a patient taking ciclosporin following a renal transplant 2 years previously. Note the marked enlargement distal to LL6 but also signs of enlargement affecting the other papillae.

fibrous swelling of the gingivae, particularly emanating from the dental papillae, which may have a fibrous, pink, and uninflamed appearance (Figure 3.3). However, the enlargement is a major impediment to successful plaque control that can result in secondary gingival inflammation, and it also creates a cycle of poor plaque control resulting in increased enlargement, which in turn further impairs plaque control. Studies on the pathogenesis of this condition have demonstrated that phenytoin can, in susceptible individuals, induce fibroblast proliferation, and it has been proposed that mechanisms causing the enlargement relate to altered fibroblast metabolism. The prevalence of gingival enlargement in patients taking phenytoin has been described variously from 10 to 50% in different studies. The presence and severity of the enlargement has been related to the presence of plaque, the serum concentrations of the drug, and the potential adverse effects of phenytoin on folate metabolism. The management of this condition is primarily aimed at addressing the plaque control and surgical removal of the enlarged tissue by gingivectomy (see Chapter 11). However, in the presence of persisting phenytoin medication, there is a considerable risk of recurrence of the condition.

Although there are many reports of marked spontaneous improvement following withdrawal of the drug and replacement with a different anticonvulsant therapy, considerable caution needs to be exercised when considering this treatment given the serious implications of loss of control of seizures in the patient whose epilepsy is currently well controlled. In severe cases, the dental practitioner may need to liaise closely with the attending neurologist in order to discuss whether substitution of the drug with another anticonvulsant would be appropriate and beneficial.

Ciclosporin

Ciclosporin is an immunosuppressant drug that is particularly widely used for the suppression of graft rejection following transplantation of organs, most notably kidneys but also any other organ transplant procedure. The gingival enlargement seen with ciclosporin is often less notably fibrous than that of phenytoin-induced gingival enlargement and is reportedly responsible for the most severe gingival overgrowth of all three classes of drugs implicated (Figure 3.4). It is also exacerbated in patients who have had renal transplants by the fact that many of them are also prescribed a calcium channel blocking drug that appears to have synergistic actions in causing gingival overgrowth. The prevalence of gingival overgrowth in patients taking ciclosporin may be as high as 30–40%, and because of the severity of the response, this is a troublesome and disfiguring side effect of this medication. An alternative graft rejection-preventing drug, tacrolimus, has become widely used and is not usually associated with risk of gingival enlargement. However, given the various serious implications of destabilizing the prevention of graft rejection with a patient following organ transplantation, it is not usually advisable or possible to substitute ciclosporin for tacrolimus in a patient in whom graft rejection is currently being managed successfully. Again, treatment therefore depends on maintenance of good plaque control and surgical management of the enlarged gingival tissue as appropriate. Recurrence of gingival enlargement following corrective surgery is a common problem, and considerable emphasis needs to be placed on achieving excellent standards of plaque control and regular dental care to minimize this risk.

Calcium channel blocking drugs

The calcium channel blocking drugs are very widely used medications for the control of hypertension and also in the management of coronary artery disease. Their primary action is to cause vasodilation. In recent years, calcium channel blockers (including nifedipine, amlodipine, felodipine, verapamil, and diltiazem) have become one of the most widely prescribed classes of drugs for the primary management of hypertension. The reported prevalence of gingival enlargement associated with the calcium channel blockers is highly variable, ranging between 5 and 40% of patients being affected in different studies according to the different criteria used for diagnosis. The appearance of the enlarged gingivae is often less fibrous and more vascular than that involving phenytoin, and it is also often of less severity (Figure 3.5). As with the other drugs implicated in drug-induced gingival enlargement, there are many reports of marked spontaneous improvement to the gingival condition following withdrawal of the drug. For patients with simple hypertension who are taking calcium channel blocker monotherapy for their management, physicians are often

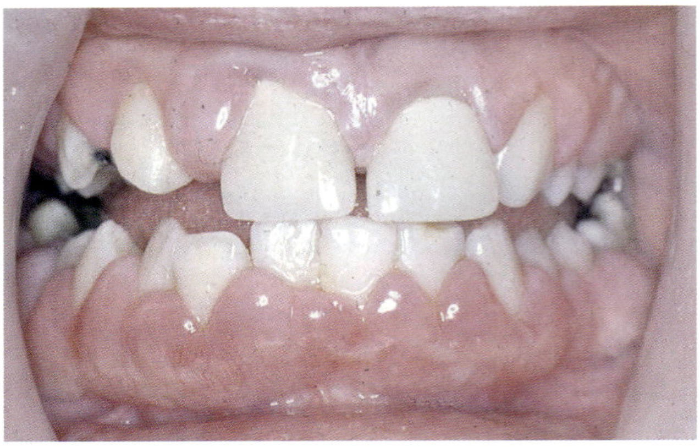

Fig 3.5 Calcium channel blocker-induced gingival enlargement in a patient taking nifedipine for hypertension.

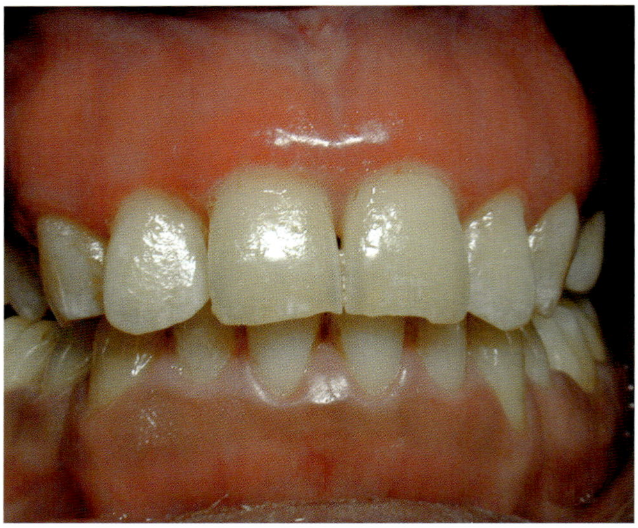

Fig 3.6 Characteristic shiny red appearance of gingivae in xerostomia, in this case due to habitual mouth breathing.

cooperative in trying a different type of antihypertensive treatment, such as an ACE inhibitor, to replace calcium channel blocker therapy following a request from the dentist. Clearly, in cases in which a number of different classes of antihypertensive have been required in order to achieve proper hypertensive control, removal of the calcium channel blocker would be much less appropriate. Given the success of calcium channel blocker drugs as first-line treatment for hypertension in recent years, calcium channel blocker-induced gingival enlargement is an increasing problem and one that will likely increase even further in the future. Again, emphasis on good plaque control and debridement of the false pocketing, together with surgical management where required, is normal treatment that can be very successful but that is also often associated with recurrence in due course.

Xerostomia

Xerostomia, or dry mouth, results in reduced or lack of salivary flow and can result in increased gingival disease due to the reduction in salivary antibacterial factors present in saliva. This is most commonly seen in patients who are mouth breathers, where habitual open-mouth posture leads to drying of the anterior gingival tissues, particularly in the upper anterior region (Figure 3.6). This typically results in a shiny, fiery red gingivitis that is also often associated with a hyperplastic response of the gingiva, where patients typically remark on the unsightly appearance of the gingivae, together with profuse gingival bleeding on minor trauma such as toothbrushing and eating. Xerostomia is a classic feature of some systemic diseases and is also associated with a number of medications in widespread use. Sjögren's syndrome is an autoimmune syndrome combining rheumatoid arthritis with xerostomia and dry eyes. In this case there can be marked failure of salivary secretion, and excessive gingival inflammation may typically be seen. A wide range of drugs have also been reported to cause xerostomia, including β-blockers, tricyclic antidepressants, antipsychotic drugs, antihistamines, and many antihypertensive drugs.

Other salivary gland disease, particularly gland damage following radiotherapy for neoplasms, may also result in profound xerostomia. In all cases, management of xerostomia tends to be symptomatic and may involve the use of salivary substitute that in the management of gingival disease seen with xerostomia is dependent on a very high standard of plaque control, which may occasionally require supplementation with local antiseptic agents such as chlorhexidine rinses or gel.

Systemic factors that increase susceptibility to periodontitis

Diabetes mellitus

There are two types of diabetes mellitus (DM): type 1 DM, which is due to failure of insulin secretion because of autoimmune damage to the beta islet cells of the pancreas, and type 2 DM, which is due to the body developing resistance to the effects of insulin. Both type 1 DM and type 2 DM are reported to have similar effects on periodontal tissues. However, type 2 DM is by far the most common condition and a very important cause of increased periodontitis.

There is a well-documented worldwide epidemic of type 2 DM, with alarmingly high prevalence rates of the condition reported throughout the world. This epidemic has been increasing dramatically and is one of the major public health challenges in medicine in the early 21st century. In the United Kingdom, the overall prevalence rate of type 2 DM is approximately 5% of the adult population, but the prevalence in patient cohorts older than 50 years may be greater than 10%. One major concern regarding the current type 2 DM epidemic is that many of the cases (perhaps up to 50%) of this condition are undiagnosed. The complications of DM include increased cardiovascular disease, peripheral vascular disease, ocular disease, neurological disease, renal disease, and periodontal disease. The magnitude of the risk of these complications is related to the level of glycaemic control of affected patients. Consequently, the challenges of DM include appropriate screening to identify those patients who are affected, appropriate glycaemic control to minimize the risk of severe side effects, and the prevention and management of the side effects of the condition, including periodontal disease.

Glycaemic control

DM causes elevated blood glucose concentrations, which result in the complications of DM. DM can be diagnosed by the physician by performing a fasting blood glucose test, which assesses the patient's ability to appropriately metabolize circulating glucose following a controlled oral dose. However, a better estimate of a patient's level of glycaemic control over a period of months can be obtained by estimating the percentage of glycated haemoglobin (HbA1c) in circulation. International guidelines suggest that an HbA1c level of 7% or less is advisable as a target for glycaemic control in DM patients. Above this level, the risk of complications of DM increases exponentially. However, it has been suggested that an appropriate target for HbA1c levels should be slightly lower—6.5%. Many patients with DM are quite knowledgeable about their HbA1c levels, which are regularly tested by their physician. It is useful for the dentist to have some note of a patient's level of glycaemic control, as measured by HbA1c, in assessing the likely impact of a patient's DM on periodontal health. Because of the exponential relationship between glycaemic control and risk of complications, a small change in HbA1c (e.g., 0.5%) may substantially increase the risk of these complications.

Diabetes mellitus and periodontal disease

The effects of DM on periodontal disease have been widely described in the literature. DM has been consistently found to increase both the extent (the number of teeth affected) and the severity (the amount of periodontal destruction occurring) of periodontitis. The magnitude of the effect will vary from patient to patient, according to their glycaemic control, but in many studies the overall effect of DM is to increase the risk of periodontitis by twofold or greater. In some cases, DM results in multiple and recurring periodontal abscesses. However, this is not universally the case and any increased progression of periodontitis in middle-aged patients may be associated with the onset or the presence of DM. The gingival appearance in these patients is not markedly different from that seen in other patients with periodontitis and, in particular, is not specifically associated with exaggerated gingival inflammatory response.

In addition to the well-documented effects of DM on risk of periodontitis, there is also increasing evidence that control of periodontal disease in patients with DM may result in some improvement in glycaemic control. Systematic reviews suggest that rigorous successful periodontal therapy in patients with DM may on average result in a lowering of HbA1c levels of approximately 0.5%. This is considered to be a highly significant clinical benefit in many patients.

Summarizing these observations, the following important points can be made regarding DM, the periodontal patient, and the dentist:

- Patients with DM are at increased risk of periodontitis, particularly when their glycaemic control is poor.
- Patients with periodontitis may suffer from DM and, in particular, many may have undiagnosed DM.
- Vigorous periodontal treatment may be beneficial to glycaemic control in a patient with DM.

Treatment of periodontitis in patients with DM

DM may potentially impair the healing responses throughout the body, and this may also apply to treatment outcomes in periodontitis. However, in most cases, it is reported that patients will respond to conventional therapy. In cases in which a poor response to treatment is seen in a patient with DM, adjunctive antibiotics may be considered, although this should not be used as a first line of treatment. In all cases in which it is known that glycaemic control is less than optimal, patients should be encouraged to try to achieve an appropriate level of diabetic control. As with all conditions, it is of particular importance to recognize that patients with DM are at higher risk for future periodontal disease, and preventative advice and prompt early intervention are advisable. Newly-diagnosed DM patients should be educated about the implications for their future dental health, particularly because evidence suggests that this knowledge is often lacking. Close liaison with appropriate physicians is always advised in these cases, and any opportunities to educate both diabetes patients and their physicians on the importance of oral health should be explored.

Diagnosis of DM during periodontal examination

As noted previously, many patients who suffer from type 2 DM may be undiagnosed. Therefore, it is likely that in many dental patients with moderate to severe periodontitis, underlying undiagnosed type 2 diabetes may be contributing to their condition. It does not seem appropriate to arrange for diabetic screening of all patients with periodontitis, but in susceptible patients, particularly those older than age 45 years, it may be wise to request screening from their general medical practitioner if their periodontal condition has deteriorated significantly in the recent past. Studies support the usefulness and benefit of requesting diabetic screening in patients with periodontitis who have other identifiable risk factors for type 2 DM. The major risk factors for diabetes include age, obesity, and a family history of diabetes. The increasing prevalence of obesity internationally is seen as a major cause of the dramatic increase in prevalence of type 2 diabetes globally. Obesity is typically quantified using body mass index (BMI), which is calculated by dividing the patient's weight in kilograms by his or her height in metres squared. Many patients are able to give reasonably accurate estimates of their weight and height, but BMI can be more accurately calculated if these are measured professionally. A BMI of 18–25 is considered normal, whereas a BMI of 25–30 is considered overweight. A BMI greater than 30 is considered obese. Given the high prevalence rate of periodontitis in middle-aged patients, it is likely that opportunistic screening of periodontal patients with other diabetic risk factors for undiagnosed diabetes may have important implications for both their general health and their future periodontal health.

Effects of treatment on glycaemic control

As noted previously, the rigorous management of periodontal disease in a patient with DM may help the patient's glycaemic control. The implications of this should be explained to the patient, and all measures required to manage the periodontal condition should be implemented as thoroughly as possible.

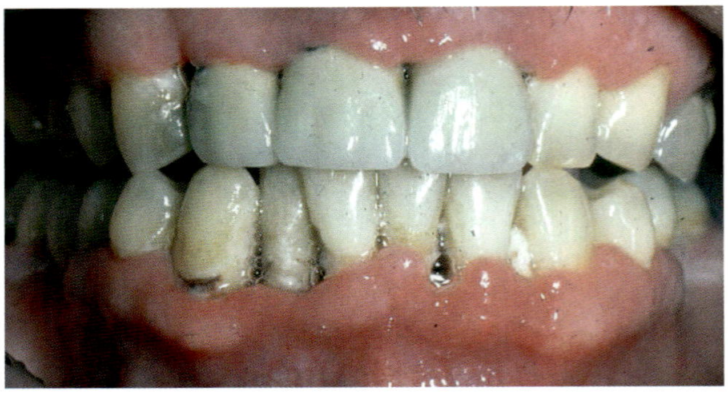

Fig 3.7 Recurrent necrotizing periodontitis in a patient with HIV infection (and with poor oral hygiene). Note the "punched out" loss of interdental papillae and loss of periodontal attachment interdentally.

HIV infection

Many patients with diagnosed HIV infection will suffer from periodontitis, as will many patients without HIV infection. In most cases of HIV-infected patients who are being successfully managed by antiretroviral therapies, the effects on periodontitis may be negligible, and patients can be managed using conventional methods. In a small group of patients with HIV infection, particularly those whose infection is not yet under control by appropriate therapy, the HIV infection may predispose to recurring acute necrotizing ulcerative periodontitis. Necrotizing periodontal disease is characterized by ulceration of the gingivae, resulting in classic punched-out ulcers of the dental papillae that may be covered by a greyish slough and are associated with aetiological factors including poor plaque control and cigarette smoking (Figure 3.7). During its acute phase, the gingivae are painful, although systemic effects are minor or absent. The condition will typically resolve within a few weeks, particularly if appropriately treated with gentle debridement of the lesions, oral hygiene instruction, and a short course of systemic antimicrobials such as metronidazole (200 mg TDS for 3 days). In patients with necrotizing periodontitis, recurrence is common if adequate treatment measures are not implemented. Recurrences will result in further destruction of the superficial periodontal tissues with consequent loss of normal gingival architecture. Recurrent, persisting or unresponsive necrotizing periodontitis is a well-recognized feature of HIV infection, although appropriate periodontal treatment is usually successful in stabilizing the condition. However, the tissue damage is irreversible, resulting in considerable disfiguring gingival destruction.

Although severe necrotizing periodontal disease is relatively uncommon, it should not be assumed that a patient with necrotizing periodontal disease has undiagnosed HIV infection unless there are other signs of local or systemic illness suggestive of an immune-compromised individual.

Case report

A 20-year-old man attended the emergency department at a dental hospital complaining of sore gums. On examination, the patient had the characteristic features of early necrotizing gingivitis and was referred for periodontal care, which initially included gentle debridement with ultrasonic scalers and prescription of a course of metronidazole. The patient was a heavy smoker of approximately 25 cigarettes a day and had poor oral hygiene with abundant plaque and calculus deposits evident. He had a very busy, stressful job. During a series of three visits at 2-week intervals, the patient was followed up for review, when it was noted that the necrotizing periodontal disease had failed to resolve and had caused further destruction. On the last of these review visits, considerable recent weight loss in the patient was noted, and the patient complained of feeling generally tired and "under the weather." On this visit, a specialist periodontal opinion was sought and it was considered, given the apparent failure to respond to normal treatment measures and the associated illness, that an underlying systemic condition, particularly HIV infection, was a possibility. The patient was sent for routine haematological testing, together with CD4:CD8 lymphocyte ratios, and a review appointment was arranged for 1 week later where it was planned that, if appropriate, the patient may be referred for counselling and HIV testing. On the day of the review appointment 1 week later, the patient's representative rang to apologize that he was not well enough to attend the review appointment because he had developed a severe chest infection and was unable to get out of bed. The patient's general medical practitioner had visited the patient on more than one occasion and prescribed antimicrobials. However, the patient had failed to respond to this treatment. Given the previous history, the dentist advised the patient to go to the emergency clinic at the local hospital, and the dentist contacted the casualty consultant to discuss previous findings and possible diagnosis.

Three months later, the patient contacted the periodontal department requesting a further review of his periodontal condition. When he attended, it was noted that the necrotizing periodontitis was now arrested and there were no further ulcerating lesions. The patient reported that on admission to the hospital emergency clinic, he was admitted and treated in the intensive therapy unit of the hospital for an atypical pneumonia. He remained there for 10 days, before receiving further care on the hospital wards. He was diagnosed as suffering from AIDS, and antiretroviral therapy had been initiated. At the periodontal review appointment 3 months later, the patient was well and was gaining weight.

Although this case was not documented by clinical photos at the time, it is intended as an illustration that careful, appropriate periodontal diagnosis may occasionally have important and, in this case, possibly life-saving implications. An important clinical note in this case is that the diagnosis of necrotizing periodontal disease per se was not sufficient to consider investigation for an underlying systemic cause, but (1) the unresponsive nature to the normally extremely successful periodontal treatments instigated and (2) the visible and dramatic decline in the patient's general health together allowed a prompt hospital diagnosis and implementation of life-saving treatment.

Neutrophil disorders

The neutrophil is the "front line" cell for the protection of the body against bacterial infection, and most systemic defects of neutrophil function are associated with increased

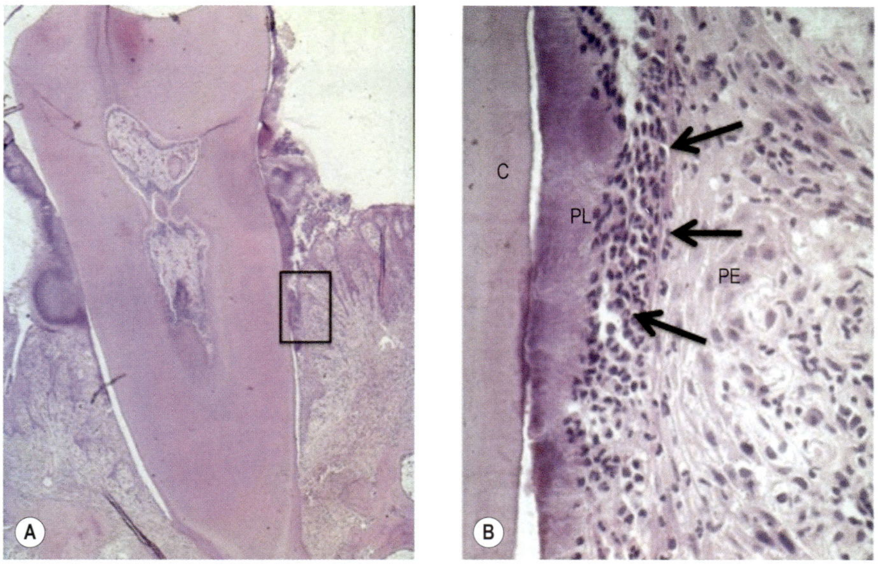

Fig 3.8 Histological pictures of an advanced periodontal lesion. (A) Tooth showing severe attachment loss and deep pocket. (B) Detail of periodontal pocket highlighted in panel A. Neutrophils have migrated into the pocket to effectively "wall off" the subgingival plaque (arrows). C, cementum of tooth; PE, pocket epithelium; PL, subgingival plaque.

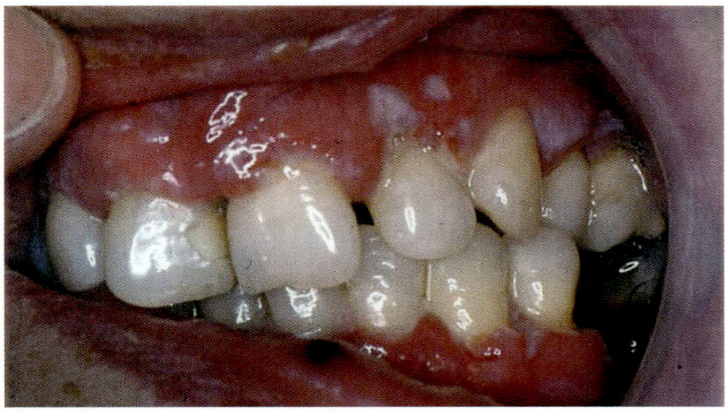

Fig 3.9 Periodontal disease in cyclic neutropenia. Note the ulceration at the gingival margins and extending to the attached gingivae, together with marked inflammation, swelling, and redness.

susceptibility to periodontitis (Figure 3.8). These conditions are generally uncommon but can often result in dramatic and rapid periodontal breakdown, which may even affect the deciduous dentition. Probably the most common cause of transient neutropenias is the use of cytotoxic chemotherapeutic agents in the management of malignant disease. Cancer patients undergoing chemotherapy typically receive repeated doses of such agents, which may result in transient neutropenias or a more prolonged, established neutropenia. This is because the very rapid half-life and turnover of neutrophils in the body (<24 h) makes them the most susceptible normal cells to cytotoxic agents. Patients who receive prolonged chemotherapy in this way may often show signs of increased periodontal breakdown as a result of this treatment. There are many other, mainly uncommon, causes of either transient or more prolonged neutropenia or neutrophil dysfunction, including cyclic neutropenia (Figure 3.9), aplastic anaemia, and a number of specific single gene disorders in which periodontal breakdown in the deciduous dentition is a prominent feature, which are discussed in the next section.

Genetic diseases

There are a number of inherited diseases that can have profound effects on the periodontal tissues and that are the result of single point genetic mutations that are transmitted by classic Mendelian genetic inheritance patterns. These are all exceptionally rare, and the average dentist would be unlikely to come across more than one or two of these cases during his or her professional career. These include a range of conditions that affect the function of the neutrophils where high susceptibility to other bacterial infections is also seen.

In Papillon–Lefèvre syndrome (resulting from a mutation of the cathepsin C enzyme), severe periodontitis affecting both deciduous and permanent dentitions is associated with hyperkeratosis of the palmar and plantar surfaces of the hands and feet.

Leukocyte adhesion deficiency (resulting from a mutation in the gene for the β-integrins) is a condition in which neutrophils are unable to interact normally with endothelial cells and thus are unable to migrate from the blood into the surrounding tissues. These patients suffer from severe recurring bacterial infections and typically have severe periodontitis affecting both deciduous and permanent dentitions.

Chédiak–Higashi syndrome (resulting from a mutation of the *LYST* gene, which makes a protein involved in transporting material to lysosomes within the neutrophil) is also characterized by severe recurring bacterial infections and severe periodontitis affecting both deciduous and permanent dentitions.

In addition to genetic diseases that affect periodontal disease, other genetic diseases that affect connective tissues have been reported to result in severe periodontitis. These include hypophosphatasia, which is due to a mutation to the gene that codes for the tissue nonspecific alkaline phosphatase protein and results in bone mineral defects and profoundly impairs formation of dental cementum, resulting in severe periodontitis and early loss of teeth. Ehlers–Danlos syndrome is a group of connective tissue disorders that result in hyperextensibility of joints and other severe connective tissue disorders, and one type of this disease is associate with severe periodontitis.

Again, it is emphasized that these conditions are exceptionally rare and unlikely to be encountered in a general dental practice setting.

Nutrition and periodontitis

Although there is significant interest in the potential role of nutritional factors in the aetiology of periodontal disease, to date the evidence of their importance is unclear. Severe malnutrition in areas of sub-Saharan Africa is associated with sporadic cases of noma (also known as cancrum oris). In this condition, severe immunosuppression causes necrotizing periodontitis to progress to massive necrosis of the orofacial tissues. The effects of frank vitamin C deficiency—scurvy—on the periodontal tissues have been recognized for many years, resulting in swollen haemorrhagic gingivae and rapid periodontal breakdown. However, there is little evidence of the postulated benefits of vitamin C or other antioxidant supplements in the prevention of periodontal disease.

Vitamin D, and its active metabolite 1,25 (OH_2) cholecalciferol, plays an important role in both control of bone metabolism and regulation of the immune system. Vitamin D synthesis is particularly dependent on exposure to sunlight, and it has become increasingly clear that relative vitamin D deficiency is extremely common in people who live in temperate climates, particularly during winter when sunlight exposure is decreased. There is evidence that relative vitamin D deficiency may be associated with increased risk of periodontitis. In addition, one study has suggested that vitamin D deficiency is associated with poorer outcomes of periodontal surgery. However, much work is required to determine if these factors do have significant effects on periodontal disease susceptibility and progression. In particular, there is little evidence to support the role of nutritional interventions or supplements in the management of periodontal disease in those who are adequately nourished.

Other medications

A number of other medications are being increasingly used for the management of a range of medical conditions that may have effects on periodontal disease. Most of these possible actions have not been fully investigated, but their possible effects might be inferred by their mechanisms of action, such as their anti-inflammatory properties. For example, statins (HMG–CoA reductase inhibitors) are widely prescribed for the lowering of cholesterol. Statins are known to have anti-inflammatory properties independent of their effects on cholesterol levels, and there are a few reports suggesting that they may have beneficial effects on periodontal disease.

A range of "biological" anti-inflammatory treatments are increasingly being used for the management of chronic inflammatory diseases such as rheumatoid arthritis. These groups of drugs are specific inhibitors of inflammatory cytokines, mainly anti-TNF-α but also anti-IL-1, IL-6, and anti-RANKL, which inhibits osteoclast formation and activity. Theoretically, these agents may all have important effects on periodontal disease, although further work is required to establish what, if any, are these effects.

Table 3.1 Summary of systemic factors that may influence presentation or progression of periodontitis

Factors	Effects
Factors affecting mainly gingival inflammation	
Pregnancy	Increased gingivitis Pregnancy epulis formation
Other hormonal factors Contraceptive pill Puberty	Similar but lesser effects on pregnancy
Drug-induced gingival enlargement Phenytoin Ciclosporin Calcium channel blockers	Marked increase in gingival volume, particularly at the papillae, associated with plaque control and drug dose
Xerostomia Mouth breathing Salivary gland disease Many medications	Fiery red gingivitis
Factors affecting mainly periodontal disease progression	
Diabetes mellitus Type I (insulin dependent) Type 2 (insulin resistant)	Very common; increased extent and severity of attachment loss Recurring abscesses
HIV infection	Recurrent necrotizing periodontitis
Neutrophil disorders Chemotherapy for malignancies Other drug-induced neutropenias Cyclic neutropenia Aplastic anaemia Other genetic disorders of neutrophil function	Increased periodontal breakdown Periodontitis in deciduous dentition
Genetic disorders Affecting neutrophil function Papillon–Lefèvre syndrome Leucocyte adhesion deficiency Chédiak–Higashi syndrome etc. Affecting connective tissues Hypophosphatasia Ehlers–Danlos syndrome type VII	Severe, rapidly progressing periodontitis Periodontitis in deciduous dentition
Nutritional factors Severe malnutrition Vitamin C deficiency	 Noma

Summary

It is clear that systemic factors play a very important role in the presentation and progression of periodontal diseases. These factors are summarized in Table 3.1. Although many of these factors are very rare, a number of others, most notably diabetes, pregnancy, and calcium channel blocker drugs, are commonly seen in dental patients. As patients keep their teeth longer, and remain in reasonably good health to old age, it is likely that the effects of these systemic factors on periodontal disease will take on even more importance in the future.

Chapter 4

Periodontal diagnosis

Risk factor assessment

Introduction

As noted in Chapter 3, a patient's susceptibility to periodontal disease may be profoundly affected by a range of different factors in addition to the presence of plaque. Identifying the factors that regulate the susceptibility to periodontitis has attracted considerable research activity in recent years. Identifying these risk factors may have important implications for the clinical management of individual patients.

First, it may be possible to identify patients who are at higher risk of future disease before this has become established, allowing the implementation of an appropriate preventative regime. Second, the assessment of a patient's risk of future disease may affect treatment planning decisions because these may influence likely outcomes of treatment. Third, some, but not all, risk factors may be modifiable by intervention, resulting in a reduced risk of future disease. Finally, a better understanding of how different risk factors may act to cause increased susceptibility to disease in some patients may in the future result in the development of novel treatments aimed at controlling or removing these risk factors.

About risk factors

The terminology used to describe the factors that are associated with increased risk of disease is somewhat confusing and inconsistent. However, in general, the term "risk factor" is used to describe something that is causally related to increased risk of disease, whereas the term "risk marker" is a factor that, although associated with increased risk of disease, is not necessarily causally related. For example, age is a well-recognized marker of disease in that there is an increased prevalence of periodontitis in older people. However, this is not necessarily because getting older increases one's susceptibility to disease but, rather, because periodontal attachment loss is cumulative, so more people in older age groups are likely to have the disease. Therefore, demonstrating an association between the presence of a factor and increased risk of disease is only the first stage in demonstrating a true causally related risk factor.

An association between two measurements does not necessarily demonstrate that one is causing the other. An association is merely a statistically significant relationship between the two measurements. Associations may be due to one factor causing the increased risk of disease—for example, the presence of plaque being associated with an increased likelihood of developing periodontitis in the future. Second, an association may be the result of the presence of a shared risk factor that results in an increase in both conditions. For example, an association between periodontal disease and risk of cardiovascular disease may be partly explained by the fact that smoking is a recognized causal risk factor for both conditions. Third, some associations may be spurious. Thus, the relationship between two factors may be mathematically associated but the factors may have no real or biological link to each other. There are many classic examples of spurious correlations, many of which are amusing and can be readily found by a quick Internet search.

To demonstrate the causal relationship between the presence of a risk factor and increased risk of disease, a number of other criteria can be applied to test the causal relationship, including the following:

- There should be a longitudinal relationship such that the presence of a risk factor in a prospective study results in the subsequent increased susceptibility to disease development.
- There should be a dose–response relationship; for example, the more someone smokes, the more likely he or she is to develop periodontitis.
- There should be a biologically plausible mechanism to explain the association.
- Removal of the risk factor results in lowering of risk of disease in the future.

The latter criterion is perhaps the most important and most convincing way of demonstrating a causal relationship between a risk factor and increased disease susceptibility.

Another important aspect of understanding risk factors is that their effects can be quantified. It is thus potentially possible to describe the fact that the presence of a risk factor increases the risk of disease by a certain magnitude. For example, current smokers are more than twice as likely to suffer a myocardial infarction than are people who have never smoked. In risk factor studies, the effect of the factor is quantified in terms of relative risk. Thus, a relative risk of 2 signifies a doubling of the overall risk of future disease. In cross-sectional and retrospective studies, this is calculated as an "odds ratio," which is a statistical approximation to the relative risk of the factor. In epidemiological terms, the importance of a risk factor is determined by (1) the frequency of the presence of the risk factor, (2) the magnitude of the relative risk of the factor, and (3) the overall prevalence of disease.

For example, the importance of smoking as a risk factor in periodontal disease can be shown by the frequency of smoking in the population (e.g., ~25% of the population), the relative risk of smoking in developing periodontal disease (estimates up to approximately five times), and the overall prevalence of periodontitis in the population (e.g., ~15%).

In studies of the main risk factors for periodontal disease, it is not always possible to estimate the magnitude of the risk because of the fact that many risk factors are not simply "present" or "absent" but, rather, may vary in effects according to the size of the factor. For example, as discussed in Chapter 3, the magnitude of the effect of diabetes mellitus on risk of periodontitis varies dramatically according to the level of glycaemic control of individual patients.

Risk factors for periodontal disease

The following are the main risk factors that have been shown to increase susceptibility to periodontitis:

- Smoking
- Genetic factors
- Systemic factors
- Specific bacteria
- Psychosocial factors

Smoking

It is well established that smoking is one of the most important risk factors for periodontitis. The magnitude of the effects of smoking on periodontitis varies considerably among different studies. In patients who regularly smoke more than 10 cigarettes daily, it has been estimated that the relative risk of periodontitis may be as high as fivefold. The effect of smoking is both time and dose dependent, such that the longer a patient has smoked and the more the patient smokes, which can be estimated in terms of "pack-years," the greater the risk of periodontitis. It appears that the effects of smoking are largely due to a systemic effect resulting in an impaired inflammatory response, with, for example, reduced neutrophil numbers and function at the inflammatory site. Studies of the direct local effects of smoking on the plaque microflora are equivocal, although some studies have suggested an increased number of pathogenic bacteria present in plaque of smokers. It is interesting to note that although the effects of smoking on periodontitis have been described for many years, until approximately two decades ago it was thought that the main effect of smoking on periodontitis risk was that smokers tended to have poorer oral hygiene. In fact, current studies are unequivocal in demonstrating that smoking is a major risk factor for periodontitis independent of any effects on dental plaque. In addition, as discussed in Chapter 9, smoking markedly impairs periodontal treatment outcomes.

The clinical appearance of periodontal disease in smokers is usually characterized by reduced gingival bleeding, and often the gingivae have a relatively pink and uninflamed appearance because of the suppressive effects of smoking on the inflammatory response. However, the amount of periodontal breakdown seen is markedly increased.

Smoking is arguable the most important modifiable risk factor in periodontitis—possibly even more important than plaque control. Smoking cessation strategies are therefore an important part of periodontal treatment and are discussed further in Chapter 7. In assessing the importance of smoking as a risk factor in individual patients, a full smoking history should routinely be taken from all patients. This should include questions about whether the patient is a current or previous smoker, how much the patient smokes, and how long the patient has smoked. Similar information should be obtained from past smokers, along with the date when they quit.

Systemic factors

The major identified systemic risk factor in periodontitis is diabetes mellitus (DM). This is because of the high prevalence of DM in the population and the magnitude of the effect of the condition on periodontitis. This topic was discussed in detail in Chapter 3.

Genetic factors

There is clear evidence that genetic factors may play an important role in determining the susceptibility to periodontitis, as they do with other common chronic diseases. The evidence that genetic factors play an important role in determining susceptibility to periodontitis includes the following:

- Evidence for familial tendency particularly in aggressive disease
- Evidence for racial predilection in aggressive disease
- Twins studies
- Association with specific genetic polymorphisms

As discussed in Chapter 3, a number of very rare genetic mutations result in risk of severe periodontitis that may affect both permanent and deciduous dentitions. However, in most patients, such inherited gene mutations do not occur. The major effects of genetic factors on risk of periodontitis occur through normal genetic variations seen among all individuals. These normally occurring genetic variations are known as polymorphisms, which are common genetic variations that result in subtle genetic differences among all individuals. Particular interest in periodontal research has focused on the role of genetic polymorphisms of genes associated with control of the inflammatory response, such as cytokine genes. Genetic polymorphisms particularly of the interleukin-1 genes have been associated with risk of periodontitis, although data from different studies are conflicting and equivocal.

Knowledge of the role of genetic polymorphisms in many other common chronic diseases suggests that the effect of any individual gene variant is likely to be very small, and consequently genetic determination of susceptibility may be due to the combined effects of a wide range of different polymorphisms in many different genes.

The clinical implications of the current knowledge of the genetic susceptibility to periodontal disease are still relatively limited. At clinical history and examination of a new patient, a family history of periodontitis should be taken, but its interpretation can be difficult. The existence of other family members with a history of periodontitis is not always useful in demonstrating a genetic basis for periodontitis, given the high prevalence of periodontitis, continuous changing patterns in diagnosis and periodontal management in dental practice over many years, and a lack of knowledge of severity of reported disease in other siblings. In aggressive periodontitis, particularly localized aggressive periodontitis, there is a much stronger pattern of familial inheritance, and it is wise to recommend to a newly diagnosed patient with localized aggressive periodontitis that his or her siblings also be screened for the possible presence of this condition.

Specific bacteria

Extensive research has been performed to assess the importance of specific bacteria as risk factors for periodontitis. It is well established that a specific group of bacteria, usually described as those of the "red complex," are strongly associated with periodontitis. These organisms include *Porphyromonas gingivalis*, *Tannerella forsythia*, *Fusobacterium nucleatum*, and *Treponema denticola*. Research suggests that the presence of some of these specific bacteria is associated with future risk of disease progression.

The most compelling evidence for the role of a specific bacterium as a risk factor for the development of periodontitis is from studies of a North African population that, unusually, has a high prevalence of the bacterium *Aggregatibacter actinomycetemcomitans* (*Aa*), and particularly a specific strain of *Aa* referred to as the JP2 clone. In seminal studies of the presence of the *Aa* JP2 clone in adolescents in Morocco, it was found that the presence of this specific bacterial strain resulted in a 13-fold increase in the risk of subsequent development of aggressive periodontitis over 3 years. In addition, other strains of *Aa* were also strongly associated with future risk of aggressive periodontitis, although the relative risk was reduced to approximately a factor of 3. These data provide compelling evidence that in some populations the presence of specific bacteria may be causally related to disease development and progression.

These data suggest that clinical microbial testing for the presence of *Aa*, and possibly other bacteria such as *P. gingivalis*, may be a useful diagnostic aid in assessing future risk of disease. Although microbial testing by DNA analysis of plaque samples is commercially available, more research is required to demonstrate the usefulness of such testing, which is expensive to perform, in informing assessment of future risk of disease and dictating clinical treatments such as the use of adjunctive antimicrobials.

Psychosocial factors

Psychosocial factors such as stress are often reported to be risk factors for many diseases, including periodontal diseases. Studies have shown that major life events (e.g., moving and getting married or divorced) and the "daily hassles" of life (e.g., having noisy neighbours and difficult commute to work) are associated with increased risk of periodontitis. Studies suggest that these psychosocial factors may adversely influence behaviours, such as smoking more and paying less attention to oral hygiene, but also have an independent direct effect on the immune system, which can partly account for their effects on disease.

In addition, research suggests that it may not be the presence of stressors per se, which may be common to most people, but rather people's reaction to that stress and how they cope with it that may be the main determinant of the effects of psychosocial factors in risk of disease. Psychologists measure these responses to stress in terms of psychological constructs such as "coping mechanisms" and "emotional intelligence." Thus, clinically it is difficult to assess the role of stress in an individual patient by simple questions such as "Do you have much stress in your life?" Psychologists use validated inventories, which are a series of standardized questions, to assess patients' exposure to stressors, particularly the way in which different people deal with the effects that stress has on them. There is evidence that a person's coping mechanisms and emotional intelligence can be positively modified by psychological intervention, and this raises the possibility that in the future such intervention could improve responses to behavioural change (improving plaque control and quitting smoking), but this remains to be determined.

Assessing future risk

Tooth-related risk factors

So far, we have discussed risk factors that may influence the susceptibility of different patients. In addition, there are a number of factors that may influence the risk of future disease progression in individual teeth. Studies of long-term outcomes of periodontal treatment demonstrate that well-executed periodontal treatment together with a long-term maintenance programme are extremely successful in preventing future tooth loss over a number of years. However, these studies demonstrate that risk of future progression and subsequent tooth loss is seen in a minority of patients (10–20%), and certain factors present at diagnosis on individual teeth make them more or less susceptible to future problems. At a tooth level, factors that are associated with future risk of tooth loss include the following:

- Extent of existing pocketing
- Tooth mobility
- Furcation involvement
- Maxillary teeth
- Posterior teeth

These factors are considered at initial clinical examination, treatment planning, and reassessment, as discussed in Chapters 1, 6, and 9. In assessing the prognosis of a tooth, however, it should be recognized that although, for example, the presence of a furcation lesion may markedly increase the relative risk of tooth loss (e.g., by three or four times), the absolute risk of tooth loss in most patients, even where these factors are present, is still quite low. The distinction between relative and absolute risk here is an important one and can be illustrated by the following analogy:

If a person buys a single ticket for a national lottery, imagine that his chances of winning the jackpot are 1:15,000,000 ("absolute risk" of winning). If the person buys three tickets, he increases his chances of winning by threefold (a relative risk of ×3). However, his absolute risk of winning remains very small at 1:5,000,000.

Because the absolute risk of tooth loss after treatment may be less that 5% over 10 years, the absolute risk of tooth loss even in a furcation area still remains quite low.

Calculating risk

In assessing a patient's future risk of disease and prognosis of treatment, we need to assess both the patient-related risk factors and the tooth-related risk factors to inform treatment planning decisions such as need for extractions. Clinicians tend to do this on a slightly ad hoc basis, and studies suggest that they overestimate the role of tooth-related risk factors and underestimate the importance of patient-related risk factors. It is clear that assessment of future risk is potentially extremely valuable in informing future treatment plans, including need for extractions, tooth replacement, restorations, and maintenance regimes. A number of computer-driven algorithms have been devised to assist in objective risk factor assessment. Some of these are designed for self-assessment of the public, such as that on the website of the American Academy of Periodontology. Others have been devised for use by clinicians in the personal assessment of patient risk to help inform future outcomes. Risk assessment algorithms that have been extensively validated are attractive for the clinician because they tend to remove the subjective judgements that a clinician will impose on the risk factors present and that are difficult to factor together. Further validation and development of these tests is likely to be extremely useful clinically.

Periodontal disease as a risk factor for systemic disease

One of the most important areas of periodontal research is based on the finding that the presence of periodontal disease is strongly associated with risk of a number of important common chronic diseases, including cardiovascular disease, diabetes mellitus, osteoporosis, and rheumatoid arthritis. Periodontal disease has also been associated with risk of obstetric complications of pregnancy. Determining the causal nature of these associations is consequently of considerable importance, given the implication that periodontal treatment may lower the risk of other common, sometimes life-threatening conditions.

The normal rules of evaluating the association between two factors for causal links, as discussed previously, are particularly relevant to this area of periodontal research. One of the most widely studied of these associations is that of periodontal disease with risk of cardiovascular disease—notably coronary heart disease (CHD) and stroke. First, it is clear that all of these conditions have common risk factors, particularly smoking and diabetes, which could explain the association between them. However, even when these common risk factors are allowed for, there remains a positive association between periodontitis and risk of CHD. In longitudinal studies, the overall relative risk of CHD is fairly small (~1.5) compared to that of other known major risk factors. However, a 50% increase in the risk of a life-threatening condition may be of particular significance to other at-risk patients.

The definitive proof of the causal nature of this association between periodontal disease and CHD would be an intervention study to determine if treatment of periodontal disease results in a lowering of subsequent risk of CHD. Such a study would be logistically very difficult, extremely time-consuming, and likely cost millions of dollars. However, a number of studies demonstrate a plausible biological link to explain the association. It has been found that the local inflammation seen in periodontal disease can result in measurable increases in systemic inflammatory markers such as C-reactive protein and interleukin-6. Furthermore, research shows that in these patients, treatment of periodontal disease can lower the systemic inflammatory response and may also affect other directly relevant mechanisms, such as vascular endothelial cell function.

The evidence that periodontal treatment may improve glycaemic control in patients with DM was discussed in Chapter 3. Again, this effect may be the result of decreased systemic inflammation that occurs after completion of successful periodontal treatment.

In the case of obstetric complications, many studies show the association between the presence and severity of periodontal disease and risk of preterm low birth weight. Note that not all these studies have consistently found this association, including two studies that were carried out in the United Kingdom. The large intervention studies that have been carried out in this area to determine if periodontal treatment during pregnancy can lower the risk of obstetric complications have shown that although periodontal treatment is effective and can be safely carried out during pregnancy, treating the periodontal disease did not affect the risk of obstetric complications.

Overall, this is a rapidly changing research area, but the clinical implications of this work are not entirely clear. Given the uncertainty of the causal relationship between periodontal disease and these other conditions, there is as yet little evidence that providing periodontal treatment will lower the patient's risk of developing, for example, CHD or prevent risk of obstetric complications of pregnancy. The exception to this is increasing evidence that periodontal treatment may improve glycaemic control in patients with DM. Thus, although lacking an appropriate evidence base to inform our clinical decisions in this area, it seems prudent for the clinician to regard the treatment of periodontitis as an important part of maintaining general health, particularly in a patient at high risk for CHD, for example.

Summary

The assessment of the role of risk factors in periodontal disease remains a particular diagnostic challenge because it is normal for a number of both patient- and tooth-related risk factors to be present in the same patient. Risk factor analysis is an important part of diagnosis, particularly when risk factors may be modifiable. Indeed, the whole premise of periodontal treatment may be considered to be based on managing existing tooth-related risk factors. Thus, the presence of the cardinal signs of periodontal disease, including bleeding, pocketing, and the presence of plaque, is actually a rather poor predictor of future disease because many teeth with these signs do not show progression or tooth loss in the future. However, there is good evidence that the absence of pocketing, bleeding, and plaque, for example, are good predictors of future periodontal health, and this remains the primary goal of periodontal treatment.

Chapter 5

Is it periodontal disease?

Other conditions affecting the periodontal tissues

Introduction

Periodontal diseases are a group of inflammatory conditions of the periodontal tissues that are initiated by the accumulation of dental plaque at the gingival margin. As noted previously, collectively, these are extremely common conditions that will be encountered regularly on a day-to-day basis during routine practice. However, many other conditions can also affect the periodontal tissues, including conditions affecting the superficial gingival tissues and those that can cause destruction of the deeper periodontal tissues including the alveolar bone. These conditions all tend to be far less common than periodontal disease, but many of them may either reflect a serious underlying illness or have serious consequences in their own right. Thus, arguably the most important diagnostic decision to be made when assessing any periodontal pathology is "Is it periodontal disease?" In addition, because of its high prevalence, periodontal disease may often coexist with another, less common, condition of the periodontal tissues.

No clinician is expected to be intimately familiar with all of the possible conditions that may affect the periodontal tissues to allow an instant diagnosis. From a clinical standpoint, it is much more important that a clinician be able to identify the signs to arouse suspicion so that lesions may be investigated further, typically following referral to an appropriate specialist. Further investigation will involve clinical assessment together with additional investigation that, depending on the nature of the condition and the possible diagnoses considered, may require haematological assessment and/or biopsy.

A (noncomprehensive) list of many conditions that can affect the periodontal tissues is given in Table 5.1. Although this is a convenient way to learn about these different conditions, in clinical practice the features that arouse the suspicion that a patient requires further investigation for a possible nonperiodontal cause of a periodontal lesion are most important, and many of these are listed in Table 5.2. In the cases described in this chapter, emphasis is thus placed on the process of diagnosis rather than on the (sometimes very rare) diagnoses themselves.

Case 1

A 27-year-old male visited the dentist and complained of very sore gums, particularly in the upper teeth around the palatal region. He reported that this had started suddenly approximately 4 days earlier and that he had also felt slightly unwell and had a slightly raised body temperature. He was medically well and a smoker of approximately 15 cigarettes a day since he was 16 years old. He visited the dentist irregularly but had not previously noticed any problems from his gums, such as bleeding or pain.

On examination, he had generalized lymphadenopathy, and his gingivae appeared red and swollen. Some ulceration with a greyish slough was evident, particularly in the palatal gingivae in the upper teeth (Figure 5.1). Careful examination found no evidence of any other lesions affecting the oral mucosa. His plaque control was judged to be poor, and there was a marked halitosis.

After careful consideration of the clinical findings and history, a working diagnosis of acute herpetic gingivostomatitis was made. The patient was advised to take anti-inflammatory drugs, maintain fluid intake, and rest, and a follow-up appointment was scheduled in 2 weeks to assess the progress or resolution of the condition. At the 2-week follow-up, the patient reported that the condition had resolved within 3 days of his initial visit and that he was now well again and had no further oral symptoms. His plaque control was much improved, and although there were some signs of mild chronic gingivitis, there was no residual damage evident from the condition.

Distinguishing between acute herpetic gingivostomatitis and acute necrotizing ulcerative gingivitis (ANUG) can sometimes be a difficult challenge. Acute herpetic gingivostomatitis is extremely common, but ANUG is increasingly uncommon in those who are systemically healthy. Typically, with primary herpetic infection there will be other lesions affecting other parts of the oral mucosa, such as labial, buccal, and palatal mucosa, and even the dorsum of the tongue (Figure 5.2). In this case, in the absence of any other mucosal lesions, the differential diagnosis is more equivocal. First, the patient is a smoker with poor plaque control (although it is uncertain whether the plaque accumulation was largely the result of being unable to brush because of the sore gingivae), both of which are strongly associated with risk of ANUG. Systemic symptoms of pyrexia and malaise are more pronounced in primary herpetic infection and are not usually seen in patients with ANUG. Although the main sign of the condition here is the ulceration seen at the gingival margins, it does not have the typical "punched-out papilla" appearance of ANUG but, rather, is less destructive and not particularly localized to the papillae.

In this case, the diagnosis was made by weighing the different features outlined, but it was prudent to arrange an early follow-up, which helped to confirm the diagnosis and allowed implementation of any periodontal care that might

Table 5.1 Summary of conditions that may present in or affect the periodontal tissues

Condition	Features	Basis of diagnosis
	Diseases affecting mainly the gingival tissues	
Viral infections, acute herpetic gingivostomatitis	Painful ulcerated gingivae and other mucosa tissues, pyrexia, malaise	Clinical features
Trauma (mechanical or chemical)	Ulceration, soreness	History of trauma Clinical features
Lichen planus	Persisting soreness, redness (desquamative gingivitis), white striae or erosive lesions affecting other mucosal tissues	Clinical features Biopsy
Vesiculobullous lesions (pemphigus, benign mucous membrane pemphigoid, etc.)	Sore mouth and ulcerating lesions; desquamative gingivitis; irregular ulcers, vesicles, and bullae on other mucosal tissues	Clinical features Biopsy and immunofluorescence investigations
Leukaemia	Gingival redness and swelling, persisting bleeding (oozing) from the gingivae, ulceration, other signs of bruising, malaise, anaemia, and breathlessness	Clinical features Haematological investigation: full blood count, differential white cell count, and examination of blood smear
Granulomatous diseases (sarcoidosis, Crohn's disease, gingival tuberculosis)	Granular diffuse firm swelling of the attached gingivae, other mucosal lesions	History of diagnosis Clinical features Biopsy
Wegener's granulomatosis	Characteristic bright red swollen, granular "strawberry" gingivitis, pain ulceration; extraoral lesions; pulmonary symptoms	Biopsy Systemic investigation (including chest x-ray)
	Diseases affecting mainly the deeper periodontal tissues	
Endodontic lesions	Periapical or furcation lesions, pain, swelling	Clinical features Radiography Tooth vitality
Central giant cell granuloma	Localized periodontal destruction, gingival swelling	Biopsy
Malignancy (primary carcinoma of the gingivae, secondary metastases of a distant carcinoma)	Periodontal destruction, pain, redness, and swelling of associated gingivae	History of diagnosis of a primary carcinoma Radiography Biopsy
Langerhans cell histiocytosis	Single or multiple destructive bony lesions, often with periodontal pocketing	Radiography Biopsy
Hyperparathyroidism	Multiple intrabony lesions	Radiography Blood chemistry

Table 5.2 Clinical features that may suggest that a periodontal condition is not the result of periodontal disease

History: duration, onset, etc.
Pain (e.g., gingival soreness)
Clinical appearance
General health/medical history
Other intraoral lesions
Rapidly changing lesions
Lesions not localized to marginal gingivae
Vital tooth within a destructive lesion
Marked root resorption associated with a lesion
Unresponsive to plaque control
Failure to heal after tooth extraction

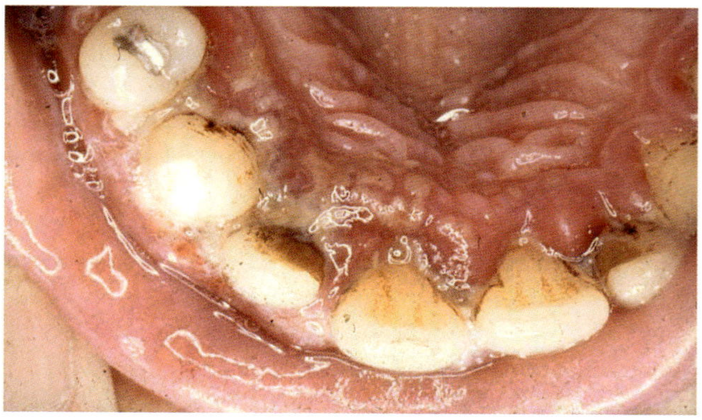

Fig 5.1 Suspected acute herpetic gingivostomatitis. The gingivae are red and inflamed, with diffuse ulceration seen at the gingival margins of the palatal aspects of the upper teeth.

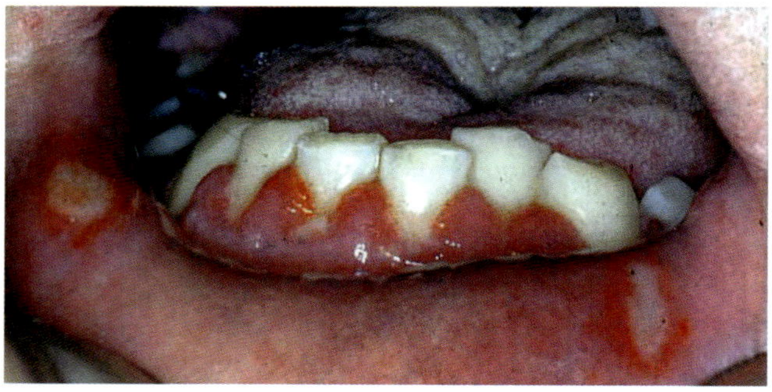

Fig 5.2 More typical appearance of acute herpetic gingivostomatitis. Gross redness and swelling of the gingivae, with discrete ulcers noted at the gingival margins of the lower central incisors, combined with characteristic ulcerative lesions on the labial mucosa.

be required following the acute condition. Although it is also possible for other acute viral infections to present with similar features, these are also self-limiting, and it would not be appropriate to carry out any laboratory testing (e.g., serum antibody titres to herpes simplex virus or direct viral identification), which would not affect clinical management.

Case 2

A 57-year-old woman was referred to the periodontist with persisting red and sore gums around the lower teeth, particularly for the past year. She had had repeated visits with a dental hygienist for scaling and oral hygiene instruction but had not noticed any improvement in her condition. Her medical history revealed that she was hypertensive and had been taking propranolol to control her blood pressure for the past 7 years. She was otherwise fit and well and a nonsmoker.

The clinical appearance of the lower gingivae is shown in Figure 5.3. The most striking feature is the fiery red gingivae affecting the attached gingivae and which in some places spares the marginal (free) gingivae. In addition, a light lacy white pattern affected the labial mucosa. The plaque control was generally good, and no increased pocketing was evident.

The fiery red appearance of the attached gingivae shown in Figure 5.3 is described as "desquamative gingivitis" and is seen characteristically in lichen planus and vesiculobullous conditions such as benign mucous membrane pemphigoid. Together with the soreness and the white lacy striae seen affecting the mucosa, this is a classic presentation of lichen planus, and the diagnosis can reasonably be made on clinical presentation without further investigation by biopsy. The patient, however, was referred to an oral medicine specialist for further management.

Although distinguishing between this condition and chronic gingivitis appears relatively straightforward, a periodontal referral clinic may see cases such as this on a regular basis. Diagnosis can be more difficult because achieving adequate plaque control can be difficult given the soreness of the gingivae, although this is not the case here. Because periodontal disease is very common, lichen planus and periodontal disease may co-present, and in these cases it is wise to implement periodontal care in addition to managing the lichen planus, although there is no evidence that controlling the periodontal disease will affect the course of the lichen planus. In this case, the patient was noted to be taking β-blocker drugs for treatment of hypertension. A number of commonly prescribed drugs, including β-blockers such as propranolol, are sometimes associated with causing a "lichenoid reaction" that clinically cannot necessarily be distinguished from true lichen planus. In this case, in which the patient had been taking her medication for 7 years and the lichen planus had only recently presented, it was considered that a relationship between the medication and the lesions was unlikely.

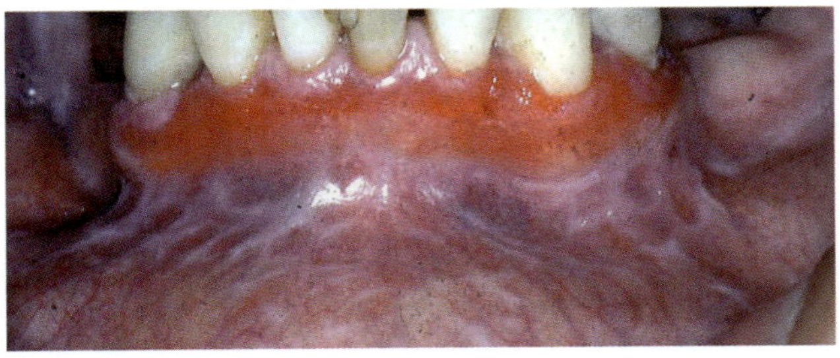

Fig 5.3 Appearance of lower gingivae showing fiery red attached gingivae ("desquamative gingivitis") and the presence of white lacy striae affecting the labial mucosa. Note how the marginal gingivae appear relatively unaffected in some areas. This is a classical presentation of oral lichen planus.

Case 3

A 59-year-old woman visited the dentist and complained of swollen bleeding gums. She reported that the gums had become progressively inflamed during the past few months, and that they sometimes started to bleed spontaneously and then continued to "ooze" for a number of hours. They felt sore, particularly on eating or brushing. She was a nonsmoker and had no history of previous serious illness. However, she did report that she was currently markedly lethargic and felt generally "under the weather."

The patient was normally a regular attender at the dentist, having a checkup at least annually. There was no previous history of periodontal problems. The patient generally brushed her teeth twice a day and used dental floss, but this had been difficult to carry out recently due to the soreness and bleeding.

On examination, the patient generally looked pale. Intraorally, the gingivae appeared swollen and inflamed and had a red appearance with ulceration evident over the attached gingivae (Figure 5.4). There was one area of interdental bleeding in the upper left region that the patient reported had been oozing for several hours after eating. A full pocket chart was not carried out due to the bleeding and the soreness, but a rotational tomogram radiograph showed no evidence of bone loss.

From the clinical presentation, it was strongly suspected that the patient may have leukaemia, and thus the patient was referred urgently for haematological investigation (in fact, the dentist telephoned the haematology department to discuss the case and organize urgent referral).

The patient was diagnosed with acute myeloid leukaemia from the haematological investigations, including full blood count, differential white cell count, and microscopic examination of a blood film (smear). Patients typically have massively increased leukaemic white cells, are anaemic, and have severely decreased platelet counts.

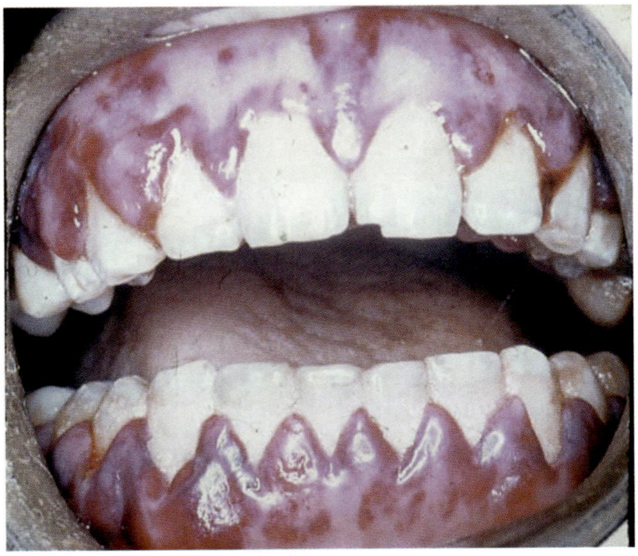

Fig 5.4 Acute myeloid leukaemia. The gingivae are red and swollen, and the attached gingivae have a diffuse ulcerated appearance. There is spontaneous gingival bleeding in the upper left region that the patient reported had persisted for a number of hours.

In some respects, the suspected diagnosis was fairly easily reached in this patient, given the very unusual appearance of the gingivae, the history of nonspecific unwellness, and the bleeding history. The severe suppression of platelet numbers results in the type of gingival oozing that lasts for many hours and is characteristic of this diagnosis and other conditions affecting platelet numbers (thrombocytopenia) or platelet function.

Although leukaemia is relatively uncommon, gingival changes are often an early presenting feature of this disease, and the dentist should always be aware of this possibility. There has been some debate about whether leukaemia should be considered a systemic secondary factor in periodontitis (discussed in Chapter 3) or whether the condition is a primary presentation of the disease. Whichever is the case, it is probably largely immaterial. The affected gingival lesions contain large numbers of leukaemic leucocytes, which presumably may preferentially accumulate there due to underlying inflammation.

Leukaemia can present in the gingivae with a range of different appearances and associated symptoms, but when the initial presentation is at the dentist's office, the establishment of possible systemic symptoms is very helpful in making the diagnosis (Figure 5.5). Patients with diagnosed leukaemia may continue to have periodontal symptoms, including gingival bleeding and redness, and may also suffer increased periodontal breakdown due to both the disease and its treatment.

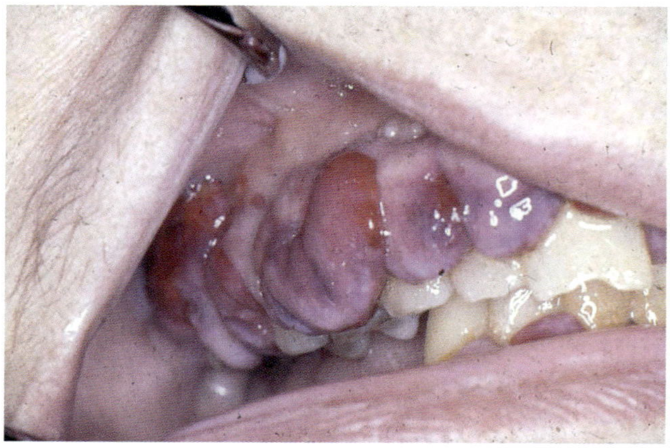

Fig 5.5 A 64-year-old woman presented complaining of swollen gums. She was noticeably breathless and had bruising in some areas on her limbs. She reported that she had stopped cleaning her teeth because they bled for many hours after brushing. The dramatic swollen appearance of the gingivae in this case is clearly unlikely to have a primarily periodontal cause. She was urgently referred for haematological investigation, where a diagnosis of acute myeloid leukaemia was made.

Case 4

A 31-year-old female patient visited her general dentist and complained of redness and bleeding of the gums and some soreness during eating and toothbrushing. The patient was medically healthy and a nonsmoker.

The clinical appearance of the patient is shown in Figure 5.6. There was a florid fiery red swollen appearance particularly of the attached gingivae, whereas the marginal (free) gingivae were in places less affected by the lesions. There were no signs of other lesions elsewhere on the oral mucosa and no history of any extra oral lesions of either the skin or other mucous membranes.

In view of the unusual appearance of the gingivae, the patient was referred to the local oral surgery department, where an incisional biopsy was carried out. The histology reported nonspecific inflammation and no characteristic signs of other pathologies. The patient was then referred to a specialist oral medicine department for further investigation and management. In view of the fiery red appearance of the attached gingivae, a possible diagnosis of a vesiculobullous disease, such as benign mucous membrane pemphigoid or linear IgA disease, was suspected (although the appearance was not typical). Thus, a further biopsy was carried out together with immunofluorescence studies to investigate the possible presence of autoantibodies to epithelial components in the tissue or the circulation. Again, these studies were negative, and the biopsy again showed only a very nonspecific picture of chronic inflammation. The patient showed no improvement with dapsone and topical steroid treatments.

Because there were radiographic signs of bone loss on some of the posterior teeth, a consultation with a periodontist was sought. A full periodontal assessment showed areas of very deep pocketing (up to 10 mm), particularly in the posterior teeth, and matching radiographic bone loss (Figure 5.7). The patient's plaque control was good, and there were no significant calculus deposits noted either supra- or subgingivally. Thus, a diagnosis of generalized aggressive periodontitis was made. It was considered that the gingival redness might be due to an additional nonperiodontal cause, but in the absence of other diagnoses and in the presence of aggressive periodontitis, it was agreed that the focus should be on managing the periodontal condition.

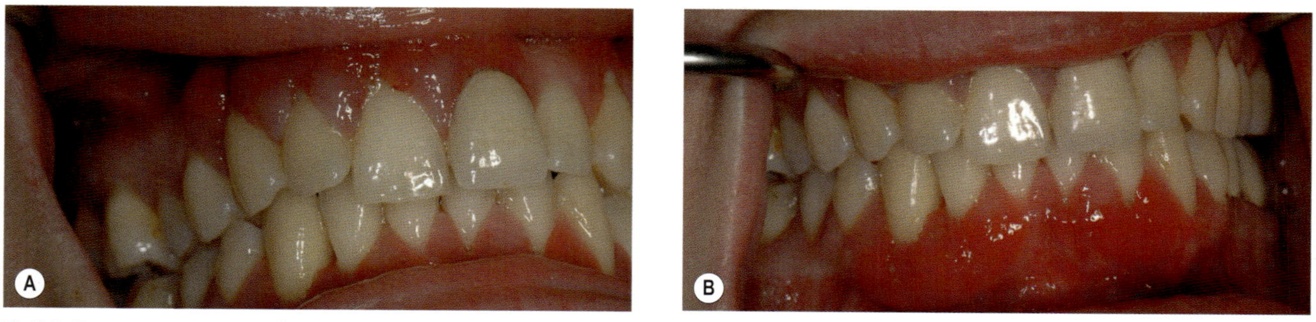

Fig 5.6 Case presentation with gingival swelling and fiery red attached gingivae, not always extending to the marginal gingivae.

The patient then received a course of nonsurgical periodontal treatment concentrating on thorough root surface debridement of all sites. This was carried out during two visits under local anaesthesia. At the end of the second appointment, the patient was given adjunctive systemic antibiotics—in this case, azithromycin 500 mg daily for 3 days—and the patient was scheduled for review in 6 weeks.

At the review appointment, the patient reported a marked improvement in her gingival condition, and a new 6-point pocket chart showed marked reduction in pocketing. On examination, it was evident that there had been considerable improvement in the gingival condition (Figure 5.8), although some localized areas of redness on the attached gingivae were still evident.

The response to periodontal treatment strongly supported the primary diagnosis of aggressive periodontitis as the cause of the gingival lesions. Continued follow-up of the patient for more than 1 year showed continuing resolution of these lesions, together with maintenance of the improvements in pocket depths achieved during the treatment.

In many ways, this is a difficult diagnostic dilemma. At initial presentation, the dramatic appearance of the gingivae did not have a typical appearance of periodontitis, and the presence of soreness and the sparing of the marginal gingivae were also suggestive of an additional underlying cause.

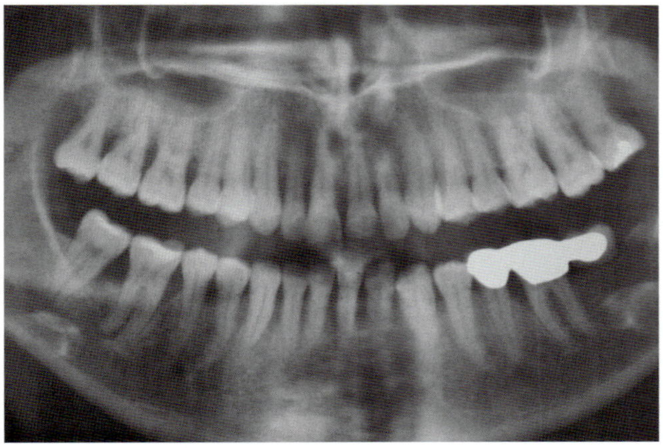

Fig 5.7 Rotational tomogram showing irregular extensive vertical bone loss.

The dramatic improvement achieved by carrying out periodontal treatment is probably the most compelling diagnostic clue. In this case, this was coupled with the fact that extensive histopathological investigation did not prove helpful. It underlines that although biopsy is a very useful diagnostic test, it is not universally useful in reaching a positive diagnosis. Many conditions may have characteristic appearance on histopathological examination, but others, notably periodontal disease, provide nonspecific information on the presence of chronic inflammation.

It is interesting to speculate in this case as to what would have happened if the initial referral had been to a periodontist. It is quite likely that periodontal treatment would have been initiated but combined with a referral to a specialist oral medicine centre. However, the response to the periodontal treatment provided was compelling evidence of the cause of this unusual diagnostic dilemma.

Case 5

A 46-year-old male patient was referred to a periodontist for investigation of uncomfortable and swollen gums, particularly in the upper anterior region, for the past 6 months. The patient reported that the gums were uncomfortable but not particularly painful and did not bleed on brushing. He was a nonsmoker. The medical history revealed that the patient suffered from sarcoidosis, particularly affecting the lungs, for the past 3 years and was currently being treated with the immunosuppressive drug azathioprine.

The clinical appearance of the gingivae is shown in Figure 5.9. There was a diffuse granulomatous appearance of the upper labial gingivae extending along the attached gingivae. The gingivae were tender to probing, but there was no periodontal pocketing or bleeding on probing.

It was decided that the appearance and features were consistent with sarcoidosis of the gingivae, in view of the known diagnosis of sarcoidosis. To confirm this, an incisional biopsy of the lesion was taken, which confirmed the presence of characteristic noncaseating granulomas with the presence of Langhans-type giant cells.

In this case, the diagnosis was suggested by the medical history and the absence of other signs of periodontal disease. In fact, it is debatable whether the biopsy was required or

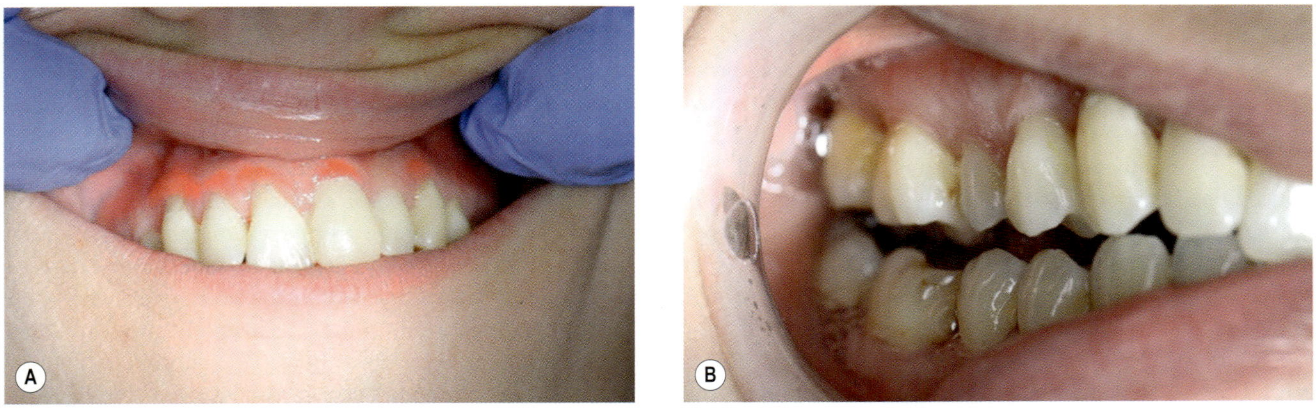

Fig 5.8 Marked clinical improvement of gingival condition at 6-week review following completion of nonsurgical periodontal treatment combined with adjunctive antibiotics. There is some localized persistence of the fiery red gingival appearance (notably in the upper anterior region), but in general the improvement is dramatic.

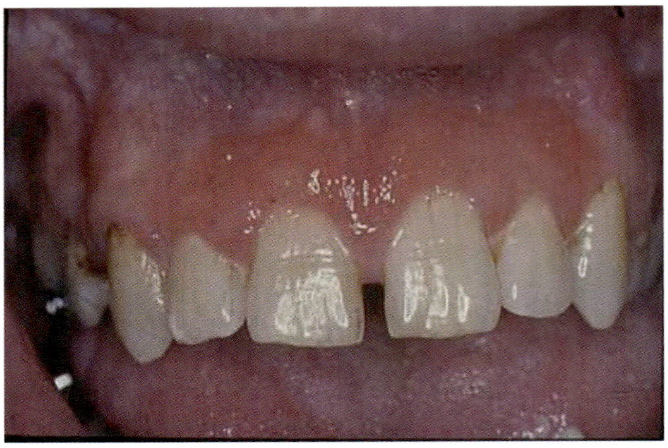

Fig 5.9 Diffuse granulomatous appearance of attached gingivae in a patient known to suffer from sarcoidosis.

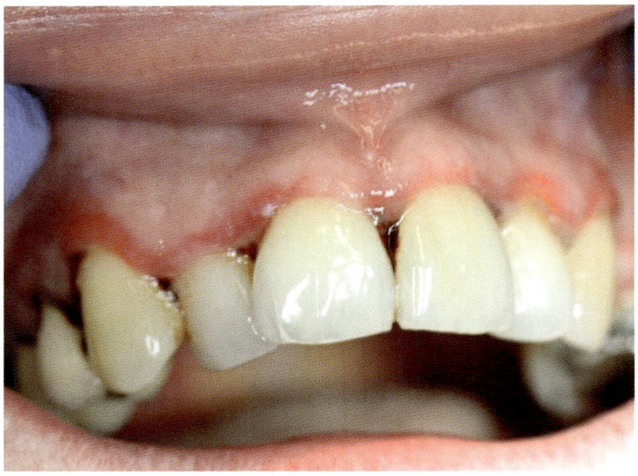

Fig 5.10 Fiery red linear inflammation of attached gingivae.

particularly informative because the diagnosis may have been made on clinical features alone. Gingival and other oral lesions are uncommon in sarcoidosis and other granulomatous conditions, including Crohn's disease and even tuberculosis. It is particularly rare for these lesions to be the initial presenting feature of the disease, but where unusual lesions such as these are seen, particularly in the absence of other signs of periodontal disease, biopsy is often informative.

Case 6

A 66-year-old woman with sore bleeding gums was referred to a periodontal clinic. The patient reported that she had noticed her gums getting sore and bleeding during the past 6 months, and they had also become red. She had also noticed that her mouth was sometimes more generally sore, particularly on eating. She had no relevant medical history and had been a regular dental attender with no history of previous gum problems. She had no history of sore eyes or other mucosal or skin lesions.

The clinical appearance of the gingivae is shown in Figure 5.10. There was a linear fiery red appearance along the attached gingivae that at times extended to the marginal gingivae. The gingivae bled on gentle probing, but no pocketing was evident. Plaque control was good. However, the

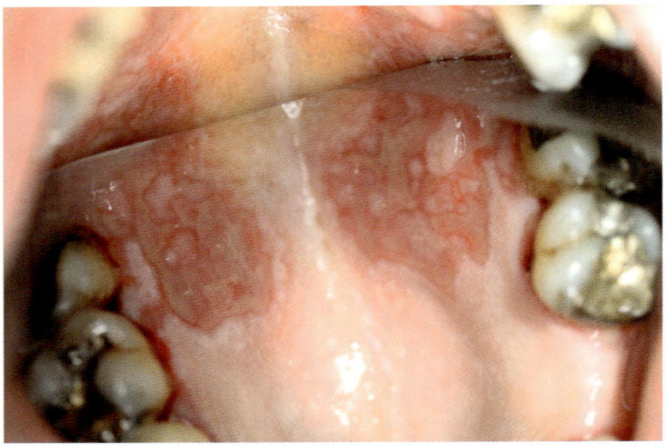

Fig 5.11 Extensive irregular palatal ulceration and visible blistering within the lesions.

most striking lesions were noted in the palate of the patient, in which there was extensive ulceration, together with obvious blister formation (Figure 5.11). On the basis of the clinical findings, a diagnosis of a vesiculobullous disorder, possible linear IgA disease, was made and the patient referred to an oral medicine clinic for further investigation, definitive diagnosis, and management.

This case is clearly not the result of periodontal disease, given the appearance of the gingivae and most strikingly the extensive extragingival lesions. Occasionally, the extensive mucosal ulceration as seen here does not result in the symptoms one would expect, and in this case the patient had only vague feelings of a sore mouth in addition to the sore gingivae.

Case 7

A 27-year-old male patient was referred to a periodontal clinic by his general dentist because of localized deep pocketing at LR6, UR6, and UL7, with a suggested diagnosis of generalized aggressive periodontitis. The patient had no symptoms and had attended only at the strong recommendation of his dentist. He had been previously referred to the same periodontal clinic 3 years previously but had failed to attend the appointment. The patient was an irregular attender at his dentist but did not report any history of any major previous dental problems. He brushed his teeth twice a day. He had nothing of relevance in his medical history and was a nonsmoker.

Clinically, the gingivae were largely uninflamed and plaque control was good. However, a 6-point pocket chart examination showed very deep pockets in isolated areas, notably UR68, UL8, LR6, and LR 46. These teeth exhibited grade I mobility. The clinical findings were consistent with the dentist's suggestion of a diagnosis of aggressive periodontitis. However, radiographic examination with a rotational tomogram showed the presence of multiple extensive radiolucent lytic lesions within the body of the mandible and in the maxilla (Figure 5.12). A likely diagnosis of Langerhans cell histiocytosis was made, and subsequent referral and biopsy confirmed the diagnosis.

Langerhans cell histiocytosis (previously called eosinophilic granuloma or Hand–Schüller–Christian disease) is a very rare condition that can affect bones throughout the

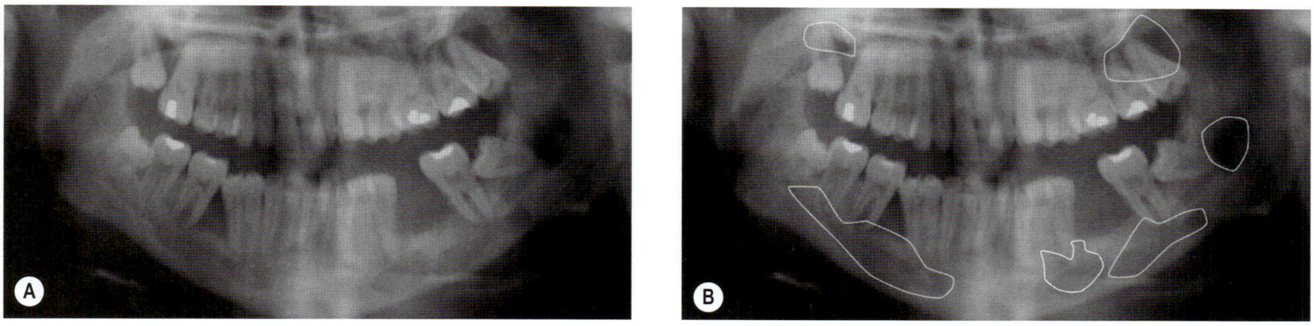

Fig 5.12 Rotational tomogram showing extensive lytic radiolucent lesions in the jaws (A) and with principal lesions outlined for clarity (B).

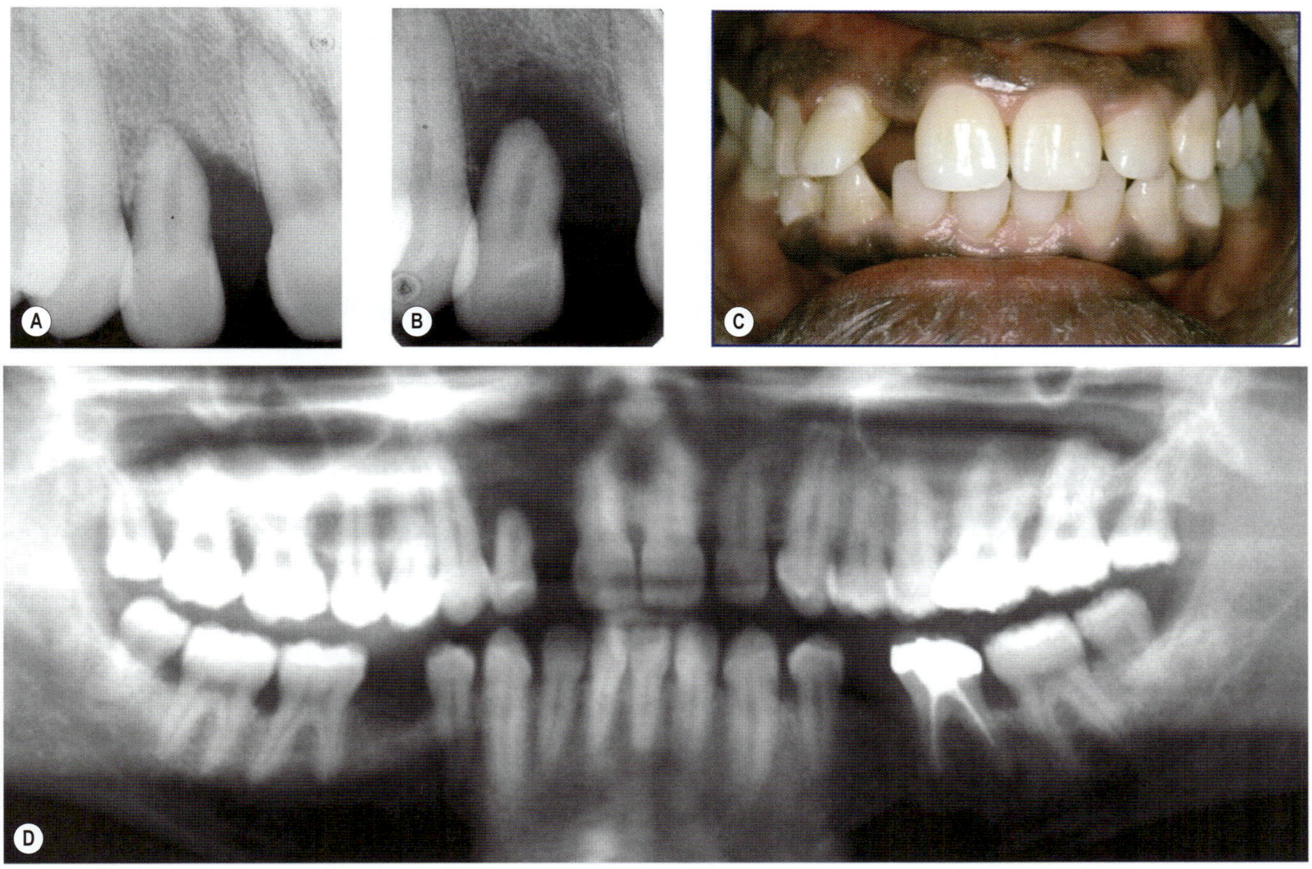

Fig 5.13 (A) Periapical radiograph at initial presentation: bone loss extends to the apex of the tooth; there is evidence of apical root resorption. (B) Periapical radiograph 6 weeks later—extensive destruction of periapical bone. (C) Clinical appearance. (D) Rotational tomogram showing evidence of periodontal bone loss particularly affecting the upper molars.

body, but when it is present in the jaws, it can clinically mimic periodontitis. Thus, although unusual, it is by no means unheard of to present with periodontal signs or symptoms. It can occur as a solitary lesion or, as in this case, may cause multiple lesions. In this case, it is likely that the extent of the lesions is particularly severe given the presence of deep pocketing 3 years previously that, because of the patient's failure to attend an appointment, was not investigated at that time. Diagnosis is based on the characteristic histology with a marked infiltrate of eosinophils.

Case 8

A 25-year-old man presented in a dental emergency clinic complaining of mobility and drifting of the upper right lateral incisor. On examination, the tooth was noted to be grade II mobile and had drifted distally. There was a very deep pocket associated with the tooth, which did not show signs of suppuration. A periapical radiograph showed a vertical bony defect mesial to the UR2 that extended close to the apex of the tooth. It appeared that there had been extensive apical root resorption of the tooth. The pocket was debrided and the patient given a prescription for metronidazole 200 mg TDS for 7 days. He was referred to the periodontal clinic for further management.

Six weeks later, the patient attended the periodontal clinic. He reported that the tooth had become more mobile and had drifted further. Otherwise, the patient had no other symptoms. He was a nonsmoker and medically healthy.

On examination, the UR2 showed marked drifting and proclination, and it was grade III mobile (Figure 5.13). Elsewhere, there was deep pocketing affecting the upper molar teeth. The gingivae were generally uninflamed elsewhere, and plaque control was good. The patient had previously lost both lower second premolar teeth but could not recall why. A new periapical radiograph showed extensive progression of the bone loss around UR2 that now extended well beyond the apex of the tooth, and the root resorption was again noted. A rotational tomogram showed extensive bone loss around the upper molar teeth and slight bone loss affecting the lower molar teeth. The UR2 was nonvital to electric pulp testing and ethyl chloride testing.

Overall, it was considered that the likely diagnosis was localized aggressive periodontitis, resulting in a perio/endo lesion of UR2. The UR2 was scheduled for extraction, and the patient arranged to receive treatment for the other pockets to include root surface debridement and adjunctive antibiotic treatment with doxycycline 100 mg daily for 2 weeks. However, in view of the severity of the breakdown and the speed of the progression of UR2, the granulation tissue in the socket of UR2 was curetted and sent for histopathology at the time of extraction. The histopathology showed nonspecific chronic inflammation consistent with periodontal disease.

In this case, although it was believed that the likely diagnosis of the UR2 was a perio/endo lesion arising primarily from aggressive periodontitis, the speed of progression, the severity of the lesion, and the associated root resorption all indicated that it would be wise to exclude the possibility of a different cause of the bone loss, specifically a single lytic lesion from Langerhans cell histiocytosis. However, the socket healed uneventfully. Despite the presence of periodontal bone loss elsewhere, and the finding that the tooth was nonvital, it was still possible that the lesion might have an extraperiodontal cause. A similar clinical presentation with a vital tooth would be a much more potentially sinister finding, suggesting a nonperiodontal cause of the lesion. However, the negative findings on biopsy, and the uneventful healing, confirm the initial clinical finding.

Perio/endo lesions may often result in symptoms of pulpitis during their development, but this was not the case here. Conversion of a periodontal lesion to a perio/endo lesion can often result in rapid changes in radiographic appearance that would not usually be seen in a periodontal lesion.

Case 9

A 15-year-old girl with drifting and mobility of the upper left first incisor, together with associated gingival swelling, was referred to the periodontist by her orthodontist. The patient had a history of active orthodontic treatment that had been completed approximately 1 year previously. In the past 2 or 3 months, the UL2 had started to drift distally, and the patient had noticed the gums swelling around the tooth.

The patient was medically healthy and had no previous history of periodontal problems. On examination, the UL1 showed distal drifting associated with swelling of the mesial interdental papilla labially and pronounced fibrous swelling palatally (Figure 5.14). There was very deep pocketing around the tooth, which was grade I mobile and gave a vital response to ethyl chloride. There was no suppuration from the pocket but slight bleeding on deep probing. Elsewhere, the periodontal tissues were clinically healthy. Radiographs showed complete bone loss around the UL1 but otherwise were normal (Figure 5.15).

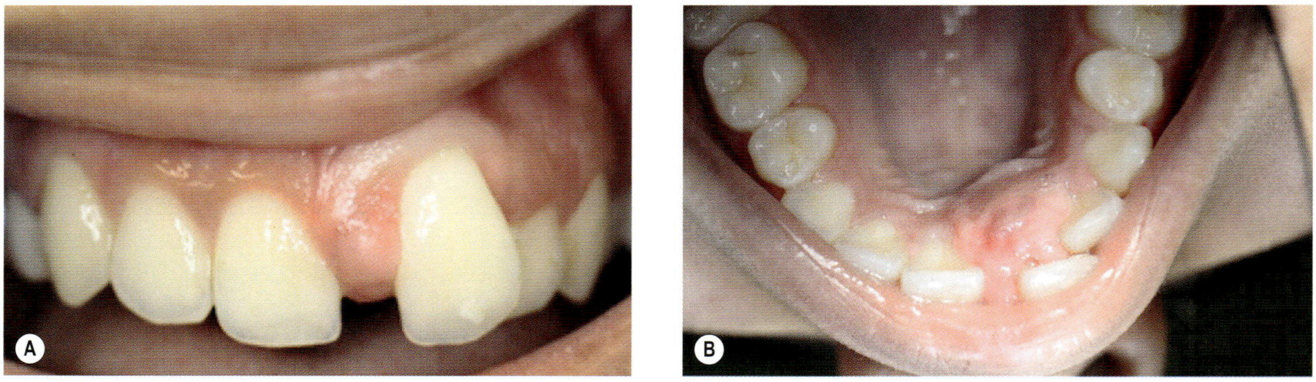

Fig 5.14 Clinical appearance showing distal drifting of UL1, fibrous swelling of mesial interdental papilla, and extensive diffuse palatal swelling. Note the absence of obvious gingival inflammation.

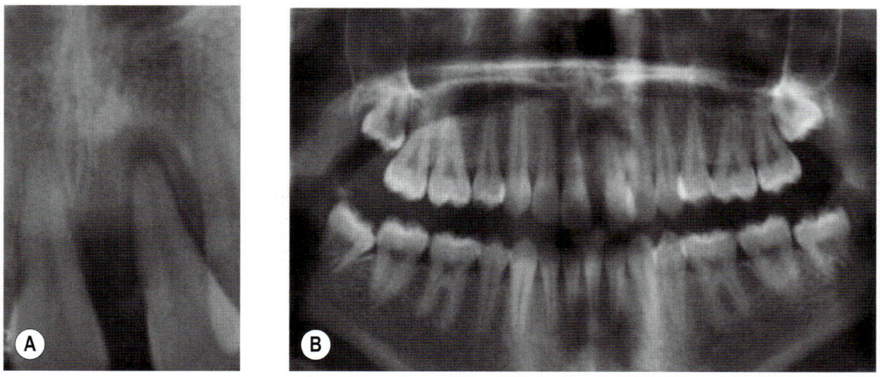

Fig 5.15 Radiographs showing complete periradicular bone loss around UL1 and normal bone elsewhere on rotational tomogram.

The possibility that this was due to localized periodontal disease is unlikely given the absence of marked inflammation and the healthy tissues elsewhere in the mouth. The vitality of the tooth is suggestive of a localized lesion resulting in tissue destruction. The patient was referred to an oral surgeon for further investigation with a tentative diagnosis of a central giant cell granuloma. Following biopsy, histopathological examination revealed the presence of a calcifying odontogenic tumour.

Summary

In this chapter, a series of cases were presented to illustrate some of the possible conditions that can present in the gingival and periodontal tissues. In particular, the chapter emphasized the approach to the clinical diagnosis process rather than concentrating on the specific diagnoses. Inevitably when presenting cases, it is not possible to present all conditions or scenarios, which is why this chapter emphasized the process of thinking behind assessing them. Most of these cases are either uncommon or extremely rare, but that does not mean that the average practitioner will not occasionally encounter some of them.

In a practice situation, it is important for the clinician to recognize the potential for an unusual diagnosis and to take prompt appropriate action to refer to a specialist for further investigation. In making a referral, it is important to communicate the nature of the referral and the specific reasons that have aroused one's suspicions, and one must not hesitate to outline one's thoughts on possible diagnosis or differential diagnosis. Most people do not mind if a potentially urgent referral turns out not to be urgent after all, but it is disappointing if the opposite occurs, where a practitioner's concerns are not acted on promptly. When a referral is considered to be truly urgent (e.g., a suspected leukaemia case), then a telephone call to the specialist is often a very good way to initiate the referral process.

Section 2

Periodontal treatment

Chapter 6

Initial treatment planning

Introduction

In order to plan any kind of therapy for a patient, we need information about the patient and his or her condition. Previous chapters discussed the assessment and diagnosis of patients with periodontal disease. For patients other than those with gingivitis or mild periodontitis, when treatment is simple and prevention oriented, by the time we are ready to plan initial treatment for our patient, we should have a wealth of information to facilitate this process. The aim of this chapter is to describe the planning of treatment for a patient with periodontal disease.

The treatment planning process

At this stage, the following should have been undertaken to inform the treatment planning process:

- Assessment of the patient's concerns, symptoms, expectations, and aspirations for treatment
- Identification of any problems such as pain that may require immediate intervention
- A general diagnosis of the periodontal condition
- A tooth-by-tooth assessment of the periodontal condition, including pocket depths, recession, mobility, furcations, and radiographic findings
- Identification of any other associated pathologies, such as caries or endodontic problems
- An assessment of the patient's disease susceptibility and identification of risk factors that may influence this, such as smoking or diabetes
- Identification of other factors that might influence treatment or treatment outcomes
- Identification of local factors that might influence plaque retention and also a functional occlusal assessment to consider possible effects on mobility, etc.

Initial periodontal treatment has sometimes also been referred to as "cause-related therapy," emphasizing the fact that the primary aim of this treatment is to eliminate or control the aetiological factors associated with the disease, to allow stabilization of the disease, and to promote healing of the tissues. Thus, at this stage, much of initial treatment planning is a relatively simple task in that initial treatment relates to the removal of the primary causative agent of periodontitis—plaque—and the correction of those factors that serve to retain plaque (calculus, overhanging restorations, etc.). Add to this smoking cessation for patients who smoke, and then the previously discussed plan would be an initial treatment plan that would serve for many periodontal patients. However, although it is common to make some of the important long-term decisions about management at reassessment following completion of initial treatment (see Chapters 9 and 15), an initial treatment plan should also consider the long-term goals of treatment, and it should be clearly explained to the patient how these will aim to address the patient's concerns and aspirations. Without this, patients often do not clearly understand the objectives of treatment, which can be demotivating at a time when motivation is most important.

Thus, the initial treatment plan will include the following:

- The immediate management of symptoms (e.g., pain and active caries)
- Achieving adequate plaque control measures by the patient
- Correction of plaque retentive factors
- Subgingival debridement
- Management of modifiable risk factors
- Reassessment, to include the definitive decision on long-term management objectives, which may include the need for extractions, restorative needs, and management of aesthetics and function

Assessing prognosis

Assessing the prognosis for specific teeth, and for individual patients overall, is inevitably an inexact exercise because it involves the assessment of a wide range of different factors that will affect the risk of tooth loss in the future. However, a judgement of likely prognosis may influence treatment planning decisions (1) by trying to control any adverse prognostic factors that are identified, (2) by affecting decisions to carry out extensive (and expensive) complex treatments, and (3) by informing decisions about extractions that may be required. As also discussed elsewhere, a wide range of different factors at both the patient level and the tooth level will affect prognosis. A judgement of prognosis is thus made by the clinician by weighing all of these factors. Studies suggest that, in general, clinicians tend to underestimate the adverse effects of patient-level factors such as smoking on prognosis while overestimating the effects of tooth-level factors.

A list of many of the factors that may influence prognosis is given in Table 6.1. Some teeth may be judged to have such a poor prognosis that they are deemed "hopeless." A hopeless tooth would generally be considered to be untreatable and may be particularly associated with grade 3 mobility, perio/endo lesions, and other pathologies such as advanced caries.

Table 6.1 Patient-level and tooth-specific factors influencing long-term prognosis

Better prognosis	Worse prognosis
Nonsmoker	Smokers
Medically fit	Medically compromised
Low susceptibility	High disease susceptibility
Good response to initial therapy	Poor response to initial therapy
Good OH	Poor compliance/OH
Shallower pockets	Deeper pockets
Horizontal-type bone loss	Vertical bone loss
Simple root anatomy; anterior teeth	Furcations and other anatomical factors (root grooves, etc.); posterior teeth
	Mobility
	Perio/endo lesions
	Other co-morbidities

OH, oral hygiene.

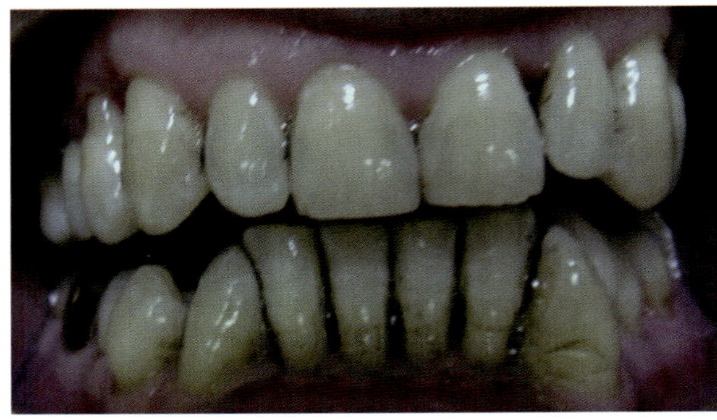

Fig 6.1 Anterior clinical view of Case 1. The gingivae are relatively uninflamed and there is some recession, particularly of the lower anterior teeth. Note also tobacco staining of teeth.

	Mobility					II								II	II		
	Recession		2	5	1	4	2					4	2	3	5	4	
BUCCAL			735	533	323	329	924	422	223	327	633	839	933	469	978	578	
DATE	4/6/2006	**8**	**7**	**6**	**5**	**4**	**3**	**2**	**1**	**1**	**2**	**3**	**4**	**5**	**6**	**7**	**8**
PALATAL	PPD		534	658	534	999	734	322	222	326	735	566	657	668	555	567	
	Furcation			> <											V	V	

LINGUAL	Furcation														V	V	
	PPD		435	533	758	789	755	545	567	657	777	999	859	789	778	547	
DATE	4/6/2006	**8**	**7**	**6**	**5**	**4**	**3**	**2**	**1**	**1**	**2**	**3**	**4**	**5**	**6**	**7**	**8**
	PPD		323	234	533	328	736	745	777	767	737	735	387	368	738	779	
BUCCAL	Recession		1	2	2	1	3	2	2	2	2	3	2	1	1	1	
	Mobility							I	II	I	I		II			I	

Fig 6.2 Six-point pocket charting with recession, mobility, and furcation involvement recorded.

Case 1

A 46-year-old man presented to the periodontist, having been referred by his general dentist. He did not have any specific complaints but was concerned about the risk of tooth loss following the diagnosis of periodontal disease by the dentist. He was medically fit and smoked 20 cigarettes a day for approximately the past 20 years.

On examination, the gingivae appeared relatively uninflamed (Figure 6.1), and the teeth showed evidence of tobacco staining. The following are BPE scores for the patient:

4*	4	4*
4	4	4*

A full periodontal examination was carried out. The 6-point pocket chart, together with recession, mobility, and furcations, is shown in Figure 6.2. There is severe pocketing of most teeth, a number of the teeth are mobile, and there are furcation involvements of a number of the molars. The plaque and bleeding charts are shown in Figure 6.3. There is plaque generally distributed at interproximal sites. However, probably related to his smoking, there is very little bleeding on probing. The radiographs showed many vertical bony defects, as seen in the periapical of UR456 (Figure 6.4). No perio/endo lesions or other pathologies were detected. Subgingival calculus was noted to be present generally during probing.

Overall, a diagnosis of generalized severe chronic periodontitis was made. This was associated with long-term heavy smoking and inadequate plaque control.

It was emphasized to the patient that the prognosis in the long term was dependent on plaque control and on being able to quit smoking. It was also noted that the prognosis for a number of teeth was uncertain given the mobility, furcation lesions, and deep infrabony pockets. After discussion with the patient, he agreed to be referred to a smoking cessation clinic.

The initial treatment plan was therefore as follows:

1. Referral to smoking cessation clinic
2. Oral hygiene instruction, focusing particularly on interproximal cleaning with interdental brushes
3. Supragingival scaling and stain removal
4. Full mouth root surface debridement under local anaesthesia in four visits
5. Reassessment

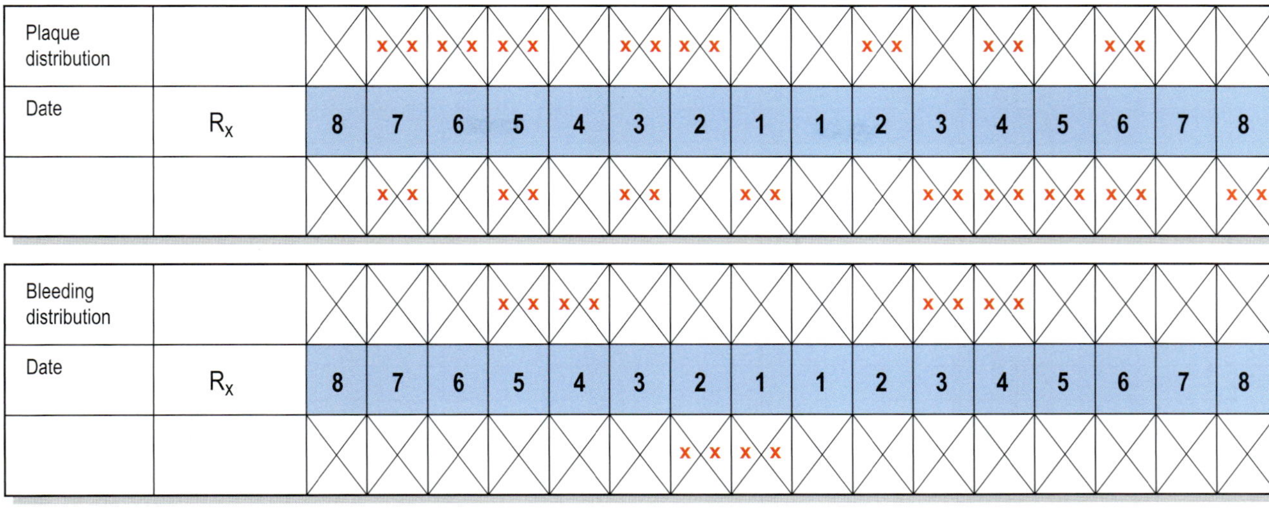

Fig 6.3 Plaque and bleeding distribution at initial assessment.

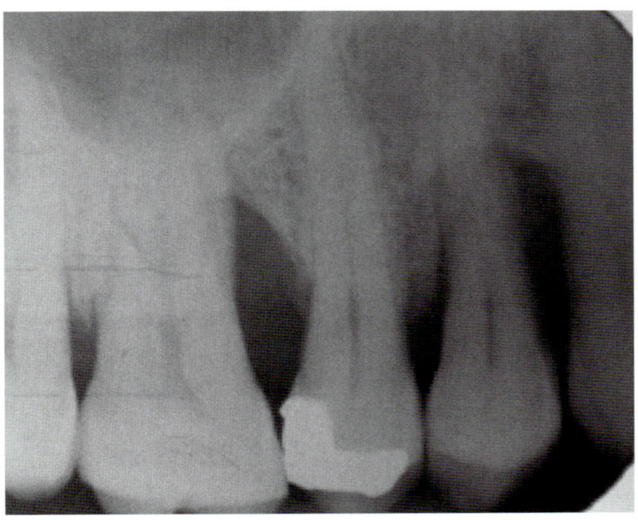

Fig 6.4 Periapical radiograph of UR456.

It was further noted that at reassessment, in addition to assessing response to treatment, consideration would be given to

- Current smoking status
- Possible further treatment needs (including surgery) of deep sites, including the infrabony lesions, particularly if the patient had quit smoking
- Review of mobile teeth

Planning extractions

One of the most important decisions that is required when planning treatment is to consider if a tooth should be extracted. In planning treatment, two aspects of this decision need to be considered: whether the tooth should be extracted and, if so, when it should be extracted.

When considering if a tooth should be extracted, a number of issues must be considered. First, the patients' wishes, their best interests, and their consent are paramount. In clinical practice, it is not uncommon for a dentist to recommend extraction of a tooth but for the patient to be reluctant to follow this advice because the tooth does not trouble him or her in any way. On other occasions, a patient readily

Table 6.2 Good and poor reasons for extracting teeth

Good reasons for extractions	Poor reasons for extractions
Pain, discomfort, or impairment of function in an untreatable tooth	Where condition is treatable
Risk of serious infection due to medical issues	Where condition is stable/not progressing
Aesthetics	The mere presence of disease per se
To avoid subsequent failure of planned definitive prosthesis/restorative treatment	Where no provision is made to replace them if indicated
Because of the patient's wishes	To prevent perceived risk of future disease

consents to extraction because a tooth is uncomfortable or painful, or the patient actively requests extraction. Second, it is necessary to consider whether a tooth can be successfully treated rather than extracted. Factors that tend to make teeth untreatable include grade 3 mobility, perio/endo lesions, and the presence of other pathologies such as gross caries and fractures.

Third, the strategic importance of the tooth should be considered against the treatment proposed; for example, if a root resection (described in Chapter 12) is considered to be the only way of saving the tooth, can the extensive treatment (and its associated cost), including endodontic treatment and surgery, be justified? Fourth, extraction and prosthetic replacement may be the most satisfactory way of treating aesthetic problems (see Chapter 15), irrespective of whether the disease might be manageable. Strategic extractions of teeth considered to have very poor prognoses might be indicated where definitive restorative treatment with prostheses is proposed, particularly where subsequent failure of a tooth might compromise a definitive prosthesis. In addition, extraction of teeth with poor prognoses might be indicated in specific medically compromised cases. For example, extraction of compromised teeth might be indicated prior to a patient commencing intravenous bisphosphonate therapy or before commencing chemotherapy such as bone marrow ablation in the management of leukaemia. A list of potentially good and poor reasons why teeth with periodontal disease are extracted is suggested in Table 6.2.

The other issue to be considered is when a tooth should be extracted during a treatment plan. Teeth that are causing significant symptoms and require extraction should be

	Mobility	X	I	I	I	2											X
	Recession	X		2	1												X
BUCCAL	PPD	X	866	748	637	758	634	627	546	535	434	312	533	333	434	334	X
DATE		8	7	6	5	4	3	2	1	1	2	3	4	5	6	7	8
PALATAL	PPD	X	958	847	844	959	644	555	435	623	524	523	622	434	335	333	X
	Furcation	X	1	2													X
LINGUAL	Furcation	X		X									X				X
	PPD	X	534	X	979	8610	845	435	424	515	413	658	X	1057	422	334	X
DATE		8	7	6	5	4	3	2	1	1	2	3	4	5	6	7	8
	PPD	X	424	X	538	869	954	344	544	434	544	438	X	969	333	423	X
BUCCAL	Recession	X		X	2	2	2					2	X	1			X
	Mobility	X		X	2	2	1	1	1			1	X	2			X

Fig 6.5 Case 2: Six-point pocket charting with recession, mobility, and furcation involvement recorded.

extracted at the initial stages of treatment. In other cases, extractions might be planned during a course of root surface debridement when a tooth may already be anaesthetized. Often, it is convenient and in the patient's interests to defer extractions until after completion of initial therapy. First, this gives the opportunity to assess the response to initial treatment, which may help inform the decision to extract. Second, it may make prosthetic replacement of teeth easier if potential abutment teeth have already been treated periodontally. However, it is important to plan ahead; thus, when it is planned to make a new prosthesis after completion of periodontal therapy, it may be helpful to extract teeth earlier to allow healing and ridge remodelling to occur.

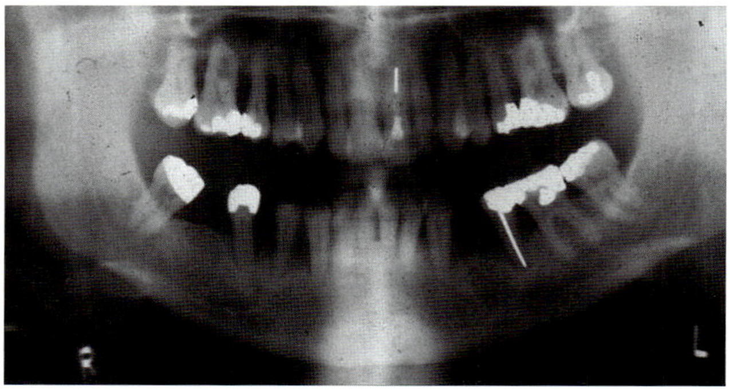

Fig 6.6 Rotational tomogram of Case 2.

Case 2

A 45-year-old woman was referred to a periodontal department by her general dental practitioner. She complained of loose teeth, particularly in the lower right region, and had had bleeding gums for a number of years. She was very concerned about the prospect of losing any more teeth. She was medically healthy and a nonsmoker. She had a plaque score of 64% and bleeding score of 75%. On examination, the gingivae appeared red, swollen, and inflamed, and deep pocketing was noted on many teeth, particularly on the right side. She had previously lost LR6 and LL4 because "they had become loose." LR45 were grade 2 mobile and had drifted distally since loss of the LR6. LL5 was also grade 2 mobile, whereas a number of other teeth showed grade 1 mobility. The clinical findings from the pocket chart, mobility, and recession are shown in Figure 6.5. The initial radiograph is shown in Figure 6.6.

The patient was diagnosed with severe generalized chronic periodontitis. The initial treatment plan included intensive oral hygiene instruction, including toothbrushing and interdental cleaning, supragingival scaling, and full mouth root surface debridement with local anaesthesia over four visits. At initial diagnosis, the LR45 and LL5 were provisionally scheduled for extraction and replacement with a removable partial denture due to their severe bone loss and mobility.

After completion of initial therapy, an excellent response to treatment was noted, including some improvement in mobility, although LR45 were still grade 2 mobile. It was decided to retain these teeth, which were originally provisionally planned for extraction, and instead a splint was fitted to manage the mobility of these teeth and the patient was scheduled for maintenance therapy.

In fact, this case is a "bit of a cheat" because we now have 23 years of follow-up data for her that show no further progression of disease. The case is described further as Case 4 in Chapter 15. It is particularly interesting to use hindsight to further consider the treatment planning decisions made during the initial treatment phase. The grade 2 mobility, drifting, and very severe bone loss on LR45 would probably suggest that these teeth would be graded "poor" or "hopeless" by most clinicians, and extraction at initial presentation together with extraction of LL5, particularly given its endodontic status (which had been obturated with a silver point, a now obsolete treatment that is known to give poor obturation of canals), might have seemed reasonable. In retrospect, the decision not to extract these three teeth appears to be a wise one.

A different hypothetical scenario is suggested in Figure 6.7. In this case, the patient had already hypothetically lost the LR45. It is likely that an objective treatment would thus be to replace the missing teeth with a cobalt chrome removable partial denture. Thus, in this scenario, extraction of LL5 and possibly LL3 would have been advisable for the long-term prognosis of the denture, even though we now know that without intervention these teeth have actually survived for more than two decades.

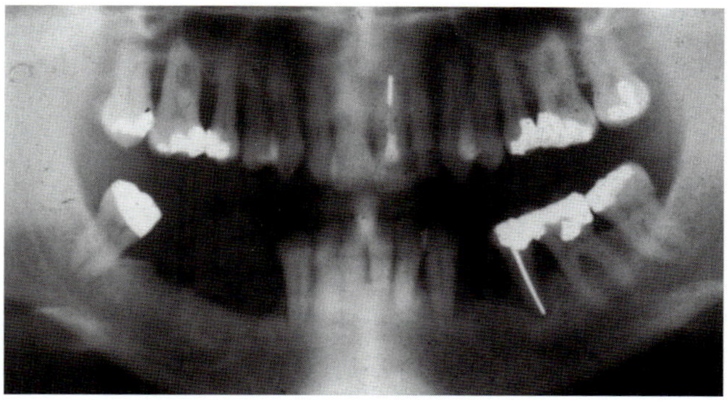

Fig 6.7 Hypothetical treatment planning scenario in which LR45 have been previously extracted.

Summary

Initial treatment planning is directed toward the control of the patient's disease and principally includes the management of plaque and calculus deposits, together with modifiable risk factors such as smoking. Although many of the decisions regarding the need for more complex treatments are ultimately taken at a later stage of therapy, these need to be carefully considered at this stage and an outline of long-term objectives must be discussed with the patient. Assessment of prognosis at this stage requires the consideration of the factors that are known to influence treatment outcomes, but it is not usually possible to predict outcomes at this stage with much precision. In particular, careful consideration of the planning of extractions is required, even if these plans must be altered as treatment proceeds.

Chapter 7

Behaviour change

Plaque control and smoking cessation

Introduction

This chapter discusses two of the most important interventions in periodontal treatment—oral hygiene instruction and smoking cessation. These interventions may also represent some of the most challenging aspects of periodontal treatment because they are dependent on achieving permanent changes in behaviour by the patient. The chapter adopts a "how to do it" presentation style rather than the illustrative individual case reports used throughout much of the rest of the book. We have done this because there are many individual factors to consider for different patients, and thus we consider that the material is more suited to the style adopted here.

Plaque control

The importance of achieving a satisfactory level of plaque control for successful periodontal treatment outcomes has been emphasized throughout this book. What constitutes a "satisfactory" level of plaque control is potentially a more thorny issue. In general, a reasonable target level of plaque control is considered to be an approximately 20% plaque score that is demonstrated over a number of visits. However, because disease susceptibility varies enormously among individuals, this level needs to be considered for each individual patient according to his or her susceptibility, such that in a highly susceptible patient the aim should be to achieve a plaque score that is as low as possible, whereas pragmatically a higher plaque score may be accepted in a less susceptible patient who shows few signs of gingival bleeding or disease even when more plaque is present.

Some plaque formation is inevitable because it is not possible, or even desirable, to have a sterile mouth, and bacteria will always colonize the tooth surface and start to form a biofilm. The emphasis is thus on control of plaque, particularly by preventing it from becoming a mature and pathogenic biofilm, and in practice early plaque formation that is controlled by high levels of oral hygiene practices at frequent intervals may be largely undetectable by clinical assessment.

The process of achieving adequate plaque control requires the following:

- Oral hygiene methods that can effectively control plaque formation
- The ability of the patient to carry out these methods
- The motivation of the patient to implement these methods on a regular basis

Oral hygiene methods to control plaque formation

Toothbrushing

The major cause of periodontal disease is the presence of and effects of bacterial plaque. Most people remove, or attempt to remove, this biofilm with the aid of a toothbrush, and many methods of toothbrushing have been described. However, no one technique is necessarily better than another in plaque removal. Therefore, if plaque is removed effectively without causing trauma, any technique is acceptable. However, when a patient's current plaque control methods are inadequate, then this is likely to require either modification or complete change in methods used.

There are two main types of toothbrushes—the manual toothbrush and the electric-operated or powered toothbrush (Figure 7.1). A manual toothbrush should ideally be small-headed with medium nylon bristles to ensure it is sufficiently manoeuvrable to reach all surfaces. Modern powered toothbrushes either are based on oscillating circular heads or based on sonic vibration of the brush bristles. It is inadvisable to be too dogmatic about what is the "best type" of brush because effective brushing has more to do with techniques rather than the tools used. Powered toothbrushes potentially have an advantage over manual toothbrushes particularly when patients have difficulties with dexterity.

The techniques for brushing teeth with manual or powered brushes are slightly different. A variety of techniques have been described for brushing with manual toothbrushes, and many of these are summarized in Table 7.1. The theoretical advantage of some of these techniques is that they are directed specifically at cleaning the gingival margin ("sulcus cleaning techniques") where plaque accumulation is most abundant and has the most severe effects on periodontal health. The theoretical disadvantages of some techniques is that they are less likely to reach the gingival margins (e.g., vertical or roll methods), are technically awkward to perform (e.g., modified Stillman technique), or may have an increased risk of causing tooth trauma (e.g., scrub technique).

The most commonly taught method in practice is the modified Bass technique (Figure 7.2), which, when using a manual brush, involves the following:

- The toothbrush is placed where the tooth and gum meet, starting on the outside surface of the teeth.
- The toothbrush should be placed at a 45-degree angle toward the gums (Figures 7.3 and 7.4).
- A circular motion should be used, cleaning two or three teeth at a time.
- The toothbrush should be moved slowly around mouth until the full arch has been cleaned.

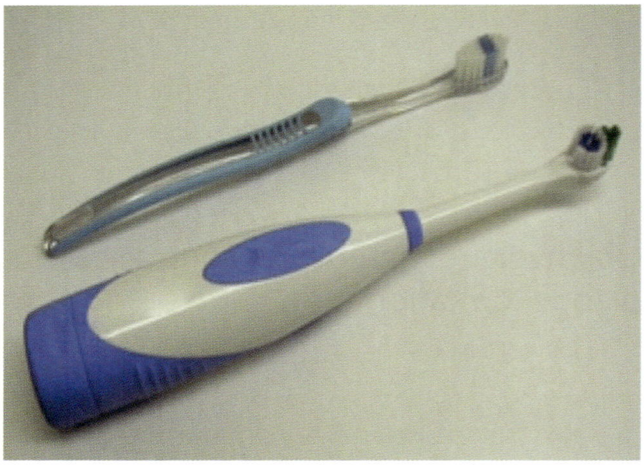

Fig 7.1 Manual and powered toothbrushes.

Table 7.1 Toothbrushing techniques

Technique	Principle	Detail
Bass technique	Sulcus cleaning	Circular vibratory motion starting at gingival margin
Stillman technique	Sulcus cleaning	Mini-scrub vibratory motion starting at gingival margin
Modified Stillman technique	Roll	Combination of Stillman technique concluding with roll of brush from gingival margin toward occlusal surface
Leonard technique	Vertical	"Up and down" brushing movement
Fones technique	Circular	Rotational movement on tooth surfaces
Rolling stroke	Circular/roll	Circular scrub of teeth when closed together; has been suggested to encourage children when starting toothbrushing
Scrub technique	Horizontal	"Back and forth" scrubbing movement

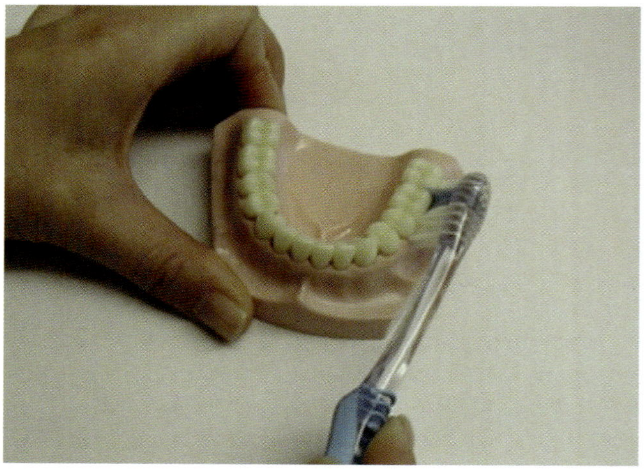

Fig 7.2 Demonstrating the modified Bass technique using a model and manual toothbrush.

- Once the outside of the teeth has been cleaned, then the inside of the teeth should be brushed using the same angulations and technique.
- Finally, the tops of the teeth can be cleaned using just the backward and forward motion.
- Once the lower teeth have been cleaned, the same technique should be applied to the upper teeth.

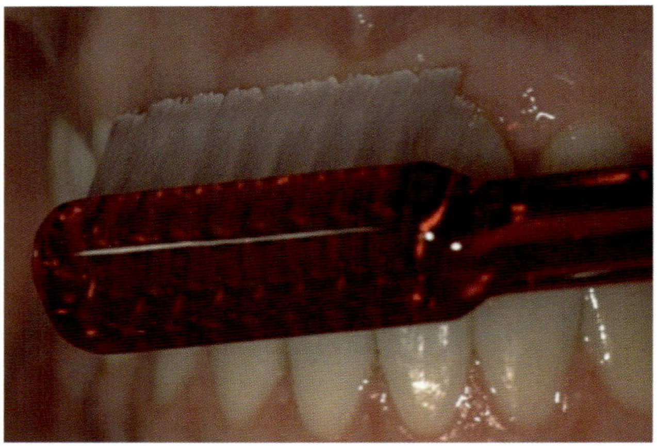

Fig 7.3 The modified Bass technique in action.

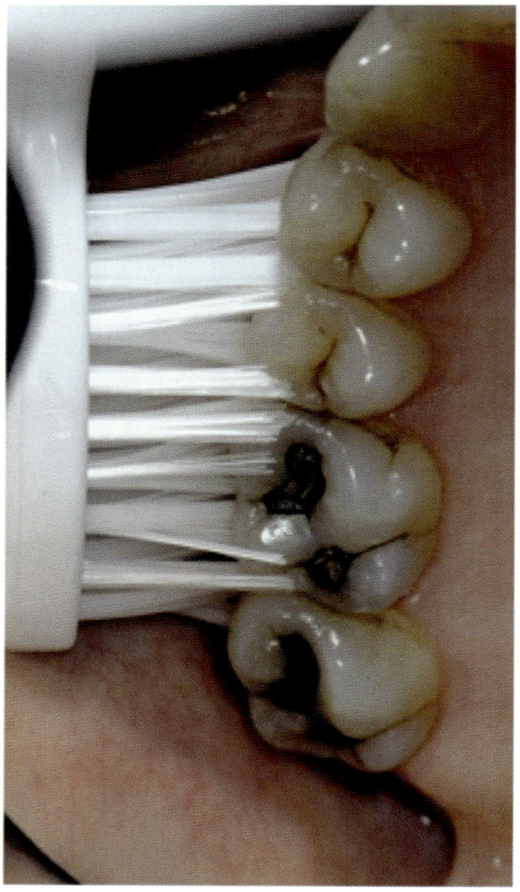

Fig 7.4 Brushing the upper premolar region buccally.

The main reasons for the popularity of this method are that it is specifically directed at cleaning the gingival margin (sulcus cleaning method) and is largely atraumatic to the tooth surfaces and gingival margins. On the other hand, some people find it technically difficult to do effectively, and in these cases an alternative sulcus cleaning technique may be preferred, such as the Stillman technique (mini-scrub).

A person should do the following when using a powered toothbrush:

- Use the same placement and angulations as with manual toothbrush for sulcus cleaning, but instead of a circular motion, each tooth should have the brush placed on it for 3 or 4 sec and then move on to the next tooth, as shown in Figure 7.5.

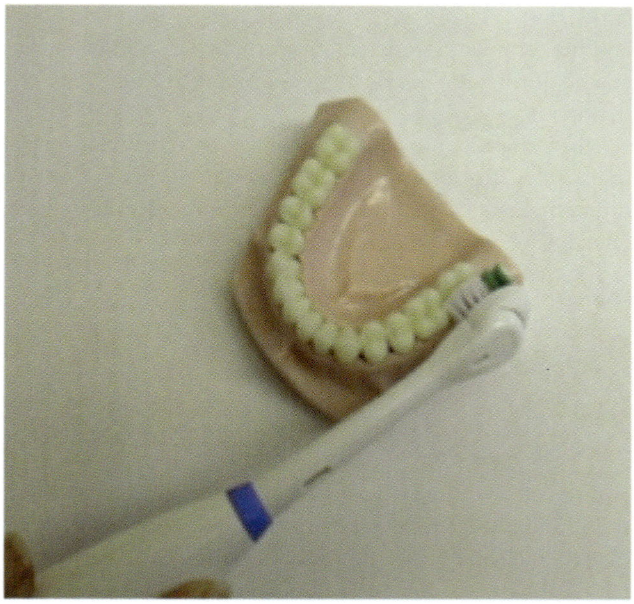

Fig 7.5 Using an electric toothbrush.

- Once the outside of the teeth has been cleaned, brush the inside of the teeth using the same angulations and technique.
- Finally, the tops of the teeth should be brushed.
- Once the lower teeth have been cleaned, the same technique should be applied to the upper teeth.

There is no reliable evidence base on which to choose one method over another, recommend the amount of time toothbrushing should take, or recommend how often a toothbrush should be replaced. In the absence of an evidence base, it is still useful to have clear advice that can be provided consistently to patients. This may include recommending a specific amount of time for brushing (usually 2 min, which may be usefully timed by the patient) and the systematic order of brushing of one arch, first buccally and then palatally/lingually, before going on to the other arch.

Toothpastes are usually used for toothbrushing. Toothpastes aid brushing because of their abrasive properties and because they make the process more pleasant and refreshing. In addition, they provide a way of delivering a range of active ingredients.

Toothpastes generally contain the following ingredients:

- Water
- Abrasives (silica or powdered calcium salts)
- Detergents
- Binding agents
- Humectants to retain moisture
- Flavouring
- Preservatives

In addition, they often contain a range of active ingredients designed to give therapeutic benefits, particularly fluoride and antibacterial agents (e.g., triclosan). In specific formulations, they may also contain the following:

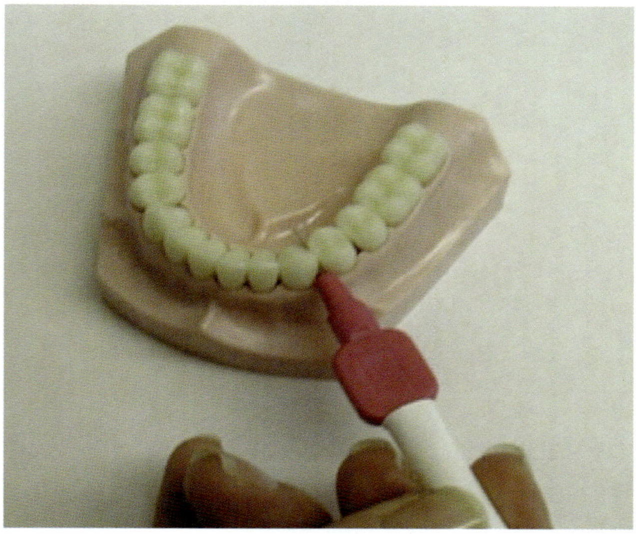

Fig 7.6 Demonstrating the use of interdental brushes on a model.

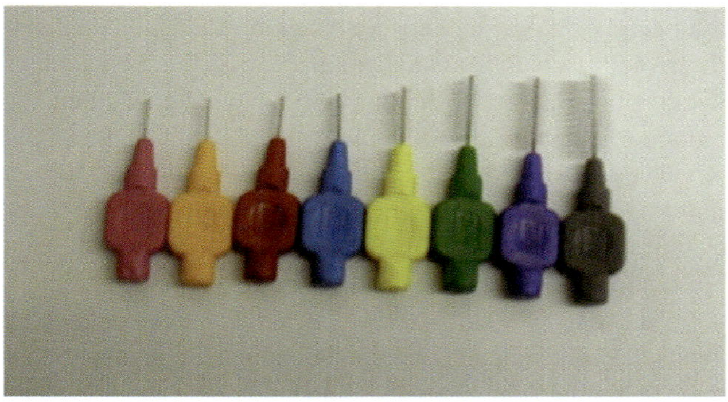

Fig 7.7 An array of interdental brushes in various sizes.

- Desensitizing agents (potassium nitrate, strontium, and arginine)
- Anticalculus agents (pyrophosphates)
- Sodium bicarbonate (baking soda)
- Enzymes—to enhance the antibacterial properties of saliva
- Xylitol—to reduce the level of cariogenic bacteria in the mouth

◇ *Interdental cleaning*

Meticulous brushing will only clean three of the tooth's five surfaces. Thus, in order to treat and prevent disease in the interproximal regions, patients need to be encouraged to use other oral hygiene aids to help clean the interdental regions.

Interdental brushes are an effective way of removing bacteria between the patient's teeth with a variety of sizes to suit the patient's needs (Figures 7.6 and 7.7).

- They are easier to use than floss, especially for patients with poor manual dexterity.
- They are economical because they can be used repeatedly.

The other commonly taught and used method for interdental cleaning is the use of dental floss. The technique for using floss should be as follows (Figure 7.8):

- Starting with approximately 30 cm of floss, wind most of the floss around each middle finger, leaving a couple of centimetres of floss to work with.
- Holding the floss between your thumbs and index fingers, slide it gently up and down between your teeth.
- Gently curve the floss around the base of each tooth, making sure you go beneath the gum line.
- At the gum line, curve floss into a C shape against the sides of both teeth and move it up and down.
- Use clean sections of floss as you move from tooth to tooth.

The ability of the patient to perform these methods

The next challenge in improving a patient's plaque control is to instruct the patient in the use of the appropriate methods of tooth cleaning. It is often assumed that when a patient fails to improve his or her plaque control sufficiently after receiving oral hygiene instruction (OHI), it is because the patient is not motivated to implement the advice he or she has been given. In fact, often it may be more that the patient either did not understand or fully comprehend the advice given or is finding it difficult to actually implement the advice. Thus, giving OHI requires the careful application of the professional's communication skills and assessing a patient's dexterity in carrying out the advice.

Communication skills are an important attribute for any healthcare professional, and it should not be assumed that they are something that one either has or does not have. Like most skills, they need to be thought about, practised, and honed. A list of some attributes of good communication skills is given in Table 7.2.

Obviously, when giving oral hygiene advice, we must always advise patients to use techniques that they are able to perform. Dentists have high levels of manual dexterity, particularly within the oral cavity. However, by no means all patients possess such fine motor skills, so the use of dental floss may be quite a challenge for some. In addition, as dentists, we must do "our bit" to help patients achieve the level of plaque control that we want them to achieve. This means not only motivation and instruction (as discussed later) but also the removal of secondary local factors that are preventing them from cleaning effectively at an early stage. Therefore, some supragingival debridement and the removal of restoration overhangs should be undertaken during the oral hygiene phase of the patient's treatment.

When instructing patients in how to effectively brush their teeth, it is good to remind them that a tooth has five different sides that all need cleaning to make oral hygiene effective:

- Outside or buccal
- Inside lingual or palatal
- Occlusal
- Front (mesial)
- Back (distal)

As mentioned previously, it is important to gear advice to the individual patient's needs, expectations, and ability to carry out sometimes complicated tasks (particularly if the patient has not done such things before). For instance, it may be more effective to deliver advice during a series of dental appointments, which allows for feedback so that the patient's understanding and compliance can be monitored. Children may benefit from advice given in a group setting, whereas adolescents may find DVDs or online material useful and motivational.

Table 7.2 Attributes of good communication skills for giving oral hygiene instruction

Be empathetic	Use the patient's name. Make it sound that you care. Avoid adversarial or critical comments
Address the patient directly	Make eye contact. Sit the patient up, or perhaps give the advice with the patient sitting in a normal chair
Avoid jargon	Use appropriate language that the patient understands
Do not overload the patient with information	Spread the instruction over a number of visits. Do not expect a patient to comprehend all the information if you give toothbrushing, flossing, and interdental cleaning advice all in one visit (and make a record of what advice is given at any particular appointment to ensure consistency)
Demonstrate	Use models and demonstrate techniques in the patient's mouth
Check for understanding	Ensure the patient has understood the information, and ask the patient to demonstrate this
Reinforce	Continue to repeat the message at subsequent visits. Be consistent with your advice. Ensure the patient understands that OHI is an important part of his or her treatment

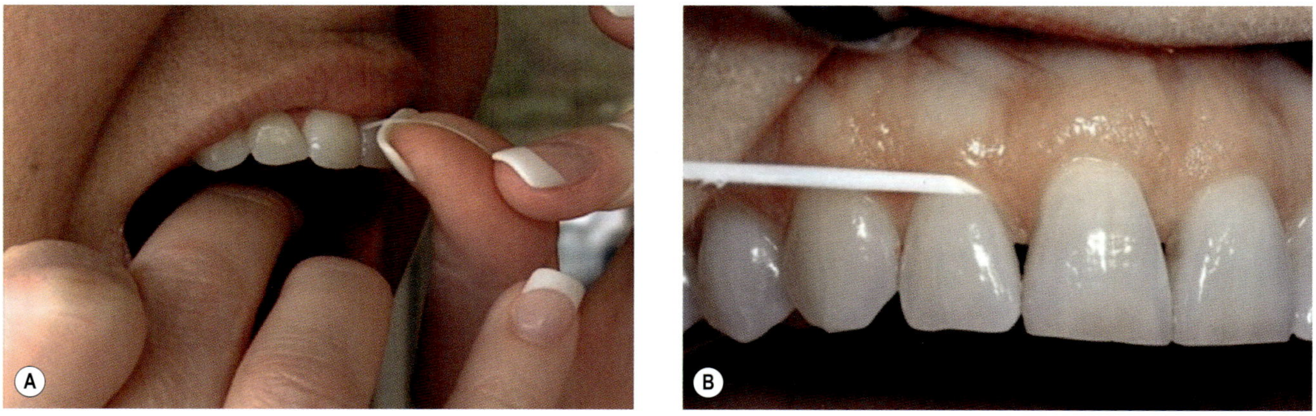

Fig 7.8 Using dental floss.

Ultimately, determining if the patient is able to implement the advice given is best judged by having him or her perform the procedures in the dental surgery setting. If necessary, the advice may need to be modified to improve patient performance. For example, the use of a powered toothbrush may be recommended if it is apparent that the patient is struggling to do the job with a manual toothbrush. Ensuring that the patient can implement the advice enables a judgement to be made regarding whether the problem is motivational or practical in cases in which plaque control remains inadequate.

The motivation of the patient

If the patient can demonstrate that he or she can actually carry out the procedures required for good plaque control, then compliance is likely to be mainly dependent on the patient's motivation to implement the behaviour change required of him or her. Psychologists have described a number of model constructs that seek to explain the factors that may influence implementation of behavioural changes. One of the most widely used concepts relates an individual patient's belief about the degree of control he or she has over what happens to him or her to affect success. This is known as the locus of control, which states the following:

- If there is a perception of a causal relationship being strong, the patient is in high internal control.
- If events are perceived as being determined by outside forces over which there is no control, the patient is in high external control.

This implies that these personality traits can markedly affect the success of plaque control measures, but it also presents the clinician with the opportunity to influence a patient's perception of the value of implementing behavioural change to motivate him or her.

In practical terms, these concepts suggest that when carrying out OHI, the clinician should try to address the following issues to motivate patients:

1. That they are affected by periodontal disease.
   Because periodontal disease is largely symptomless, particularly in its milder forms, the presence of the disease needs to be demonstrated to the patient, directly in the mouth, from radiographs, and from measurements taken such as pocket charts and bleeding scores.
2. That the condition is sufficiently serious to warrant intervention.
   The consequences of the problem need to be explained to the patient. Emphasis should be placed on consequences of relevance to the patient. Sometimes the threat of tooth loss occurring sometime in the future is not sufficient to motivate the patient because this may seem abstract or unimportant for some people. Other benefits of treatment may occasionally be more immediately motivating, such as controlling bad breath, aesthetic consequences, social interaction and bleeding gums, and managing halitosis.
3. That intervention can favourably affect the process.
   Patients can sometimes have a fatalistic view of periodontal disease, regarding the progression of disease as inevitable. These views may be reinforced by family members and friends who have also suffered the consequences of periodontal disease, and these views need to be countered. For instance, while taking indices to monitor progress through treatment, it is important that the patient is actively involved and shown this information in a way that he or she can understand and relate to. Showing the patient his or her disclosed mouth and showing areas of improvement is an excellent motivator. Demonstrating how improved plaque control has resulted in a decreased level of inflammation through a bleeding distribution chart and showing the patient where there is less bleeding in his or her mouth is also an excellent motivational tool.

Summary

Achieving an adequate level of plaque control is a challenge for many patients. Like any aspect of treatment, it needs to be approached in a logical, carefully thought out way, and where compliance is less than satisfactory, the reasons for this need to be identified and addressed, if possible.

Patients may not comply for a variety of reasons:

- Wrong or badly explained information by clinician
- Poor understanding of recommendations
- Inadequate dexterity
- Unwillingness to perform oral self-care
- Lack of motivation
- Poor dental health beliefs
- Stressful life events
- Domestic peer pressure and other negative environmental influences on behaviour change

For some patients, lack of motivation will mean that whatever is tried seems to be unsuccessful. However, if a patient continues to attend for dental treatment, this suggests that there is not a total disinterest in oral health and provides the opportunity to continue to reinforce the plaque control message.

Thus, when giving oral hygiene instruction, several principles should be followed:

- Oral hygiene advice should be tailored to the individual patient.
- The patient should be involved in the instructional process, such as using self-instruction manuals.
- Instructions should be given with demonstration in the mouth of the patient.
- Basic oral hygiene advice should be followed by an individualized maintenance programme.

Smoking cessation

Getting people to quit smoking is one of the major global public health challenges. The importance of smoking in the aetiology of periodontal disease, and its adverse effects on periodontal treatment outcomes, has been discussed elsewhere in this book. Because of these major effects on periodontal disease, getting patients to quit smoking should be regarded as an important part of periodontal treatment, in addition to the well-documented benefits of quitting on health generally. Studies suggest that dentists are often reluctant or reticent about asking about smoking and emphasizing smoking cessation, perhaps because they do not view this as within their traditional remit, but these studies also suggest that patients expect their dentist to ask about smoking habits and offer advice on smoking cessation.

The same principles of good communication skills and motivation apply to smoking cessation as they do to OHI, as discussed previously. In addition, nicotine is strongly physically addictive, which will make the smoking cessation more difficult to achieve due to the genuine physical cravings that an addicted smoker will experience when he or she suddenly stops smoking. In particular, the principle of being empathetic and supportive applies strongly, rather than adopting a somewhat judgemental or adversarial "I can't understand why you smoke so here's my advice—Take it or leave it" approach.

There is a large evidence base on the effectiveness of strategies for smoking cessation. These studies have been used by health agencies such as the UK National Institute for Health and Clinical Excellence to provide clear authoritative guidelines (NICE Guidelines) to health professionals for smoking cessation strategies. These guidelines, and similar material from other health agencies in other countries, are readily available online.

Three types of interventions for smoking cessation are usually recognized:

1. Brief intervention by a health professional within the normal practice setting, typically 5–10 min
2. More extensive counselling from trained counsellor
3. Specialist smoking cessation clinic providing one-on-one or group counselling together with pharmacological support

In general, dental professionals will mainly be involved in brief interventions, but they may also have level 2 trained counselling within a group practice environment and may refer to specialist smoking cessation clinics.

Guidelines for brief interventions can be organized around the four "A's":

- Ask
- Advise
- Assess
- Arrange

Ask: All patients should be routinely asked if they smoke, and their responses should be recorded in the patient records.

Advise: Current smokers should be advised about the adverse effects of smoking and the benefits of quitting. For a patient with periodontal disease, this should include specific information on the major impact of smoking on periodontal disease and its treatment and also the benefits of quitting on treatment outcomes.

Assess: Smokers should be assessed to determine if they are interested in quitting, and some assessment of likely degree of addiction should be made. A regular smoker of 15+ cigarettes per day is likely to have a high degree of addiction. Patients should be asked when they have their first cigarette of the day; those who smoke soon after rising have a high degree of addiction.

If a patient is interested in quitting, he or she can be encouraged by, for example, setting a date to quit or referring to online smoking cessation material for further support. If the patient is willing, then refer to a specialist smoking cessation clinic. If a smoker is not interested in quitting at the present time, this should be accepted nonjudgementally, but it should be suggested that he or she think about it for the future, leaving the door open for future smoking cessation interventions.

Arrange: Arrange to follow up those that are trying to quit, again in a supportive way. Referral to specialist smoking cessation clinics should be arranged for those who are willing to be referred.

Behavioural and pharmacological support

Because of the physical addiction of nicotine, sudden nicotine withdrawal can result in cravings, irritability, and anxiety. These symptoms usually subside within a few weeks; nicotine replacement therapies (NRTs) are widely used by smoking cessation clinics or prescribed by physicians to help manage nicotine withdrawal. For the physically addicted smoker, professional counselling or NRT can double the chance of successfully quitting, and combining behavioural support with NRT further increases successful outcomes.

As with OHI, all patients are different and may require different management strategies for their smoking. Many patients require a number of attempts before successfully quitting, whereas others simply quit one day without any support. Either way, the dental professional can play an important and supportive role in the process.

Chapter 8

Nonsurgical treatment

Introduction

Nonsurgical treatment is aimed at the removal of plaque and plaque-retentive factors from the tooth surface. Plaque-retentive factors include calculus and may also include factors such as overhanging restorations and other iatrogenic factors. Removal of plaque-retentive factors is an important part of disease control because it facilitates the establishment of regular effective plaque control measures by the patient. In addition, all patients with periodontal pockets will require the removal of plaque and calculus from subgingival sites because these areas are inaccessible for cleaning by the patient. Consequently, mechanical nonsurgical periodontal therapy is always combined with appropriate oral hygiene instruction (OHI). Successful nonsurgical therapy will result in control of the microbial plaque biofilm, which in turn results in resolution of inflammation and healing of the pocket, creating a local environment that encourages periodontal health and greatly decreases the likelihood of disease recurrence and further progression. The evidence of its clinical efficacy is overwhelming and thus nonsurgical treatment has been the mainstay of successful periodontal practice for well over half a century.

The aim of this chapter is to explain the application of nonsurgical treatment of periodontitis, focusing on the requirements for successful subgingival debridement.

What is nonsurgical treatment?

A course of nonsurgical treatment includes the following elements:

- Oral Hygiene Instruction
- Supragingival scaling to remove calculus
- Correction or elimination of other plaque-retentive factors
- Subgingival debridement

In addition, during this phase of treatment, management of other modifiable risk factors, such as smoking cessation, should be introduced. In specific circumstances, this treatment may be supplemented with adjunctive chemical antimicrobial therapy, either with antiplaque agents to help manage plaque control or, rarely, with systemic antibiotics (see Chapter 14).

As discussed in Chapter 9, a course of nonsurgical treatment should be followed up by a reassessment of the patient's response to treatment and by further decision making about appropriate further treatment needs.

At this point, it is important to note some of the terms used to describe this treatment modality. The term scaling is used to describe the removal of calculus from the tooth surface, either supra- or subgingivally. The term root planing is a more accurate description of removing both calculus and root surface irregularities during treatment, whereas the term root surface debridement (RSD) has become more widely used to describe the process of atraumatically removing plaque, calculus, and any root surface irregularities within a pocket.

By definition, RSD is a "blind" procedure. When instrumenting below the gingival margin into a pocket, it is not possible to see exactly where the tip of the instrument is located, so it is generally not possible to visualize just how successful the instrumentation has been. As such, RSD is a technically demanding procedure and requires careful, thorough instrumentation to achieve a clean root surface. In the absence of being able to visualize the root surface, one of the aims of nonsurgical treatment is to make the tooth/root surface uniformly hard and smooth, relying on feel to assess the root surface; often, the word "glassy" is used to describe how the root surface should feel after instrumentation. A WHO ball-ended probe is excellent at detecting residual calculus and root surface roughness after RSD.

Scaling technique

There are two main types of scaling instruments—hand scalers and ultrasonic scalers. The ultrasonic scaler has a tip that vibrates in the ultrasonic frequency and effectively shakes and breaks the calculus off of the root surface, partly by its direct mechanical effect but particularly by generation of a "cavitational effect" in which microscopic bubbles in the water irrigant around the tip are formed and then implode to release energy.

There is a wide array of different types of hand instruments that are designed for use either supra- or subgingivally and that have a variety of tip shapes to access all the different areas of the mouth. These instruments are summarized in Table 8.1. Those most commonly used for RSD are periodontal curettes, which either cut on both sides of the tip (universal type) or cut on one side only (Gracey type). To be effective, hand instruments need to be kept sharp by very regular use of sharpening stones or tungsten carbide "whittlers." Most hand scaling instruments are made of high-quality stainless steel or carbon steel, and they can be effectively sharpened with sharpening stones. A few instruments, particularly most periodontal hoes, have tungsten carbide tips and thus keep their sharpness longer, but because they require diamond sharpening tools, they are very difficult to sharpen once they become dull. Principles of scaling include using a finger rest that is as close to the tooth being treated as possible, keeping the cutting edge of the tip at an approximately 90° angle (the so-called "rake" angle), and always scaling in an apical-to-coronal direction. The different curves of the various instruments are designed

Table 8.1 Types of scaling instruments

Type	Description
Sickle scalers	Used only for supragingival scaling (too traumatic to soft tissues for subgingival use); triangular in cross section and pointed at the tip
Universal curettes	Used particularly for removal of subgingival deposits and root surface debridement; cutting edge on each side of the instrument tip; rounded tip and semicircular in cross section
Gracey curettes	Similar to universal curettes but have cutting edge on only one surface of the tip, making them less traumatic to the pocket soft tissues than universal curettes (but twice as many instruments required to reach all surfaces)
Hoes	Used subgingivally, particularly for extensive subgingival calculus; risk of causing root grooves; usually made with tungsten carbide tips, making them too hard to sharpen with normal sharpening equipment
Files	Sometimes used subgingivally to create a smooth root surface; difficult to use and probably of questionable efficacy
Ultrasonic scalers	Tip inserted into ultrasonic unit and vibrates at ultrasonic frequencies (25–40 kHz); much less operator fatigue compared to hand instruments; requires copious water irrigation to keep cool; increased aerosol with associated cross-infection issues to be managed
Sonic scalers	Similar to ultrasonic scalers except tip vibrates at lower, sonic frequencies; advantage that they can be driven by a normal dental unit air line rather than needing a specific unit, but generally considered to be much less powerful

to maintain a suitable rake angle for the tip of the instrument when accessing different teeth. In general, those that are designed for posterior teeth have the most pronounced curves in their shanks, whereas those for anterior teeth may be closer to being straight in line with the handle of the instrument (Figures 8.1–8.4).

There are no hard and fast rules about when to use an ultrasonic scaler and when to use hand scalers. Studies suggest that treatment outcomes of RSD are the same whether using hand or ultrasonic instruments. Consequently,

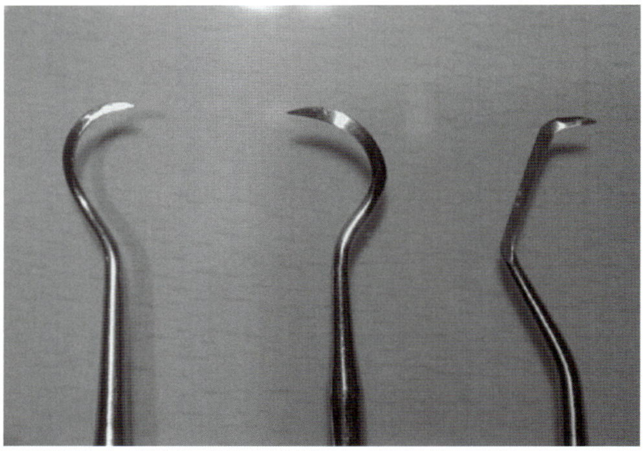

Fig 8.1 Tips of left and right Sickle scalers and the Jacquette scaler (right), which is a type of Sickle scaler used for anterior teeth. These instruments are used for supragingival scaling.

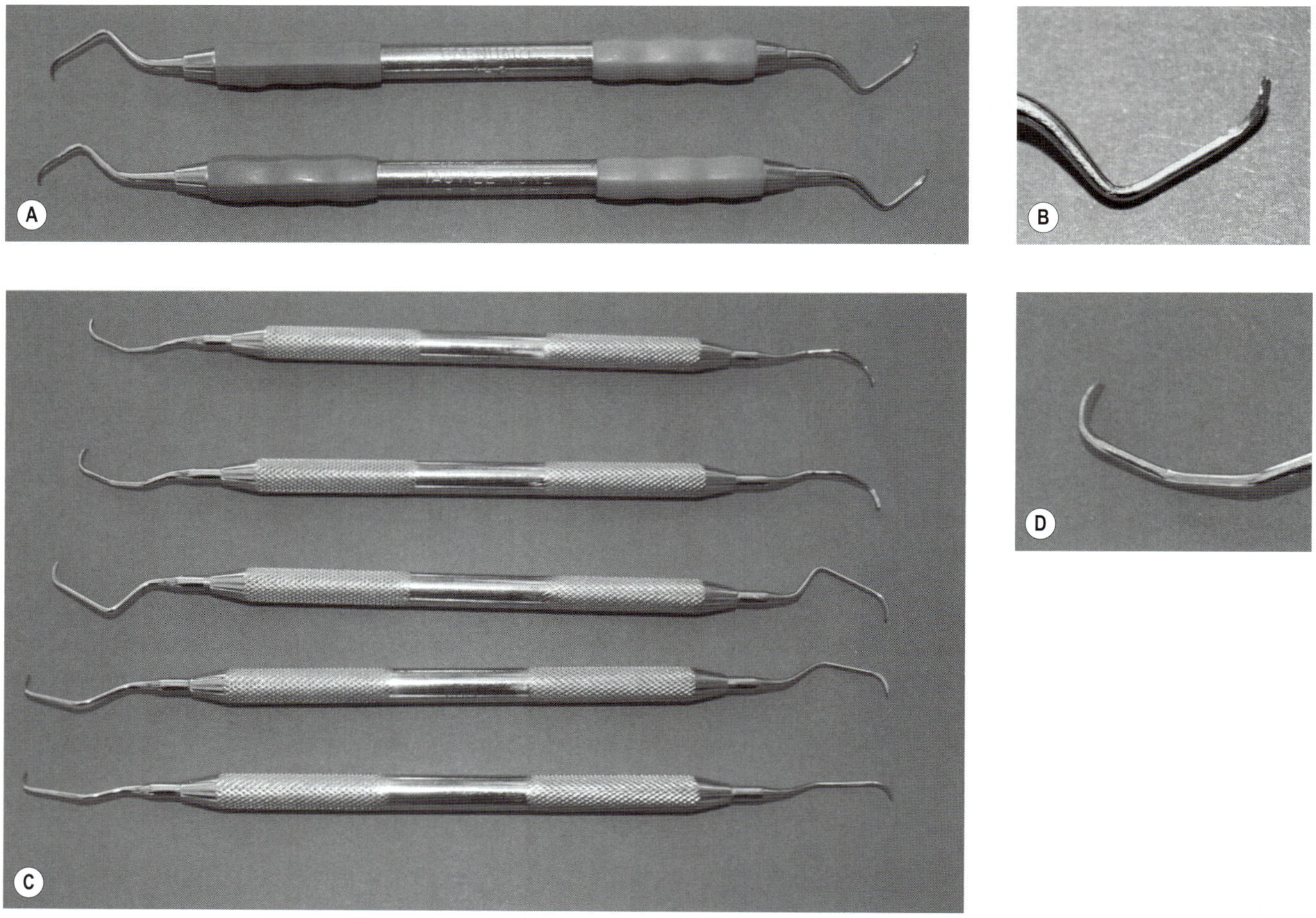

Fig 8.2 A selection of curettes used principally for subgingival areas. (A) Barnhart universal curettes, numbers 1/2 (top) and 5/6 (bottom). (B) Close-up of tip, which has two cutting sides on its blade. (C) A selection of Gracey-type curettes. From top, numbers 13/14, 11/12, 9/10, 7/7, and 5/6. (D) A close-up of the tip of a Gracey number 11 showing the single "cutting" side.

most people tend to use an ultrasonic instrument for the majority of their scaling. For RSD, especially when pockets are particularly deep, this can be finished off by hand scaling, which has the significant advantage of better tactile feedback to the operator to assess the smoothness of the root surface achieved.

The approach to a patient's nonsurgical treatment will largely depend on the number, depth, and distribution of his or her periodontal pockets. When, as is often the case, a patient will require most of his or her teeth to be debrided, typically this would be carried out over four visits. The approach would be to anaesthetize the mouth a quadrant at a time for the nonsurgical treatment, leaving a reasonable recovery period of perhaps 1 week between episodes.

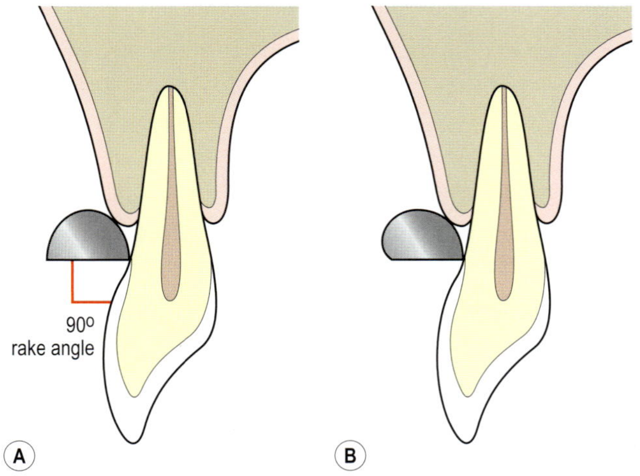

Fig 8.3 Cross-sectional diagram of the use of curettes on root surface. (A) Universal curette with roughly semicircular cross-sectional profile; the cutting edge of the instrument is at roughly 90° to the tooth surface. (B) Gracey curette with single cutting side applied to root surface.

A recent approach is to carry out debridement over one or two visits with no more than 24 hr between them and to supplement mechanical debridement with the copious use of chlorhexidine as an irrigant, gargle, and adjunct to tongue scraping. This "whole mouth disinfection" approach targets not only the pathogens within the pocket but also those in other niches throughout the oral cavity, such as the tonsils and dorsum of the tongue. Despite this vigorous approach, there appears to be little benefit in overall response, such that the approach to treatment is best left to both patient and therapist to decide. An advantage of the more traditional method of delivery is that treatment over a period of time allows patient and operator to get to know each other and for a relationship to develop, which can enhance the behavioural change aspects of both OHI and smoking cessation. However, the whole mouth disinfection approach has the advantage of being finished in far less time.

Whatever approach is decided on, adequate anaesthesia of both teeth and soft tissues must be achieved, particularly for deeper sites, using both block and infiltration anaesthesia with appropriate use of surface/topical anaesthesia, particularly when infiltrating the palatal mucosa.

Particular difficulties of root surface debridement

A number of factors make RSD a technically demanding procedure. As noted previously, the procedure is carried out blind, so the operator is ultimately dependent on good technique and careful assessment of the smoothness of the root surface. The pH within a periodontal pocket tends to be high, favouring mineralization; consequently, subgingival calculus is very hard and widespread throughout the mouth. It is also often rather diffuse, and it is easy to miss affected areas (Figure 8.5). In addition, certain root surfaces are difficult to access, including distal surfaces of molar teeth, mesial surfaces of upper first premolars with root

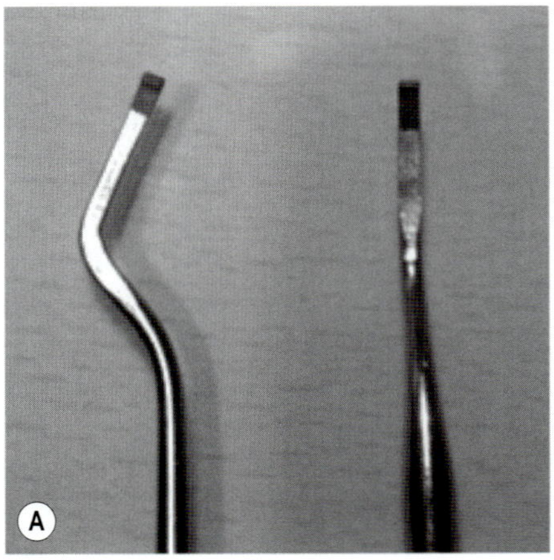

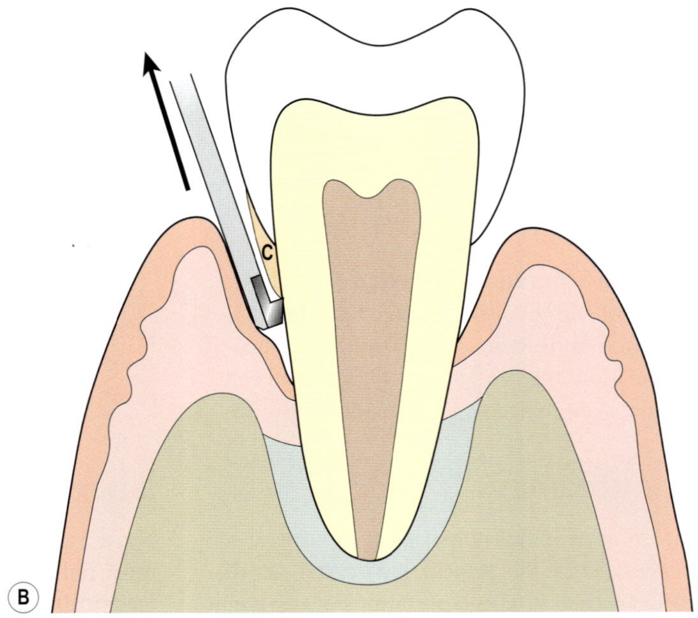

Fig 8.4 Periodontal hoes. (A) Close-up photograph of hoe tips. Note the dark appearance of the tip, which is made of tungsten carbide. (B) Cross-sectional diagram of the use of a hoe on a root surface. The instrument is positioned apically below the calculus (C) and scaled coronally.

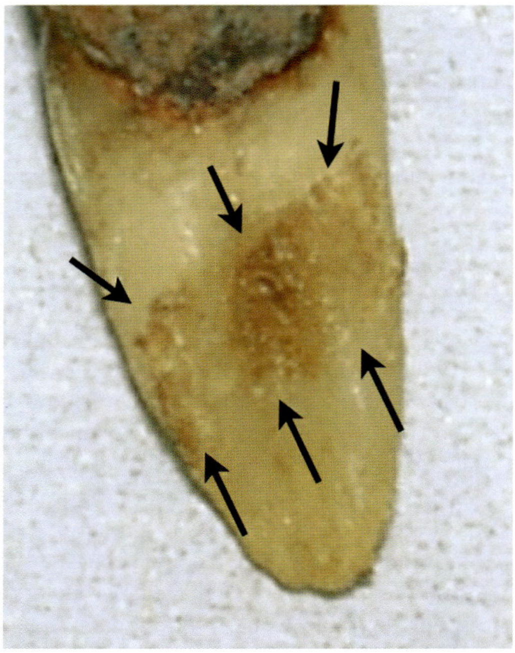

Fig 8.5 Root surface of an extracted tooth showing widespread diffuse build up of subgingival calculus (arrows).

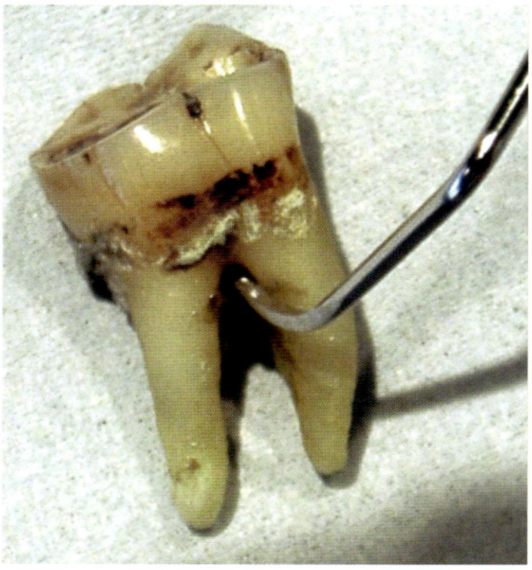

Fig 8.6 An extracted lower molar demonstrating the difficulty of debriding the furcation region with a standard curette, which is almost too wide to access the furcation entrance.

grooves (canine fossae), furcations (Figure 8.6), and other root irregularities or anomalies. Figure 8.6 shows an extracted lower molar and demonstrates the difficulties of debriding the furcation region with a standard curette, which is almost too wide to access the furcation entrance.

Treatment outcomes

Following completion of initial nonsurgical treatment, the outcome is reviewed and the patient reassessed, as discussed in detail in Chapter 9. The expectations of treatment outcome include reduction in plaque scores, reduction in bleeding and swelling, and pocket depth reductions. When inflammation is marked at the start of treatment, the improvements can be quite dramatic, which can be very motivating for the patient. Overall, studies show that pocket depth reductions and gain in clinical attachment are greatest in deep sites, and they have suggested that the average amount of pocket depth reduction seen in deep sites can be on the order of approximately 2 mm. However, this figure should be interpreted with caution because pocket depth reductions often vary considerably at different sites within the mouth of a patient and also between patients.

The clinical improvements that occur may continue for months, but most of the changes will likely occur within 6–8 weeks. The healing events occurring within the tissues can be related to the clinical changes as follows:

- Reduction in swelling—due to resolution of inflammation
- Reduction in redness—due to resolution of inflammation and increased gingival collagen production
- Reduction in bleeding on probing—due to decreased gingival blood flow and healing of sulcular epithelium
- Reduced pocket depths—due to reformation of fibrous gingival cuff, formation of long epithelial attachment, and increased gingival recession

This treatment is unlikely to have any effects on the true (histological) level of attachment or on crestal bone height; so, for example, a radiograph taken following successful treatment is likely to look the same as one taken preoperatively. Thus, treatment often does not affect the degree of mobility of a tooth. However, in some cases, some reduction in mobility is seen, probably due to the increased tooth support from a more fibrous gingival cuff around the tooth.

Figure 8.7 shows the charting of a patient before and after nonsurgical therapy. Sites bleeding on probing are shown in red. It can clearly be seen that there has been a generalized decrease in bleeding and probing depths on the order that has been observed in the literature, along with a slight increase in recession, again as may be expected given the reduction in inflammation that is shown in the new chart. It is striking that some pockets (e.g., at UR234) have shown a dramatic reduction, whereas others have not and, in some cases, appear worse at the postoperative visit. Whether this is due to true breakdown or the result of measurement error in recording the pocket depths is difficult to determine.

Figure 8.8 shows clinical pictures of a patient with severe gingival inflammation and the resolution that has occurred within 6 weeks after treatment. The reduction in gingival swelling is very marked, particularly in the lingual regions. However, some inflammation persists, and the patient's plaque control is still not optimal. In this case, a further course of RSD and OHI were prescribed after the reassessment stage.

Summary

Nonsurgical treatment is the mainstay of management of most patients with periodontal disease. Occasionally, it is technically challenging, but its efficacy has been demonstrated by many studies throughout the years. Outcomes of nonsurgical treatment need to be carefully reviewed and further treatment needs considered at that stage.

Buccal		8	7	6	5	4	3	2	1	1	2	3	4	5	6	7	8
Recession	Pre-op			111			111			001		111			111		
	Post-op			111			111		100	001	211						
PPD	Pre-op	---	856	635	734	637	828	925	525	427	986	538	935	527	728	799	---
	Post-op	---	534	422	323	333	323	324	323	223	634	324	623	324	427	573	---
Mobility	Pre-op	---		1		1		1	1	1	2	1	1				---
Furcation	Pre-op	---													1	1	---

Palatal		8	7	6	5	4	3	2	1	1	2	3	4	5	6	7	8
Recession	Pre-op																
	Post-op																
PPD	Pre-op	---	435	623	535	536	758	765	435	757	775	567	536	335	338	533	---
	Post-op	---	533	423	223	333	553	533	345	533	333	344	433	223	327	333	---

Lingual		8	7	6	5	4	3	2	1	1	2	3	4	5	6	7	8
Recession	Pre-op																
	Post-op																
PPD	Pre-op	---	333	535	555	757	333	333	333	323	333	333	537	537	477	533	---
	Post-op	---	333	723	523	575	332	322	223	223	223	353	557	557	537	534	---
Mobility	Pre-op	---		1		1								1	1		---
Furcation	Pre-op	---													1		---

Buccal		8	7	6	5	4	3	2	1	1	2	3	4	5	6	7	8
Recession	Pre-op	---		111													
	Post-op	---		111													
PPD	Pre-op	---	333	533	315	536	425	524	223	222	222	223	325	527	528	323	---
	Post-op	---	323	523	323	323	323	323	323	222	323	323	226	526	328	523	---

Fig 8.7 Periodontal charting of a patient before and after nonsurgical therapy. Numbers in red show sites exhibiting bleeding.

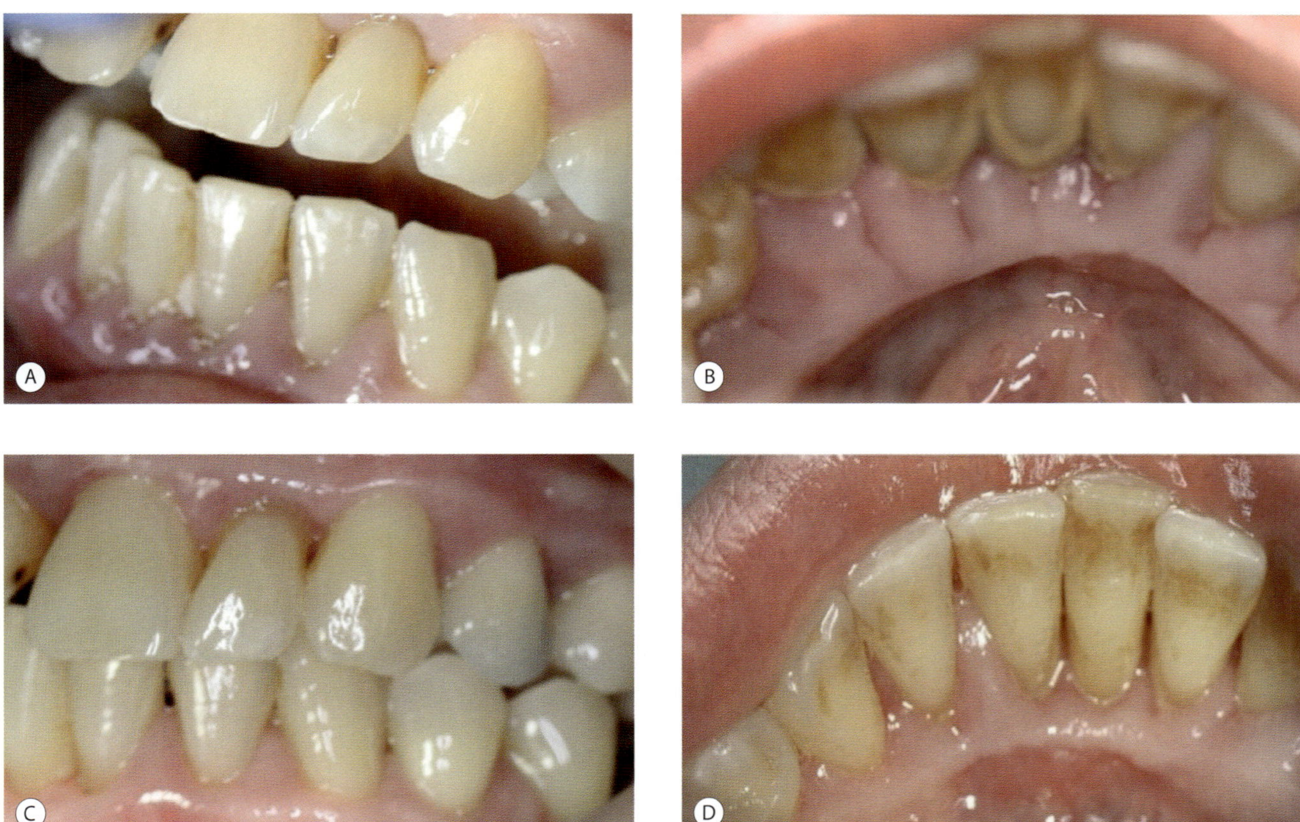

Fig 8.8 Clinical photos of patient with severe gingival inflammation, particularly associated with the calculus lingually on the lower incisors, and the improvement in swelling seen after initial therapy. In this case, some inflammation still persists, and further nonsurgical treatment is required, although the initial response to treatment is very encouraging for both patient and clinician. (Top) Preoperative; (bottom) postoperative.

Chapter 9

Reassessment

Time for decision making

Following completion of initial nonsurgical therapy, the importance of reviewing treatment responses and outcomes is well recognized, but its importance is often underestimated. Some of the most important decisions for the management of periodontal disease are typically required at this time in order to determine both future periodontal treatment needs and other important long-term goals, such as other restorative requirements.

The role of the reassessment appointment is to determine the response to the treatment that has been carried out, at both the tooth level and the patient level, and to decide on any further treatment that will be required. Reassessment is typically carried out at least 6 weeks after completion of initial treatment. Although it is known that healing events, and thus clinical improvements such as reducing pocket depths, may continue over a period of a few months, it is recognized that most of the healing will occur within approximately 6 weeks, and thus this period represents the shortest postoperative time suitable for carrying out the review of treatment response.

Reassessment (or review) is the comparison of clinical measurements before and after carrying out active treatment in order to measure treatment responses. Thus, the importance of accurate and thorough baseline assessment and diagnosis (discussed in Chapters 1 and 6) is highlighted. At the review appointment, these clinical assessments are repeated, particularly a new 6-point probing pocket depth chart and measurement of recession, plaque assessment, and assessment of bleeding. In addition, the patient is asked for his or her own assessment of treatment responses and any concerns or problems he or she may have.

Note that the Basic Periodontal Examination (BPE; and also the Community Periodontal Index) discussed in Chapter 1 is not suitable for reviewing responses to treatment, even in cases in which only mild disease was initially present. The two main reasons for this are that the index does not provide any site-specific information about changes in periodontal status and the index is not sufficiently sensitive to be able to reliably detect changes in periodontal status. An example illustrating this is shown in Figure 9.1.

Assessing treatment outcomes

The primary objective of periodontal treatment is to eliminate existing disease and to prevent future disease progression. In clinical terms, this generally means the absence of bleeding at a site, together with a pocket that is sufficiently shallow as to be possible to maintain in the future. A site that bleeds and that continues to have a deep pocket is at increased risk of further disease progression in the future, whereas the absence of bleeding and deep pockets is a good predictor of future health of a site. In practical terms, a pocket depth of less than 5 mm is considered to be maintainable in the future by adequate oral hygiene measures alone (including an appropriate professional maintenance programme, discussed in Chapter 15), and thus pocket depth reduction to 4 mm or less, together with the absence of bleeding, is considered to be a satisfactory endpoint of active periodontal treatment.

Therefore, at reassessment, any site may be judged to be as follows:

1. A "treated site"—one that is now less than 5 mm and not bleeding
2. A "responding" or "partially treated" site—one that shows improvement (pocket depth reduction) from baseline but that is still 5 mm or greater or still bleeds on probing
3. A "nonresponding site"—one that has shown no improvement from baseline or shows deterioration

It is common for there to be a mixture of all three of these outcomes in the same patient.

In addition, in assessing treatment outcomes, it is well described that different patients may show varying responses to treatment such that any particular patient may be judged to show a good overall response to treatment or a poor overall response to treatment.

To further complicate the matter, it is thus possible to see nonresponding sites in a patient who otherwise shows a generally good response to treatment or to see some sites that have responded well to treatment in a patient who otherwise shows a generally poor response to treatment.

Reasons for poor responses to treatment

Having diagnosed treatment responses at both the site level and the patient level, the next step in the reassessment process is to decide what further treatment is required, particularly for nonresponding sites. A logical approach to this process is first to decide the likely reasons for an inadequate treatment response, because this will help dictate the appropriate course of action for future management.

The main reasons for inadequate treatment responses are summarized in Table 9.1. Most commonly, inadequate responses are the result of inadequate plaque control, incomplete subgingival debridement, or because of tobacco smoking. Inadequate plaque control may be the result of poor motivation and compliance, and detecting this highlights the importance of regular monitoring of plaque by objective assessment of plaque deposits as discussed in Chapters 1 and 8. In addition, occasionally, general

Lingual	Post op	5 5 4	4 4 6	5 4 4	3 2 3
	Baseline	8 6 6	7 4 6	6 3 5	4 4 4
		7	**6**	**5**	**4**
Buccal	Baseline	7 4 5	6 2 4	5 3 5	6 3 3
	Post op	4 3 3	4 2 3	4 2 5	4 2 2

Fig 9.1 Six-point probing pocket chart of lower right sextant of a patient at baseline (prior to treatment) and at reassessment following completion of initial nonsurgical treatment. It is clear that there has been an excellent response to treatment overall. However, the BPE score for this sextant is "4" at baseline and remains "4" postoperatively because of the persisting 6-mm pocket at LR6 lingually. BPE does not provide any information about where there has been a good (or poor) response, and it completely fails to identify the generally excellent response to treatment in this sextant.

Table 9.1 Diagnosing and managing inadequate treatment responses

Cause	Comments	Further treatment options
Incorrect initial diagnosis	For example, disease too severe to be treatable; endodontic involvement or perio/endo lesion; other gingival pathology such as lichen planus; other periodontal pathology such as malignant disease causing bone loss	Implement appropriate treatment for condition
Inadequate plaque control	Poor compliance/motivation; inadequate dexterity; inability to access specific areas for OH; the presence of plaque-retentive factors such as calculus or overhanging restorations	Continue to reinforce OH procedures; correct any persisting local factors
Inadequate subgingival debridement	Difficult access for RSD—very deep sites, infrabony sites, posterior sites; the presence of difficult root anatomy such as grooves and furcations; inadequate RSD technique	Repeat RSD; periodontal surgery
Smoking	A major cause of poor patient treatment outcomes	Smoking cessation
Other	Less common causes—often difficult to diagnose except by exclusion of the above; systemic factors such as poorly controlled diabetes; possibly genetic factors; possibly associated with the presence of specific bacteria such as *Aa*	Adjunctive antimicrobial treatment; other adjunctive therapies (?)

compliance may be good, but plaque control may be inadequate at particular sites, for example, because of patient difficulties accessing posterior sites for interproximal cleaning or because of persisting plaque-retentive factors such as overhanging restorations or crown margins.

Incomplete subgingival debridement, particularly in localized areas, does not necessarily reflect on an operator's technique. Root surface debridement (RSD) is carried out "blindly" and ultimately relies on tactile assessment to determine if all deposits have been removed successfully; thus, it is not surprising that this is not always successfully achieved (see Chapter 8). In general, studies demonstrate that it is more difficult to successfully remove all subgingival deposits by nonsurgical methods in posterior sites, in deeper pockets, at infrabony sites, and where there are complicating root anatomies including furcations, root grooves, and less common root abnormalities such as enamel pearls.

Deciding that a poor response is likely to be the result of inadequate removal of subgingival deposits is an inexact science that requires a degree of clinical judgement. This is likely to be the case when root surface roughness can still be detected at reassessment or when there has been generally a good response to treatment, but some sites, particularly deeper pockets, do not respond.

Smoking is now recognized as having a major deleterious effect on both nonsurgical and surgical treatment outcomes. In some studies, persisting smoking may increase the chances of responding poorly to treatment by three- to five-fold and should thus be seen as one of the most common explanations for poorly responding patients. Fortunately, studies suggest that the benefits of quitting smoking on healing may be evident very quickly, within a few days, and are cumulative with time after quitting.

In a minority of cases, poor responses to treatment cannot be explained by one of the previously discussed three factors. These patients may present particular challenges both diagnostically and also with regard to deciding how one might manage them successfully. First, the possibility that the initial diagnosis was incorrect should be considered (see Chapters 2 and 5) and, if necessary, investigated further. In some cases, this may be the result of unreasonably high expectations of treatment responses from teeth that may have a hopeless prognosis—for example, those that exhibit grade 3 mobility. In other cases, the failure to diagnose associated endodontic involvement will account for a failure to respond to periodontal treatment. In some cases, this can easily be detected by radiography and vitality testing of teeth, but in other cases this is a particularly difficult diagnostic challenge, such as when endodontic involvement on a molar tooth is largely manifested at a furcation or when a perio/endo lesion is developing from extension of a periodontal pocket to a lateral canal without apical involvement. In these cases, vitality testing is often very informative. In less common cases, a range of other conditions risk being misdiagnosed as periodontal disease (see Chapter 5) and will of course not respond to periodontal treatment.

Despite all these possible causes for inadequate responses to treatment, a minority of patients respond poorly to treatment where none of these causes seem to apply. Although the full list of factors that determine treatment outcome is still the subject of research investigation, reasons that have been suggested for this include the presence and persistence of specific bacteria in the microflora, notably *Aggregatibacter actinomycetemcomitans* (*Aa*), an underlying systemic condition such as undiagnosed diabetes mellitus, and genetic factors, although there are undoubtedly likely to be other causes in some cases. In addition, some cases of aggressive periodontitis may generally respond poorly to conventional treatment. In clinical practice, patients who are relatively resistant (or "refractory") to periodontal treatment can only

																	B
PRESENTATION	433	524	747	523	323	333	347	633	455	434	333	423	423	635	444	334	
	8	7	6	5	4	3	2	1	1	2	3	4	5	6	7	8	
PRESENTATION	433	521	744	522	322	331	344	634	452	431	322	522	522	744	555	331	
																	P
																	L
PRESENTATION	433	226	535	335	333	212	112	212	211	111	212	222	333	736	534	445	
	8	7	6	5	4	3	2	1	1	2	3	4	5	6	7	8	
PRESENTATION	522	335	726	534	322	212	212	111	111	112	112	312	313	635	745	333	
																	B

Fig 9.2 Six-point probing pocket chart at initial presentation.

be diagnosed retrospectively (at reassessment) by exclusion of the more common causes discussed previously.

Remedies for inadequate treatment outcomes

By taking a systematic approach to reassessment outlined previously, the appropriate further treatment required can be logically identified. For example, where compliance has been poor, further treatment is primarily required to improve plaque control; it would clearly be inappropriate in such a case to plan periodontal surgery, for example. Similarly, where the patient responds poorly due to tobacco smoking, the most beneficial treatment would be to try to get the patient to quit. In both of these cases, in which compliance is compromised by poor plaque control and in which a patient does not wish to consider quitting smoking, it may well be that further treatment is largely limited to simple maintenance care, recognizing the difficulty of achieving a definitive treated outcome.

Where it is decided that poor responses are likely the result of persisting subgingival deposits, the clinician may decide to repeat the RSD procedure in those sites or may opt for a surgical approach to access deep pockets. In general, repeating the RSD is more appropriate when there are obvious deposits still to be removed, where the persisting site is relatively shallow, and on anterior sites. A surgical approach is more likely to be chosen for deeper sites, posterior sites, where there are infrabony pockets or complicating root anatomies, or where nonsurgical access is poor. There is no absolute rule about choosing between these procedures, but it is important for an active decision to be made based on the clinical assessment, avoiding the danger of continual fruitless rounds of further RSD when surgery is likely to be more successful.

When it is believed that the patient is relatively resistant to conventional treatment, it may be useful to repeat the RSD combined with a course of adjunctive antimicrobials. Given the complexities of these cases, in a general dental practice setting it might be wise to consider obtaining a second opinion from a periodontal specialist before proceeding.

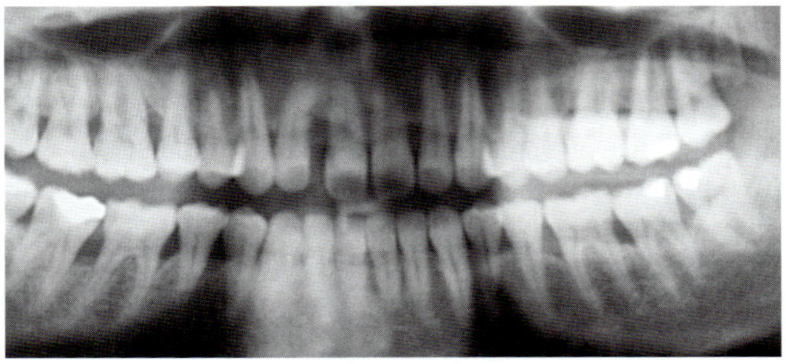

Fig 9.3 Rotational tomogram showing irregular bone loss with infrabony defects evident.

To illustrate some of these possibilities, we next discuss a number of clinical examples in which different further treatments are indicated.

Case 1

A 39-year-old woman initially presented for routine dental examination with complaints of bleeding gums and had recently noticed slight spacing in the upper anterior teeth, particularly at UR12. She was medically healthy and had never smoked.

On examination, the gingivae were slightly red and inflamed, bled readily on probing, and had a bleeding score of 55%. There were visible plaque deposits and localized supragingival calculus deposits, with a plaque score of 62%. Six-point pocket depth examination showed multiple pockets of 5–7 mm affecting particularly the molars and upper incisor teeth, and widespread subgingival calculus could be detected on probing (Figure 9.2). There was minimal or no gingival recession evident. Radiographic examination showed a pattern of irregular bone loss up to 40–50%, with vertical bony defects evident in a number of the teeth (Figure 9.3), consistent with the findings from the pocket chart. In addition, an unerupted supernumerary

UL9 was noted. There was no increased mobility and no detectable furcation lesions.

A diagnosis of severe chronic periodontitis was made, and the patient's high susceptibility to disease was noted, given the extent of the patient's lesions and her relatively young age. No other contributory risk factors were identified.

The patient received a course of initial treatment, including detailed oral hygiene instruction (OHI), supragingival scaling, and RSD of all quadrants with local analgesia over four visits. She arranged to return for reassessment 6 weeks after the last visit of RSD.

At reassessment, the patient reported that her gums felt tighter and were not bleeding. She had noticed slight generalized sensitivity to cold stimuli immediately after the treatment was completed. She had been using a proprietary toothpaste for dental sensitivity, and this was now improving slowly.

On examination, the gingivae appeared pink and healthy, and the plaque control was now good, with a plaque score of 17%. There had been a marked reduction in bleeding on probing. A new six-point probing pocket chart was undertaken and is shown in Figure 9.4. As can be seen, many of the pockets, particularly in the shallower sites, show improvements, and an absence of bleeding on probing was noted. However, some sites, particularly initially deep sites in the posterior regions, show persistence of pocketing greater than 5 mm, and it was noted that these still bled when the pockets were probed.

In this case, it was judged that compliance with OH was excellent and the patient showed an overall good response to treatment. Thus, it was likely that the localized areas of pocketing resulted from incomplete removal of subgingival deposits, although this was not obvious on clinical probing. However, access to these posterior sites was especially difficult due to their initial depth and the fact that they were partly infrabony sites. Thus, further debridement of the deep sites is indicated, either by repeating the RSD or by opting for a surgical approach to their treatment. There are no absolute rules about which of these is the correct treatment here, but in this case, it was decided to repeat the RSD on the relatively accessible anterior regions but to carry out surgical debridement of the posterior sites. The patient thus had four surgical procedures carried out for direct access for surgical debridement together with apical positioning of the flaps (see Chapter 11) to eliminate pockets. (The third molars were also extracted during the surgical procedures.)

The outcome of this treatment 6 months following completion of the surgical procedures is shown in Figures 9.5 and 9.6. As can be seen, there is an excellent outcome of treatment, with good pocket reductions and all sites less than 5 mm in depth. The patient consistently showed plaque scores of less than 20%. Thus, the patient can be regarded at this stage as successfully treated, and she was placed on a regular maintenance programme for future follow-up (further follow-up of this case is discussed in Chapter 14).

Case 2

A 53-year-old man presented complaining of a loose upper right second molar tooth. He was medically healthy but a cigarette smoker of approximately 25 cigarettes a day since he was approximately age 16 years. He was an irregular attender at the dentist, usually only attending if he had specific problems. Although he believed that he had neglected his teeth previously, he was concerned about tooth loss and keen to avoid having to wear dentures in the future.

On examination, the gingivae looked pink, fibrous, and largely uninflamed. There were generalized plaque deposits and widespread supragingival and subgingival calculus deposits. The plaque score was 62%, but generally little gingival bleeding on probing was evident, with a bleeding score of 32%. The UR7 was grade 3 mobile, and suppuration

POST INITIAL THERAPY	334	623	726	333	212	232	225	421	333	322	223	212	334	614	324	344	B
PRESENTATION	433	524	747	523	323	333	347	633	455	434	333	423	423	635	444	334	
	8	7	6	5	4	3	2	1	1	2	3	4	5	6	7	8	
PRESENTATION	433	521	744	522	322	331	344	634	452	431	322	522	522	744	555	331	
POST INITIAL THERAPY	422	622	633	312	222	212	333	522	332	321	223	423	622	635	544	333	P
POST INITIAL THERAPY	422	335	624	224	333	111	111	111	111	111	112	212	222	635	544	335	L
PRESENTATION	433	226	535	335	333	212	112	212	211	111	212	222	333	736	534	445	
	8	7	6	5	4	3	2	1	1	2	3	4	5	6	7	8	
PRESENTATION	522	335	726	534	322	212	212	111	111	112	112	312	313	635	745	333	
POST INITIAL THERAPY	422	236	624	334	222	211	111	111	111	111	111	212	223	624	655	344	B

Fig 9.4 Six-point probing pocket chart at reassessment compared to initial presentation.

	8	7	6	5	4	3	2	1	1	2	3	4	5	6	7	8	
6/12 POST SURGERY	X	412	333	212	333	222	324	422	323	212	212	212	233	333	323	X	B
POST INITIAL THERAPY	334	623	726	333	212	232	225	421	333	322	223	212	334	614	324	344	B
PRESENTATION	433	524	747	523	323	333	347	633	455	434	333	423	423	635	444	334	B
	8	7	6	5	4	3	2	1	1	2	3	4	5	6	7	8	
PRESENTATION	433	521	744	522	322	331	344	634	452	431	322	522	522	744	555	331	P
POST INITIAL THERAPY	422	622	633	312	222	212	333	522	332	321	223	423	622	635	544	333	P
6/12 POST SURGERY		333	422	212	222	212	323	422	322	322	222	333	322	313	222		P
6/12 POST SURGERY		334	424	113	223	111	111	111	111	111	111	222	212	333	333		L
POST INITIAL THERAPY	422	335	624	224	333	111	111	111	111	111	112	212	222	635	544	335	L
PRESENTATION	433	226	535	335	333	212	112	212	211	111	212	222	333	736	534	445	L
	8	7	6	5	4	3	2	1	1	2	3	4	5	6	7	8	
PRESENTATION	522	335	726	534	322	212	212	111	111	112	112	312	313	635	745	333	B
POST INITIAL THERAPY	422	236	624	334	222	211	111	111	111	111	111	212	223	624	655	344	B
6/12 POST SURGERY	X	222	322	233	212	111	111	111	111	112	112	222	222	333	344	X	B

Fig 9.5 Six-point probing pocket chart 6 months after completion of repeating RSD in anterior sites and the surgical treatment in all posterior areas.

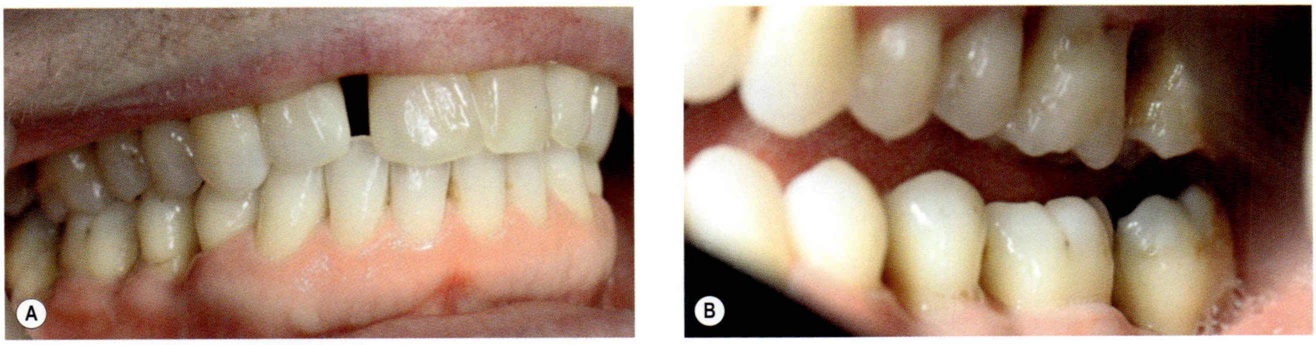

Fig 9.6 Case 1. Clinical appearance of patient 6 months following surgical treatment. Note the healthy appearance of gingivae (A) and the gingival recession around surgical sites in molar regions resulting from the apically positioned flap procedures (B).

was evident from this tooth. Elsewhere, there were generalized pockets of 5–7 mm, but no further mobility was noted (Figure 9.7).

Given the extreme mobility of the UR7, it was decided to extract this tooth and a course of periodontal treatment was proposed. The importance of achieving good plaque control was emphasized, and particularly the role of smoking as a causative factor of the disease and its potential deleterious effects on treatment outcome were emphasized. The patient agreed to consider trying to quit smoking but declined referral to smoking cessation services.

The patient received a course of nonsurgical periodontal treatment over six visits including OHI, supragingival scaling, and four visits of RSD with local analgesia, reinforcing OH techniques at each visit.

At reassessment, there had been a marked improvement in oral hygiene, with a plaque score of 23% and no detectable calculus deposits. However, a new 6-point pocket chart showed very little change in pocket depths throughout the mouth (Figure 9.7). From this chart, it can be seen that although there were some small variations in pocket depth from baseline, these are quite likely to be at least in part due to inevitable inconsistencies in pocket depth measurement. Overall, the patient responded very poorly to treatment, despite the marked improvement in plaque control seen. By far the most likely cause of this is the continued heavy smoking by the patient.

The patient reported that he did not feel ready to try to quit smoking at the present time but agreed to continue to consider it in the future. Further management of such a case is a particular challenge. It is unlikely that further improvements in plaque control will improve the situation given the absence of response to treatment so far. Surgical treatment would be very unwise because it is clear that smoking significantly impairs these treatment outcomes and because the likely primary cause of treatment failure here is due the smoking. In such a case, it is essential that the implications of and rationale for any further treatment be explained to the patient, emphasizing the primary importance of smoking cessation for an improved outcome. In this case, the patient

POST INITIAL THERAPY	X	X	666	822	X	425	616	846	533	434	634	X	445	546	837	X	B
PRESENTATION	X	989	667	734	X	555	625	747	536	425	636	X	536	457	737	X	
	8	7	6	5	4	3	2	1	1	2	3	4	5	6	7	8	
PRESENTATION		1089	746	835	X	435	525	736	555	355	646	X	636	528	757	X	P
POST INITIAL THERAPY	X	X	537	836	X	334	424	725	425	425	635	X	726	535	648	X	
POST INITIAL THERAPY	X	777	X	434	X	313	413	211	111	122	414	X	436	667	648	X	L
PRESENTATION	X	676	X	555	X	323	423	222	212	112	323	X	536	768	757	X	
	8	7	6	5	4	3	2	1	1	2	3	4	5	6	7	8	
PRESENTATION	X	747	X	424	X	212	322	211	111	222	212	X	425	637	637	X	B
POST INITIAL THERAPY	X	836	X	413	X	211	312	111	111	112	212	X	415	626	728	X	

Fig 9.7 Case 2. Six-point probing pocket chart at presentation and 6 weeks after initial therapy.

was placed on a maintenance programme of regular repeat scalings every 3 months, but always with the aspiration that he may manage to quit smoking in the future. This is obviously a severe compromise on normal treatment objectives but may represent a realistic expectation in the poorly responding smoker. It should be emphasized that this approach is in no way a "punishment" for the patient's failure to quit but, rather, it represents a realistic assessment of achievable goals given the circumstances and avoids the performance of extensive procedures that would likely have little chance of success.

Note that not all smokers fail to respond to treatment in the way discussed here. In these "responding cases," different decisions about further treatment may reasonably apply.

Case 3

A 24-year-old male patient was referred by a general dental practitioner to a periodontal specialist because of severe periodontitis. The dentist had carried out initial diagnosis and nonsurgical treatment and was concerned about lack of response to initial therapy. The patient was medically healthy and a nonsmoker. There was no family history of periodontal disease, and no other systemic complicating factor was identified.

At initial assessment, it was noted that there was severe pocketing affecting most teeth, and radiographs showed severe bone loss of approximately 70% in most areas and endodontic treatments of UL1, LR1, and LR2. Bone loss on LR2 extended close to the apex of the tooth (Figures 9.8 and 9.9). The lower incisors exhibited grade 2 mobility, and many of the remaining teeth showed grade 1 mobility. The plaque control was noted as "quite good," and there were no detectable supragingival or subgingival deposits.

At reassessment by the periodontist, the poor response to initial therapy was evident, with very little reduction in pocket depths (Figure 9.10). The plaque score was 18%, although some interdental deposits were still evident. A diagnosis of generalized aggressive periodontitis was made, together with a likely perio/endo lesion at LR2.

In this case, there is clearly an overall lack of response to treatment, and the likely causes of the failure to significantly improve the clinical condition concern the diagnosis and factors related to the high susceptibility of the patient to the disease. As discussed in Chapter 13, generalized aggressive periodontitis is typically treated with adjunctive antimicrobials, particularly where there is a relative lack of deposits initially. In addition, the prognosis for many of the teeth is poor from the outset, and it is thus not surprising that the response to treatment is therefore inadequate. In such a

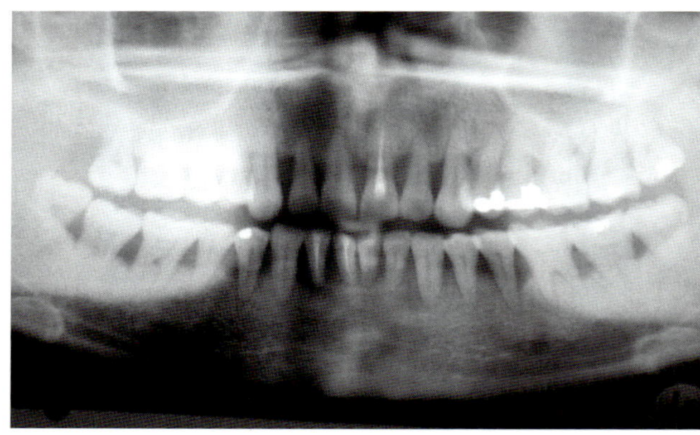

Fig 9.8 Case 3. Rotational tomogram showing severe generalized bone loss.

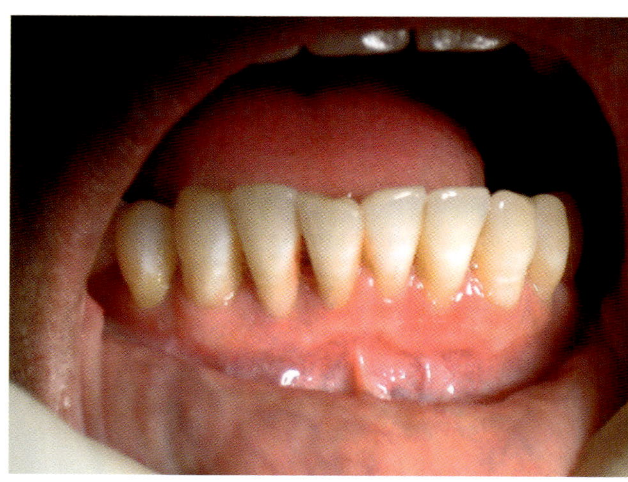

Fig 9.9 Case 3. Clinical appearance after initial therapy.

POST INITIAL THERAPY	X	756	466	648	747	636	777	857	745	835	447	968	835	666	857	745	B
PRESENTATION	X	666	577	658	857	749	868	968	756	946	779	869	947	857	777	855	
	8	**7**	**6**	**5**	**4**	**3**	**2**	**1**	**1**	**2**	**3**	**4**	**5**	**6**	**7**	**8**	
PRESENTATION	X	567	455	648	766	668	777	7410	777	967	678	758	848	948	758	646	
POST INITIAL THERAPY	X	566	334	438	446	638	677	659	645	835	646	655	748	947	846	533	P
POST INITIAL THERAPY	555	667	857	655	867	545	879	889	848	746	355	544	556	666	643	534	L
PRESENTATION	556	757	1068	647	969	646	1078	978	859	836	446	556	458	667	744	533	
	8	**7**	**6**	**5**	**4**	**3**	**2**	**1**	**1**	**2**	**3**	**4**	**5**	**6**	**7**	**8**	
PRESENTATION	455	646	959	535	946	537	957	888	869	745	534	444	559	637	534	444	
POST INITIAL THERAPY	335	546	935	524	936	448	868	788	857	655	434	544	449	537	633	444	B

Fig 9.10 Six-point probing pocket chart at reassessment by the periodontist.

case, it is often difficult to decide which teeth to extract initially given the uncertainty of treatment outcome, and thus it is reasonable to make a final decision on this following reassessment. Given the patient's reluctance to lose any teeth requiring prosthetic replacement, it was thus decided to re-treat the patient with adjunctive antimicrobials together with a new round of RSD. In this case, the patient was treated with a course of doxycycline 100 mg daily for 3 weeks on completion of the new round of RSD. The patient showed a remarkable improvement in pocket reduction, accompanied by extensive gingival recession; in the short term at least, all teeth were retained.

Summary

The reassessment appointment is a key moment in periodontal therapy requiring the use of clinical diagnostic skills to assess initial treatment outcomes both at a tooth-by-tooth level and from one patient to another. A careful consideration of the likely reasons for particular outcomes is a valuable approach to dictating future treatment needs on a rational basis. The cases discussed here illustrate this process but represent only some of the likely scenarios that the clinician is likely to face.

Chapter 10

Surgical treatment of periodontal pocketing

Introduction

In Chapter 9, reassessment of the patient following completion of initial periodontal therapy was discussed. It was noted that in cases in which deep pockets persist, it may be necessary to carry out further root surface debridement either by repeating the nonsurgical treatment or considering a surgical approach to debridement of the periodontal defect. This chapter explains the indications for surgery for the treatment of periodontal pocketing and discusses the basic techniques that are used to carry out this treatment. Periodontal surgery is often regarded as within the particular domain of the periodontal specialist, and it is described in considerable detail in a number of comprehensive periodontal textbooks and surgical atlases. Therefore, here we have placed the emphasis on understanding the decision-making processes involved in electing for surgical treatment, and the basic procedures involved, rather than providing a detailed manual of surgical procedures.

Indications for surgery

Further active periodontal treatment is generally indicated when deep pockets persist following initial therapy. Often, the persistence of deep pocketing may be the result of difficulty in completely debriding the root surface nonsurgically, and in these cases either more nonsurgical treatment or surgery may be chosen. There are no absolute guidelines in deciding which cases should be treated surgically, and in making the decision, the clinician needs to consider the likely reasons for persistence of pocketing, the appropriate remedies, the potential advantages of surgical treatment, the likely outcomes, and the patient's wishes and best interests. The potential advantages and disadvantages of surgical treatment of pockets compared to nonsurgical therapy are listed in Table 10.1.

In particular, surgery allows direct access for root surface debridement so that the root surface can be directly visualized, along with its possible anatomical anomalies (e.g., grooves and furcations) and calculus deposits, enabling accurate debridement to be achieved by direct vision. Therefore, despite the many varieties of surgical techniques that have been described, direct access to the periodontal defect remains the main indication for periodontal surgery. A surgical approach does allow the alteration of the soft tissue to facilitate oral hygiene through gingival recontouring and/or pocket elimination. It is also possible to modify the contour of the bone and alter osseous defects and to re-establish the anatomical architecture of the bone.

Periodontal surgery may therefore be indicated when there are persisting deep pockets in the presence of good plaque control. Choosing a surgical approach in these circumstances is more likely for treatment of posterior sites, in deeper pockets, where there are infrabony pockets, where there are complicating root surface anomalies, and where there are soft tissue anomalies. Choosing a surgical approach (rather than a nonsurgical approach) is less likely for less deep pockets, suprabony sites, anterior teeth, and where there are obvious residual calculus deposits that can be readily detected and removed by further nonsurgical root surface debridement. The clinician needs to weigh these different factors when making a decision (with the most important aspect being that an active decision is made based on the available evidence rather than simply repeating the nonsurgical treatment as a default position).

Contraindications for surgery

The major contraindication for surgery is poor oral hygiene. This should be regarded as an absolute contraindication for surgery. Surgery is far more likely to fail in the plaque-infected dentition, and consequently surgery is not advised in these circumstances. Studies suggest that in the presence of poor plaque control, the outcome of surgery may be worse than if nothing is done. Probably the only other absolute contraindication for surgery is lack of patient consent.

There are also a number of relative contraindications for surgery—that is, those that do not absolutely rule out surgery but indicate that surgery should only be carried out with caution, recognizing the risks involved. These include the following:

- Smoking
- Medical issues
- When postoperative recession is likely to be problematic aesthetically
- When the patient shows an overall lack of response to nonsurgical therapy (where antimicrobials might be used; discussed in Chapter 13)
- Patient preference

Surgery is more likely to fail in smokers than in nonsmokers, so careful informed consent must be established if surgery is performed in a smoker, such that the risks are fully explained. Uncontrolled medical conditions such as angina, hypertension, diabetes, or recent stroke or infarct may also tend to contraindicate surgery. Patients with bleeding disorders may require special management and represent a serious contraindication if not managed appropriately.

It is also vital to manage patients' expectations so that they will not have unrealistic expectations of the outcomes of their surgery. They should be counselled regarding possible adverse effects, such as postoperative pain and swelling and the possibility of gingival recession and root sensitivity. It should be remembered that periodontal treatment does not exist in a vacuum and that periodontal and restorative treatment will need to be coordinated particularly with regard to the timing of fixed prosthodontics where good temporization is key prior to surgery, whereas definitive restoration should be delayed until after a period of months (usually up to 6 months) for the final postsurgical gingival contour to be established.

Surgical techniques

As with all types of surgery, a detailed knowledge of the surgical anatomy of the jaws is necessary before picking up a scalpel. In particular, knowing the blood supply will inform flap design and management, particularly to optimize healing and to minimize risk of loss of tissue. As has been stressed throughout this chapter, the objective of surgery is to visualize the root surface(s) to enable effective debridement and possible management of the bone and soft tissue. Consequently, flap design should mirror this, but only soft tissue that is needed to expose the root surface should be reflected. Such a conservative approach will greatly help with postoperative healing, and not reflecting the flap beyond the mucogingival junction where appropriate will minimize postoperative recession.

Table 10.1 Advantages and disadvantages of periodontal surgery compared to nonsurgical treatment

Advantages of surgery	Disadvantages of surgery
Provides direct visualization of defect	More traumatic for the patient
Improves access to the defect	Causes more postoperative recession than nonsurgical treatments
Allows correction of root surface anomalies such as root grooves	Requires operator with specific surgical skills and experience
Allows direct exploration of a defect and detection of unexpected anomalies (e.g., lateral perforation of a post)	Not suitable in some medically compromised cases, particularly those with bleeding disorders
Allows recontouring/repositioning of soft tissues to facilitate plaque control/improve aesthetics	
Allows surgical elimination of pocket, including bone recontouring of infrabony defects	
Allows use of regenerative techniques on some occasions	

The following are the principal stages of periodontal surgical techniques:

1. Cutting and elevating full thickness mucoperiosteal flaps, usually both buccally and lingually.
2. Removal of all granulation tissue within the defect.
3. Thorough debridement of the root surface.
4. If necessary, correction of root surface anomalies and bone recontouring.
5. Replacing the flap and suturing.

As previously mentioned, a wide variety of surgical techniques and modifications have been described; the new student of periodontal surgery should be forgiven for being confused by the myriad different names and descriptions. More frustratingly, there is scant clinical evidence that one technique is superior to another. However, in principle, these different techniques can be classified into two main approaches to surgical treatment of pocketing, namely "pocket correction" techniques and "pocket elimination" techniques.

Pocket correction techniques depend on the principal advantage of periodontal surgery—direct access to the root surface—to treat the pocket by achieving effective root surface debridement and hence allowing the pocket to heal. A flap is raised, specifically to allow direct root surface access, and is replaced as closely as possible to the original level of attachment to promote healing that will minimize recession (Figure 10.1). This procedure is also known as open flap debridement, and one of the modifications of this technique is referred to as the modified Widman flap technique, which is widely discussed in the literature. Healing, resulting in pocket reduction, is as described with

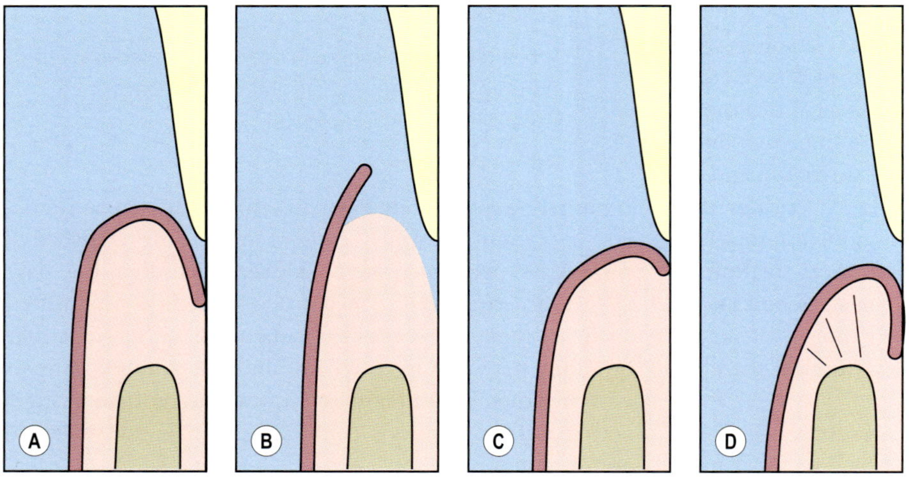

Fig 10.1 Diagrammatic representation of the principles of pocket correction surgery (open flap debridement). (A) Deep pocket; (B) flap raised to expose defect; (C) after debridement of defect, flap replaced as close as possible to original level of attachment; (D) healing after 2 or 3 months—pocket reduction results from formation of fibrous gingival cuff, long junctional epithelium, and some gingival recession.

nonsurgical treatment (see Chapter 8), involving tightening of the gingival fibrous cuff and formation of a long junctional epithelium, and it is associated with some recession.

Pocket elimination techniques, specifically the apically positioned flap procedure, aim deliberately to cause gingival recession in order to remove the subgingival component of the attachment loss, thus leaving the area more readily cleansable by supragingival plaque control. Again, a flap is raised, but prior to closure any infrabony pockets are eliminated using a handpiece and surgical bur, and the flap is then repositioned apically on the crestal alveolar bone prior to suturing. The effect of this is to surgically reduce the pocket depth at the expense of increased gingival recession (Figure 10.2). This technique is widely used for the treatment of deep pockets on posterior teeth, but due to its effects on recession, its applications in areas that are aesthetically important are severely limited.

Case 1

Following nonsurgical treatment, a patient has a persisting pocket of 7 mm at the mesial of UR5, both buccally and palatally (Figure 10.3). Given the isolated deep pocket and infrabony component of the defect, a decision has been made to surgically expose the root surface for further debridement. Using a small scalpel, the initial incision is an inverse bevel incision made as shown in Figure 10.4, keeping the blade at approximately 10° to the long axis of the tooth,

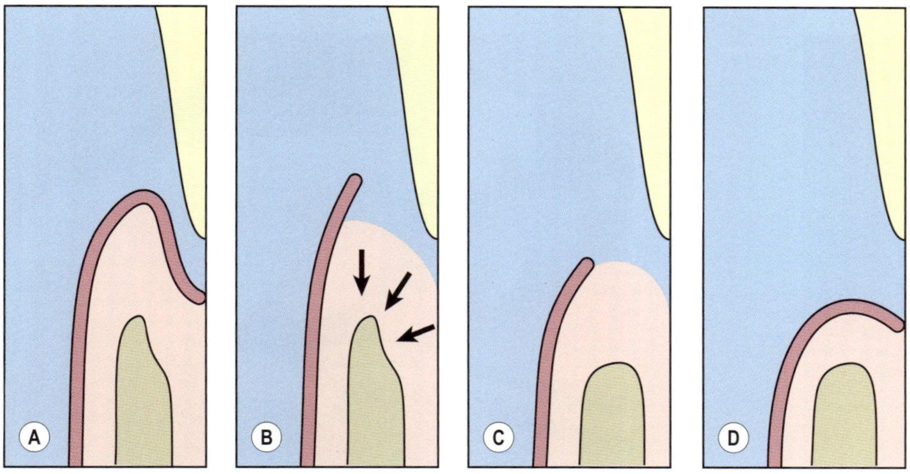

Fig 10.2 Diagrammatic representation of the principles of pocket elimination surgery (apically positioned flap). (A) Deep pocket with infrabony component; (B) flap raised to expose defect, including infrabony component (arrows); (C) debridement of defect and recontouring of bone to remove infrabony component surgically and create bony anatomy to facilitate flap position; (D) flap replaced apically and sutured in place to eliminate existing pocket. (Note recession deliberately caused to eliminate pocket.)

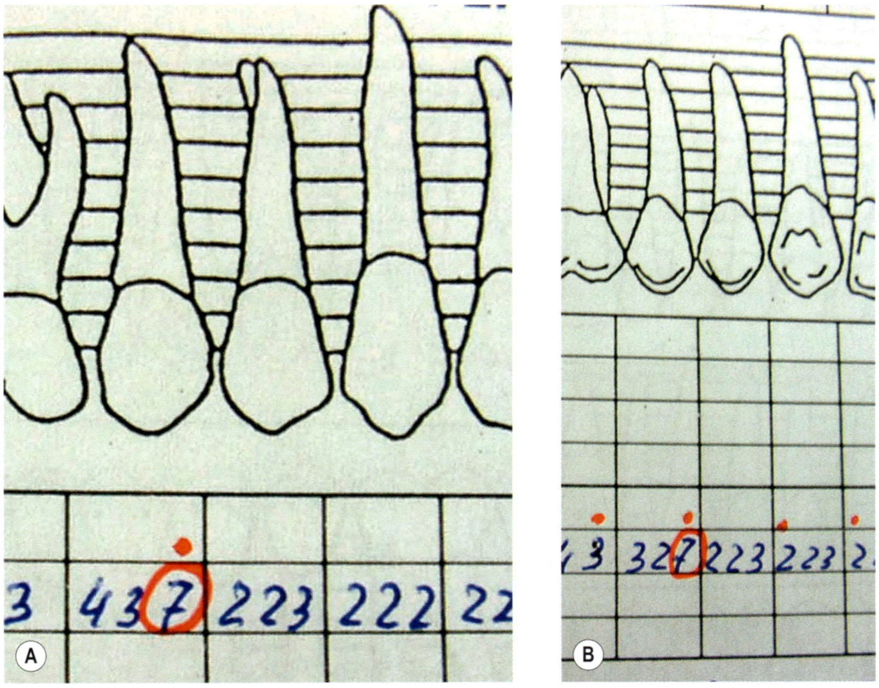

Fig 10.3 Detail of pocket chart showing isolated persisting 7-mm pocket (A) buccally and (B) lingually at reassessment following nonsurgical treatment.

approximately 1 mm from the gingival margin. This is shown diagrammatically in Figure 10.5, effectively excising the pocket lining to expose the periodontal lesion. The inverse bevel flap is the normal primary incision for most periodontal surgical techniques to facilitate excision of the pocket lining, although occasionally, particularly for regenerative surgical techniques (see Chapter 12), a crevicular incision is employed to preserve all available tissues.

The incision is developed carefully to allow full access to the lesion, moving the blade mesially and distally from where it started just to the mesial of the interdental papilla, taking care to preserve as much of the papilla as possible. A similar incision is made on the palatal aspect of the tooth, carefully incising and reflecting the flap initially with the blade and then with a retractor or even something more delicate, such as a flat plastic, taking care not to place any tension on the flap during the reflection to avoid tearing (Figure 10.6).

One dilemma is whether to use a relieving incision on the buccal aspect or to keep the flap as an envelope. The key is access: if it is possible to access the defect without placing a relieving incision, then the potential for postoperative scarring is avoided. Once both buccal and palatal incisions have been sufficiently developed so as to expose the root surface, without placing tension on the flaps, the area is cleared of granulation tissue through sharp dissection and then through use of sharp curettes. Note that each time a new incision is made, it is recommended to use a fresh blade; also, curettes must be sharp.

Once the granulation tissue has been removed, the root surface is exposed and can now be debrided (Figure 10.7). It is now possible to carry out any other modifications to

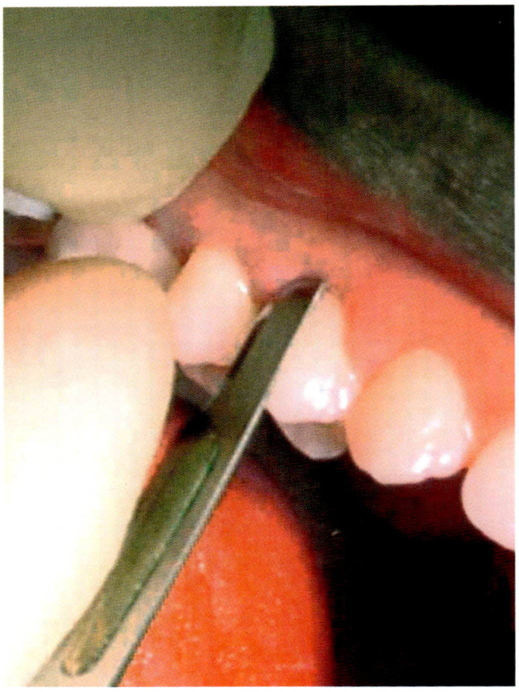

Fig 10.4 Case 1: Initial incision of inverse bevel flap for treatment of mesial defect of UR5.

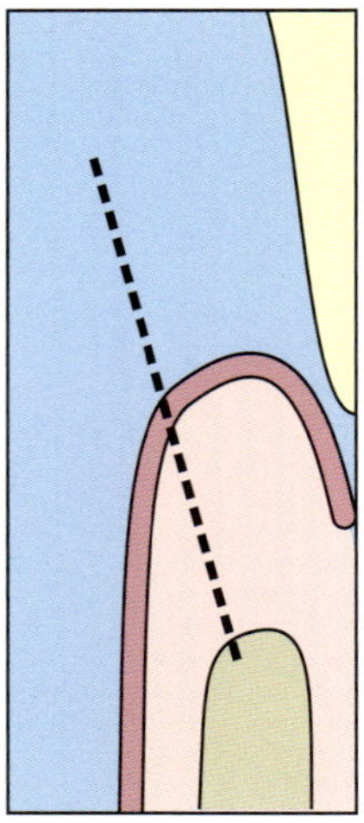

Fig 10.5 Diagram of inverse bevel flap incision. The incision is made at approximately 10° to the tooth, extending approximately 1 mm from the gingival margin down to the alveolar bone.

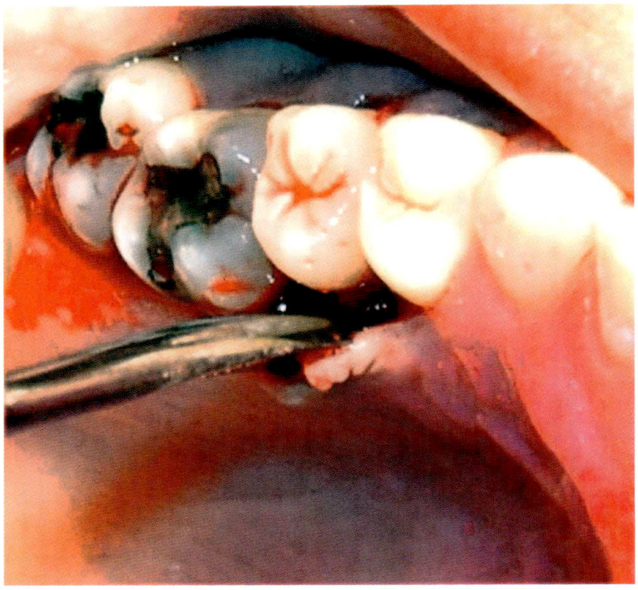

Fig 10.6 Palatal flap incised and elevated.

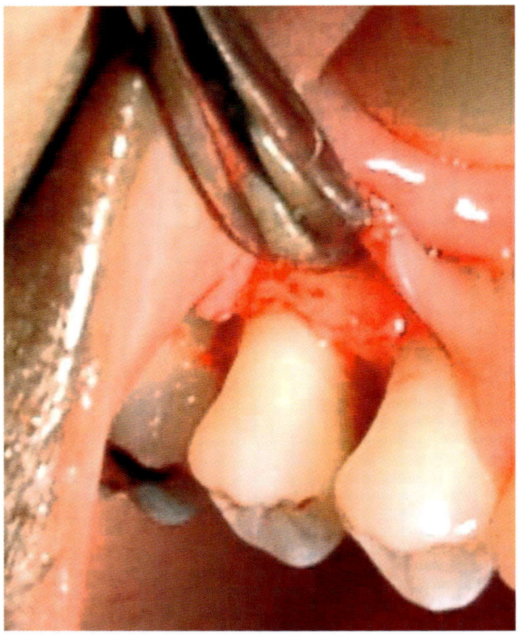

Fig 10.7 Buccal flap elevated to allow access to the root surface in the infrabony defect on mesial of UR5.

the bone, etc., as necessary. Once completed, the buccal and palatal flaps are sutured in place with simple interrupted single sutures in each papilla. In this case, a braided silk suture is shown (Figure 10.8). Other suture options include the use of resorbable materials or monofilament materials

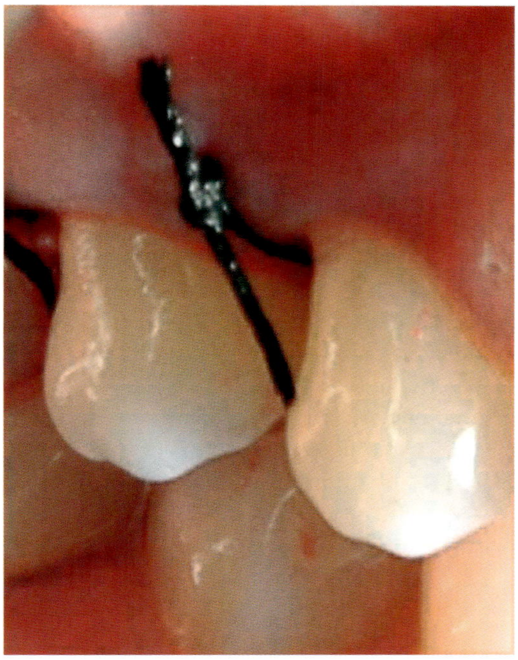

Fig 10.8 Simple interrupted black silk suture placed in the papilla.

such as ePTFE. Once sutured, the flaps are held in place for 5–10 min with damp gauze to facilitate initial fibrin clot formation. Suturing buccal and palatal flaps together allows primary healing to occur. Flaps are said to be replaced and will generally heal through formation of a long junctional epithelium. This epithelial attachment, although not replacing the attachment apparatus that has been lost through disease, is a stable and injury-resistant tissue.

Case 2

Figure 10.9 shows a patient with localized pocketing in the UR34 region. The patient has excellent plaque control and was scheduled for surgical debridement of the region. After raising a buccal flap, a significant (and unexpected) buccal groove was found to be present on the buccal surface of the UR4, which was subsequently recontoured prior to suturing of the flap.

Postoperative management

Following completion of the surgical procedure, patients must receive careful written postoperative instructions reinforced by verbal instructions.

Although as operators, we often make light of surgery, particularly in the case of consenting patients, it must be remembered how traumatic such procedures are for patients.

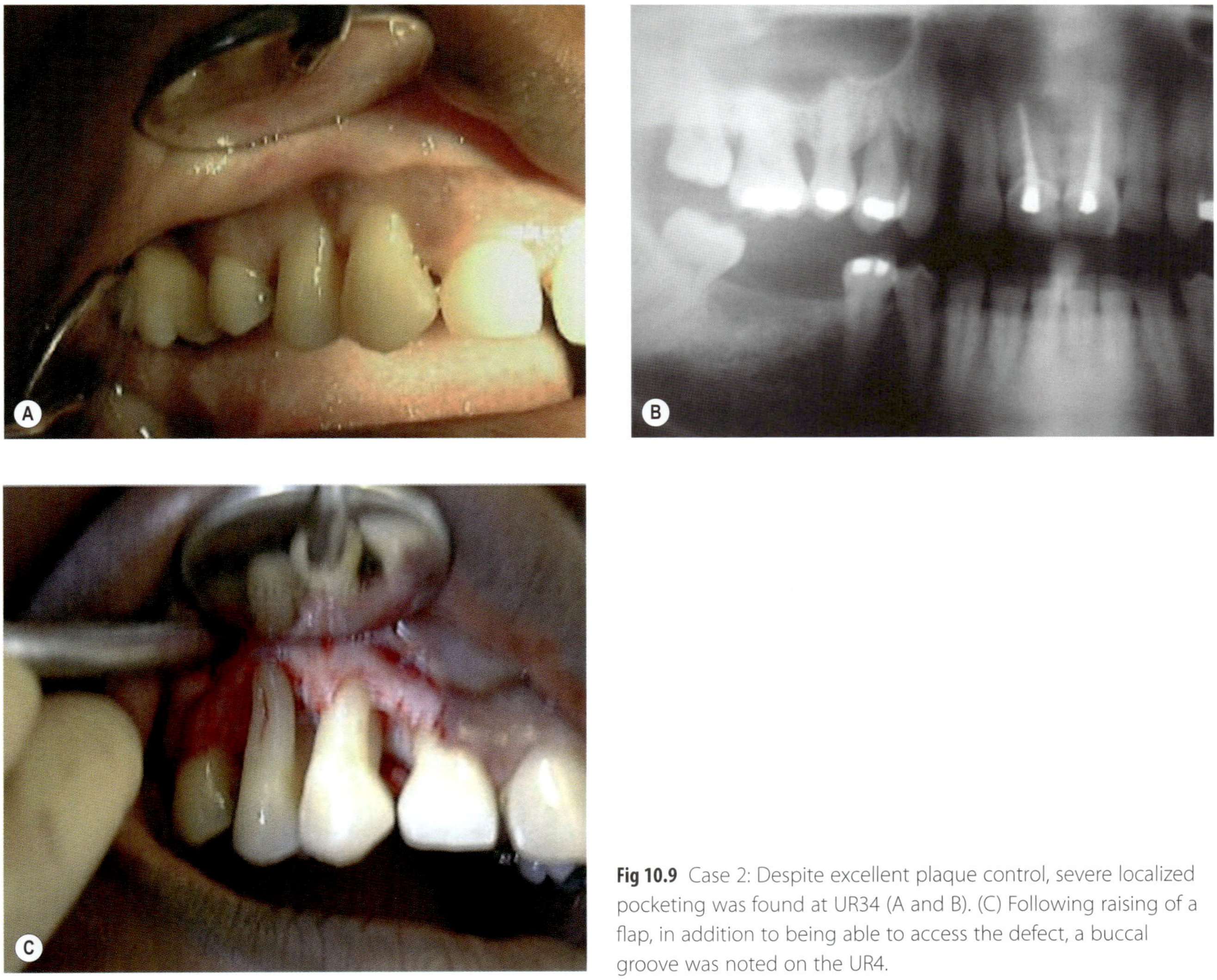

Fig 10.9 Case 2: Despite excellent plaque control, severe localized pocketing was found at UR34 (A and B). (C) Following raising of a flap, in addition to being able to access the defect, a buccal groove was noted on the UR4.

Appropriate analgesia should be prescribed postoperatively, usually paracetamol or over-the-counter NSAIDs such as ibuprofen, to minimize patient pain and discomfort. In addition, patients should be instructed to rest. They should not eat or brush on the area of surgery for up to 14 days (or until told to do so). To reduce plaque formation, a 2% chlorhexidine mouthwash should be used twice daily, whereas patients should continue their normal oral hygiene regime elsewhere in the mouth. Patients should also eat a soft diet for at least 24 hr postsurgery, and if they smoke, they should be advised not to do so in the immediate postsurgical period.

Obviously, patients will be encouraged to contact the operator should they have any concerns during this period. Postoperative reviews should initially take place at 7–10 days, when the surgical area should be be assessed for signs of healing and the surgical site gently cleaned with a cotton bud soaked in 2% chlorhexidine solution. Sutures can also be removed if necessary. Sutures are generally removed after 1 week, when the wound is properly stabilized without the need for the sutures and the sutures become only local irritants. After 14 days, following further review, the patient can probably resume normal, gentle cleaning. The frequency of visits after 14 days depends very much on the individual patient's healing and his or her ability to maintain good oral hygiene. Reassessment can take place at approximately 3 months, and if successful, the patient can enter a maintenance programme.

Summary

Surgical treatment of deep periodontal pockets can be extremely effective, particularly for persisting deep pockets after initial therapy. As emphasized throughout this chapter, the main aim of simple open flap debridement surgery is to expose the root surface so that it can be effectively debrided. There are of course many other types of surgical procedure that are described in the following chapters. However, this simple aim should be borne in mind when considering the necessity for surgery and the technique to be employed.

Chapter 11

Other surgical procedures

Introduction

The most common indications for periodontal surgery are to access the root surfaces for debridement under direct vision or to carry out a resective or regenerative procedure (see Chapters 10 and 12) during the treatment of periodontitis. However, there are a number of other distinct clinical situations in which periodontal surgery may also be indicated:

- If the gingiva is partly or completely covering the crown of the tooth/teeth, surgical reduction of the gingiva may be needed to facilitate oral hygiene.
- If the gingiva is partly or completely covering the crown of the tooth/teeth, surgical reduction of the gingiva may be needed to access the tooth for restoration.
- To provide adequate sound supragingival tooth tissue to ensure restoration retention, and resistance without encroaching on the biologic width.
- To address aesthetic concerns, particularly when an excess of gingiva is shown.
- To separate or remove a root from a multirooted tooth.

This chapter discusses some of the surgical procedures used to manage these conditions.

Gingival procedures to remove excess gingiva (gingivectomy)

Gingival overgrowth is not an uncommon clinical finding, and there are a number of reasons why this might occur (Table 11.1). Some patients who present with gingival overgrowth would benefit from a surgical gingivectomy, which aims to excise excess gingival tissue without the removal of alveolar bone. This procedure is applicable only to patients with either excessive gingival tissue or suprabony pockets with adequate keratinized gingiva. This is traditionally carried out using a reverse bevel incision or, more commonly, an inverse bevel incision. The advantages and disadvantages are detailed in Table 11.2.

Case 1: Drug-induced gingival enlargement

A 36-year-old male patient presented with concern about his gums looking very swollen. Medical history revealed that he was diagnosed with hypertension 4 years ago, and he had been taking amlodipine 10 mg and bendroflumethiazide 2.5 mg per day. He reported that his "gum problem" started 1 year after initiating his medication.

The patient has been visiting his dentist regularly and has been receiving scaling without local anaesthesia every 6 months.

The attached and free gingiva were grossly overgrown and bled readily upon probing (Figure 11.1). The interdental papillae exhibited a nodular appearance, and supra- and subgingival plaque and calculus were present, particularly interdentally. The BPE score was as follows:

3	4	3
4	4	4

Little alveolar bone was evident on the panoramic radiograph (Figure 11.2), and a diagnosis of drug-induced gingival enlargement was made. The patient received a course of initial periodontal therapy to improve his oral hygiene and removal of plaque and calculus deposits. Following completion of this treatment, the plaque scores improved to an acceptable level; however, the gingival enlargement remained, and a surgical phase of treatment was planned.

The width of gingival tissue to be removed by the combination of these incisions is preplanned by "sounding out" the underlying bone crest and ensuring that a width of keratinized gingiva of at least 3 mm remains. To remove and thin the excess gingival tissue in this case, a gingivectomy was performed using an inverse bevel incision combined with an intracrevicular incision (Figure 11.3). A third incision was performed with an Orban interdental knife along the alveolar crest in order to separate the secondary flap around the cervical area from the bone crest (Figure 11.4). The secondary flap was removed with a curette (Figure 11.5).

The flap was closed with interrupted sutures, and postoperative healing was uneventful (Figure 11.6). The final outcome is shown in Figure 11.7.

◇ ***Could this have been carried out by alternative surgical methods?***

An alternative technique to a reverse bevel or inverse bevel would be to remove the excess gingiva using electrosurgery. This involves a loop or needle electrode with a current that allows both cutting and coagulation simultaneously, which controls bleeding while recontouring the gingiva. Disadvantages are that the procedure has an unpleasant smell and cannot be used in patients with unshielded cardiac pacemakers. In addition, removal of too much tissue by electrosurgery risks causing some necrosis of underlying tissue. Laser surgery may also be useful in managing these cases.

Crown lengthening surgery

The aim of crown lengthening surgery is to expose adequate tooth structure for restorative or aesthetic reasons by

Table 11.1 Causes of gingival enlargement

Drug induced
Anticonvulsant medication (phenytoin)
Calcium channel blockers (nifedipine, amlodipine, verapamil, diltiazem)
Immunosuppressant medication (ciclosporin)
Plaque induced
In some systemic conditions, gingivitis caused by plaque accumulation can be more severe (diabetes, puberty, pregnancy)
Idiopathic
Fibrous hyperplasia of the gingiva (may be familial)
Blood dyscrasias
Acute monocytic, lymphocytic, or myelocytic leukaemia

Table 11.2 Advantages and disadvantages of different flap techniques for a gingivectomy

Technique	Advantages	Disadvantages
Reverse bevel	For smaller areas of enlargement Simple flap design Less time-consuming surgical procedure	Postoperative discomfort Intraoperative and postoperative bleeding No primary wound closure and healing by second intention Need to have good width of attached gingiva No bone recontouring possible
Inverse bevel	Can be used for larger areas of enlargement More complex technique technically Primary wound closure and healing	Less postoperative discomfort Less intra- and postoperative bleeding

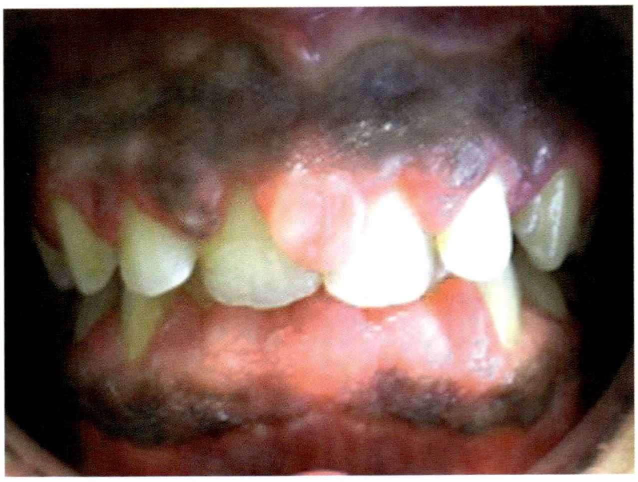

Fig 11.1 Case 1 on presentation. Gross gingival enlargement was seen.

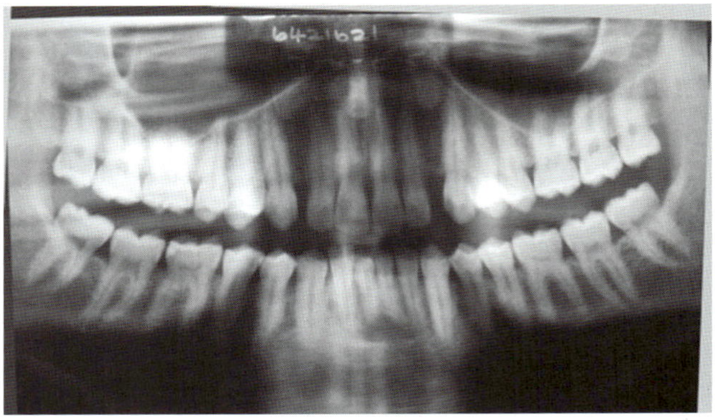

Fig 11.2 Case 2 panoramic radiograph showing minimal alveolar bone loss.

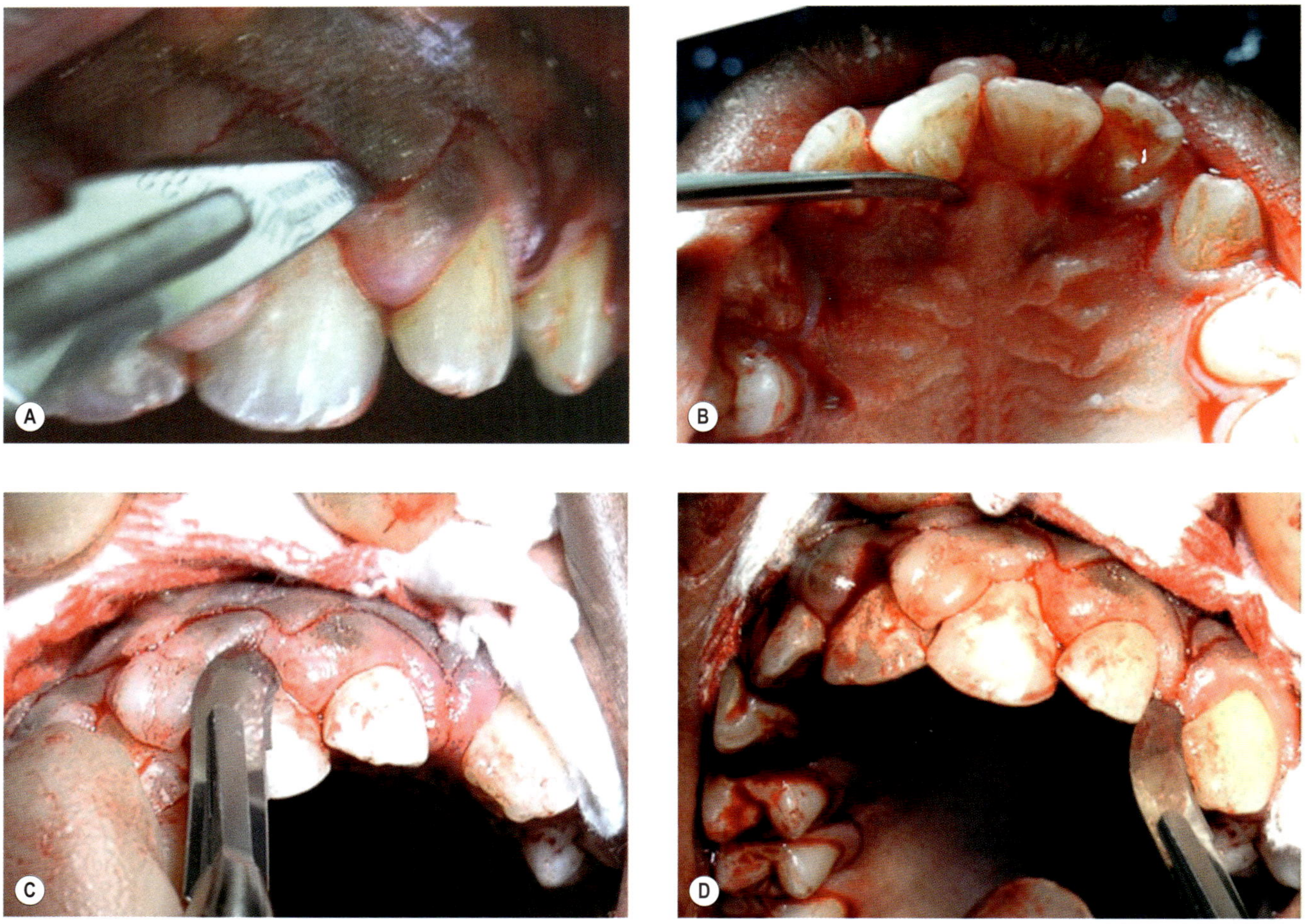

Fig 11.3 An inverse bevel incision was made to approximately the position of the cementoenamel junction, buccally (A) and palatally (B), combined with an intracrevicular incision (C and D) to allow excision of the desired width of gingiva.

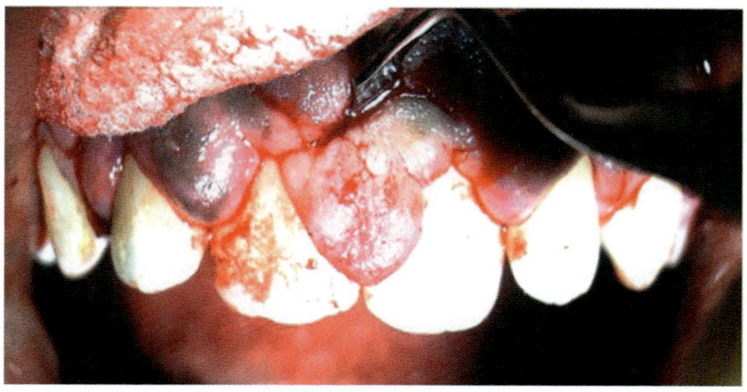

Fig 11.4 A third incision was performed with an Orban interdental knife along the alveolar crest.

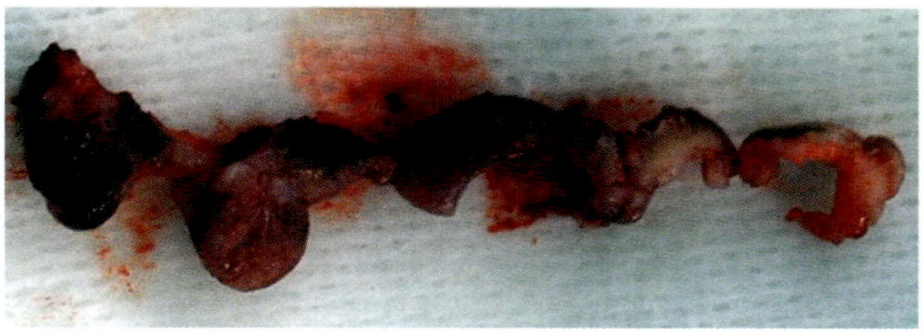

Fig 11.5 The secondary flap was curetted away from the tooth and shows the amount of gingival tissue excised.

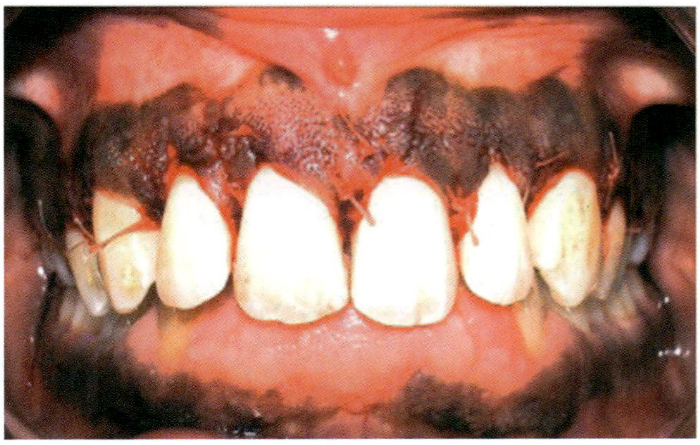

Fig 11.6 The flaps were closed with interrupted sutures.

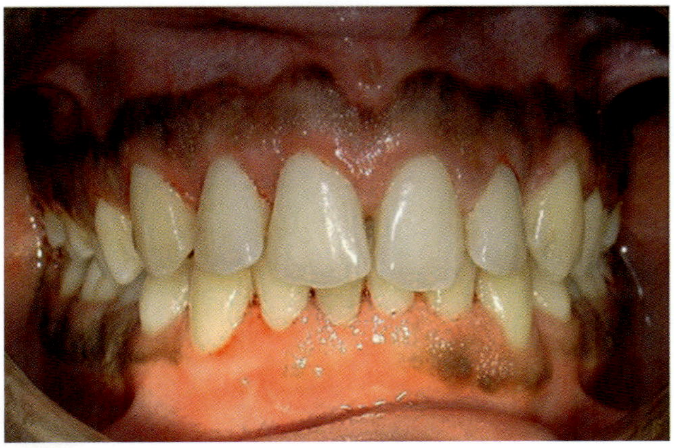

Fig 11.7 Case 1, 2 months after surgery.

removing supporting periodontal structures to gain sound tooth structure above the alveolar crest. There are several possible techniques depending on the particular clinical indication and whether the procedure is applied to a single tooth or multiple teeth.

Main indications

- To increase clinical crown height to allow predictable restoration of the tooth
  - In cases of excessively short clinical crowns (e.g., tooth surface loss)
  - When little sound remaining tooth structure remains
  - To allow restoration margins to be placed on sound tooth structure without encroaching on the biologic width
- To access subgingival caries
- Aesthetic reasons
  - "Gummy" smile
  - Uneven gingival margins
- To access endodontic perforations near the alveolar bone crest
- To access root resorption in the cervical one-third of the tooth root
- Subgingival tooth or cusp fracture in the cervical one-third of the tooth root

What is the biologic width and why is it important?

Biologic width is defined as the distance from the crest of the alveolar bone to the base of the gingival sulcus, and it includes the connective tissue attachment and the epithelial attachment. Gargiulo based the concept on a histological study that determined the average connective tissue, epithelial attachment, and gingival sulcus dimensions and their relationship with the alveolar bone crest. The average dimension of the connective tissue attachment was 1.07 mm, that of the epithelial attachment was 0.97 mm, and that of the gingival sulcus was 0.69 mm; therefore, the "biologic" width averaged 2.04 mm (Figure 11.8).

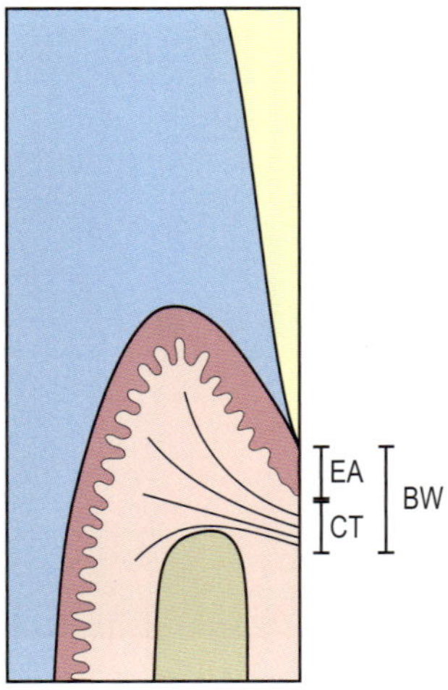

Fig 11.8 The biologic width (BW) is made up of connective tissue (CT) and epithelial attachment (EA) parts.

It is extremely important to understand and clinically manage the biologic width when planning the location of restoration margins from the alveolar bone crest. If restorations are placed where the margins impinge on the biologic width (i.e., <3 mm from the restoration margin to the alveolar bone crest), inflammation and attachment loss will occur with increased pocket depth and/or recession. If the minimum space cannot be maintained during restoration placement, additional measures such as surgical crown lengthening should be performed to ensure this space is created.

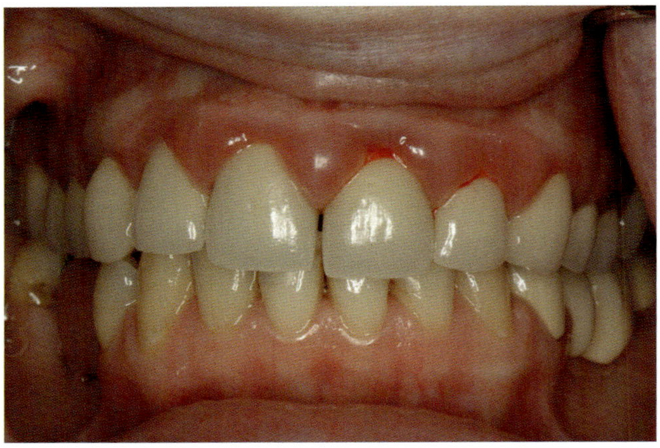

Fig 11.9 Case 2 on presentation, with swollen gingivae associated with the crown margins and immediate bleeding following periodontal probing.

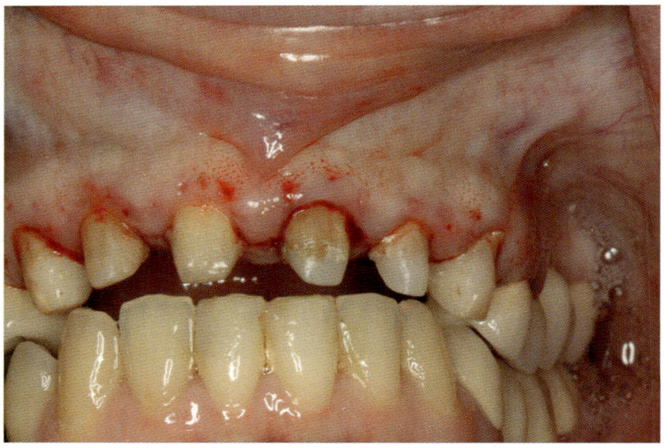

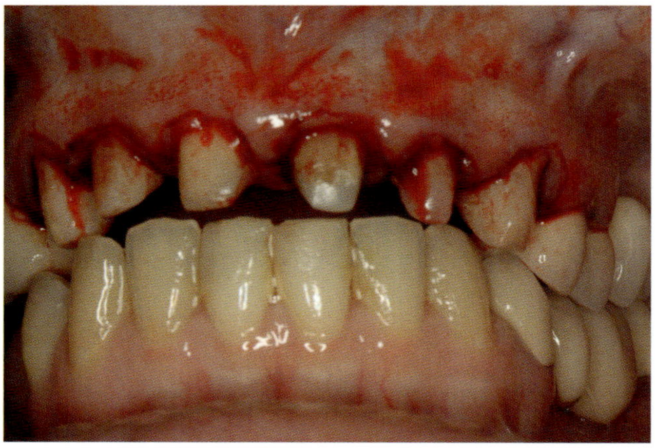

Fig 11.10 (top) and Fig 11.11 (bottom) Intracrevicular (top) and inverse bevel (bottom) incisions were made to raise a full-thickness flap to allow access to the alveolar bone crest.

Case 2: Biologic width invasion

A 32-year-old female patient presented complaining of "sore, swollen, and bleeding gums" that she had experienced following crowns being placed on her upper anterior teeth 2 years previously. Clinical examination showed that the margins of the crowns placed on these teeth were subgingival, and the gingivae were inflamed and bled immediately on probing (Figure 11.9). Probing depths of 2–4 mm were present. After oral hygiene instruction and scaling around the subgingival restoration margins, the gingival inflammation had not completely resolved. Under local anaesthesia, the bone crest was sounded out using a

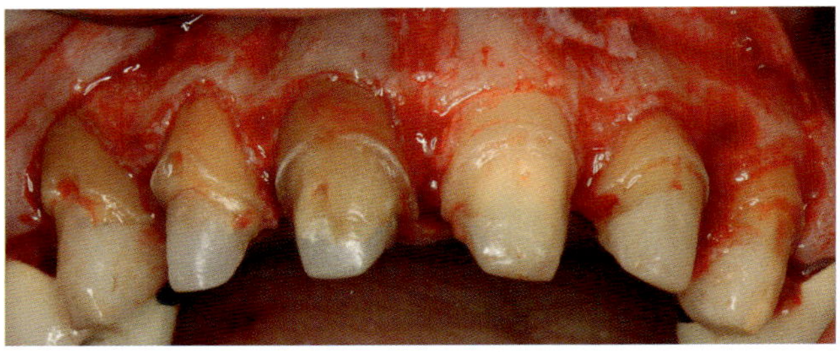

Fig 11.12 Alveolar bone was removed buccally to ensure at least 3 or 4 mm from the bone crest to the proposed restoration margin.

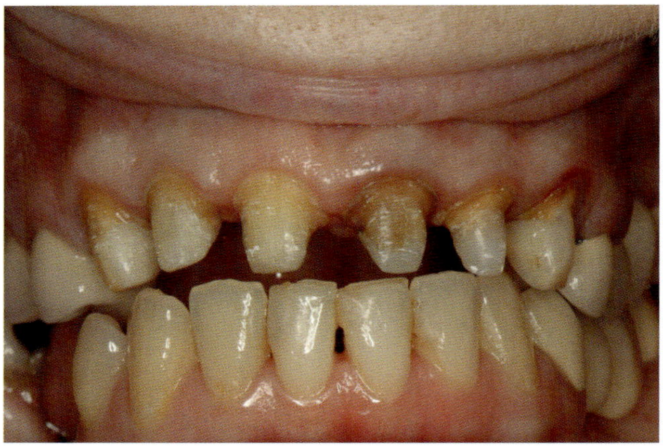

Fig 11.13 After 6 months of healing, the gingival margins were stable and clinically healthy.

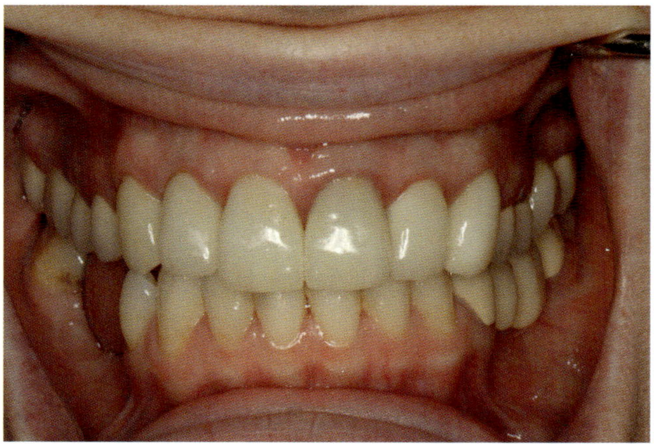

Fig 11.14 Final restorations.

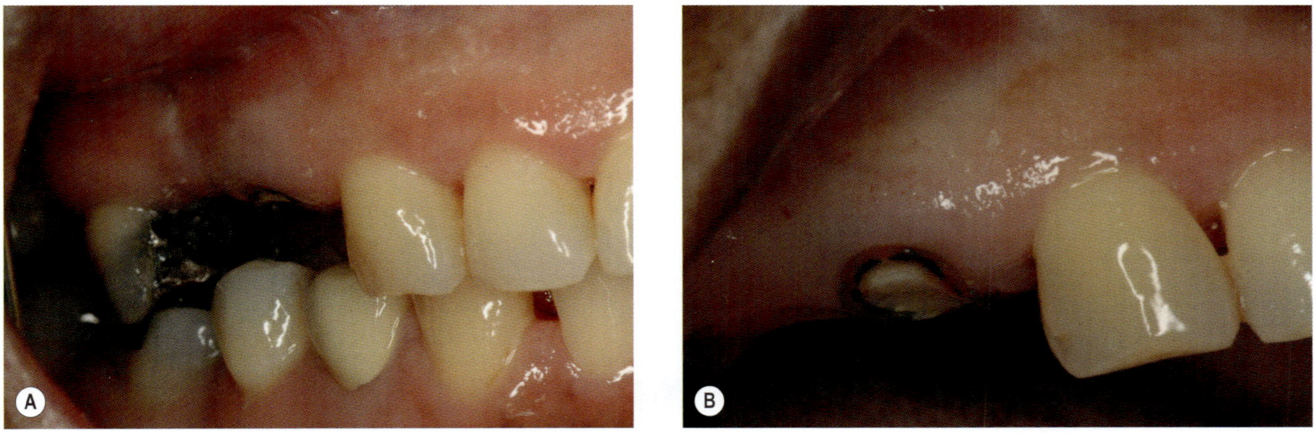

Fig 11.15 Case 3 on presentation showing the 24 fractured at gingival level.

periodontal probe, and a distance of approximately 3 mm from the osseous crest to the gingival margin was determined buccally, suggesting the likelihood that the biologic width was being violated.

The patient had an adequate width of attached gingiva; therefore, a surgical crown lengthening procedure was undertaken. The existing crowns were removed. The removal of existing restorations allows easier access to interproximal areas and visualization of the bone crest.

Inverse bevel and intracrevicular incisions were made from 13 to 23 buccally and palatally, full-thickness mucoperiosteal flaps were raised, and a cuff of 2 mm of gingiva was removed (Figures 11.10 and 11.11). Bone crest was removed until an approximately 3- or 4-mm distance from the alveolar bone crest to the restoration margin was gained (Figure 11.12).

Laboratory-fabricated provisional restorations were placed, and after allowing 6 months for healing and stabilization of the gingival margin (Figure 11.13), the new restorations were fitted (Figure 11.14).

Case 3: Fractured tooth with lack of crown height

A female patient presented after her 24 tooth had fractured while eating, and the patient was very concerned because she had already had 25 extracted after the restoration failed.

On examination, the 24 was fractured at gingival level (Figure 11.15) and had a temporary restoration and satisfactory root canal filling present.

Surgical crown lengthening was performed to allow adequate crown height with a margin on sound supragingival tooth tissue (Figure 11.16) by raising a full-thickness mucoperiosteal flap and removing sufficient crestal bone to ensure adequate supragingival tooth was available for restoration with a cast post and core incorporating a ferrule (Figure 11.17).

◈ *What other treatment options would be possible?*

- The tooth could have been extracted if there had been an unfavourable crown : root ratio or an adequate root canal treatment was not possible.
- Orthodontic forced tooth eruption aims to expose more tooth structure while maintaining the position of the gingival line and the alveolar bone. This is a conservative but time-consuming process; however, it is particularly useful for isolated teeth requiring crown lengthening.

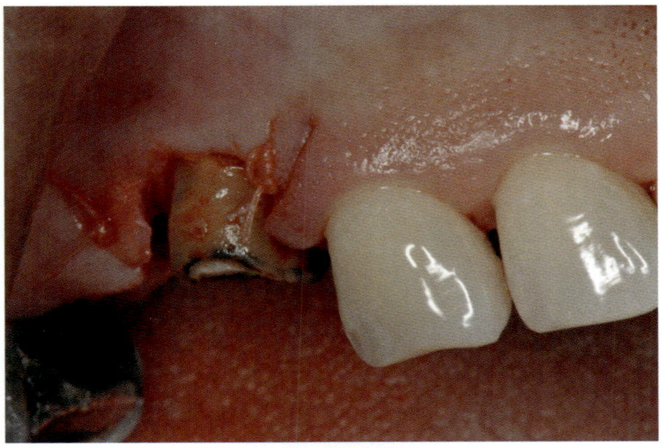

Fig 11.16 The amount of supragingival tooth tissue gained after crown lengthening surgery.

◈ *Treatment timing*

An integrated periodontal and restorative treatment plan is essential to obtain optimal results.

In nonaesthetic areas, it is advisable to re-evaluate 6–8 weeks postsurgery, whereas in the aesthetic zone, 5 or 6 months is advisable to ensure stability of the gingival margin before provision of the final restoration. When the restoration is placed, the margins should be supragingival or at the gingival margin, with careful attention given to not traumatizing the gingiva during the preparation and impression stage. Tissue retraction should be cautious, particularly with a thin gingival type, to avoid tearing of the sulcular epithelium and encroachment into the biological width.

Root resection procedures

Root resection involves sectioning and the removal of one or two roots of a multirooted tooth, usually in grade II or III furcation-involved molar teeth. Although the survival rate of root resected teeth has been reported to be between 30 and 90%, there are situations—particularly when the tooth is of strategic importance or when other techniques such as implant placement would not be straightforward—in which this technique may be indicated. The procedure is technique sensitive (which may account for the large variability in survival rates quoted in the literature) and considered more favourable in lower molars and where there is more than 50% of alveolar bone remaining.

Failures occur due to endodontic reasons, caries, root fractures, or, most commonly, periodontal reasons, which is not surprising because of the inherent periodontal susceptibility in these patients.

Case 4: Root resection

Case 4 presented with a localized periodontal defect associated with the 46. The tooth had probing depths of up to 10 mm distally, and occasional suppuration was noted. A periapical radiograph (Figure 11.18) showed bone loss of up to 90% of the distal roots and into the furcation, with good bone levels mesially. The tooth had a large amalgam restoration coronally and had a very delayed response to electric pulp testing.

A diagnosis of a periodontal–endodontic lesion was made, and a root canal treatment was performed on the 46 (Figure 11.19). Because the mesial root had good attachment levels that would support the tooth after surgery, a root resection of the distal root was planned.

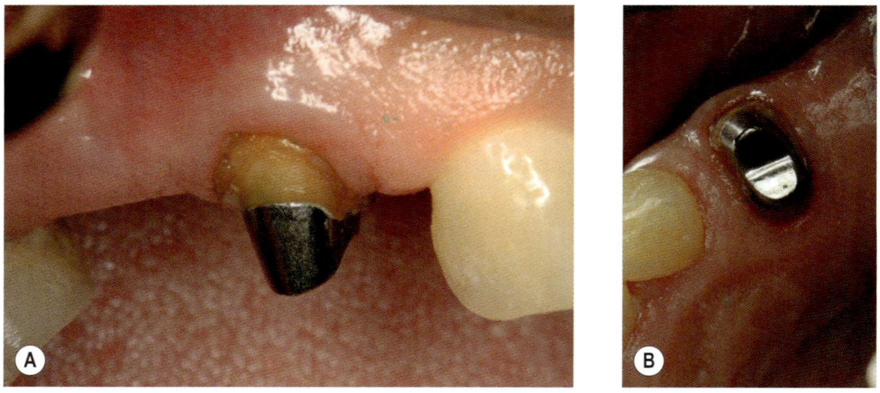

Fig 11.17 Case 3. The cast post and core with restoration margins supragingivally.

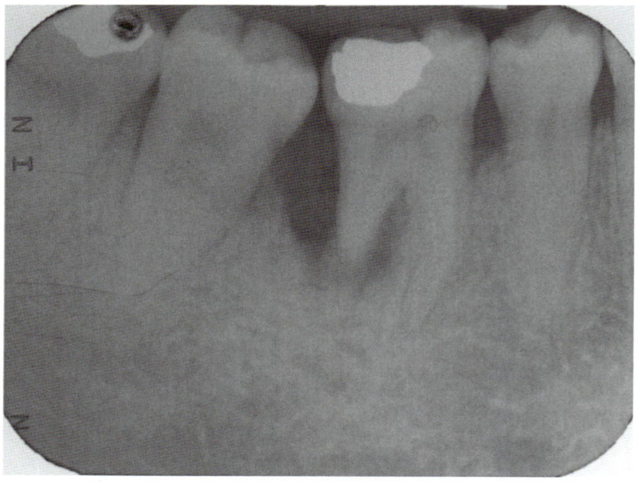

Fig 11.18 Case 4 periapical radiograph showing extensive bone loss associated with the distal root of 46.

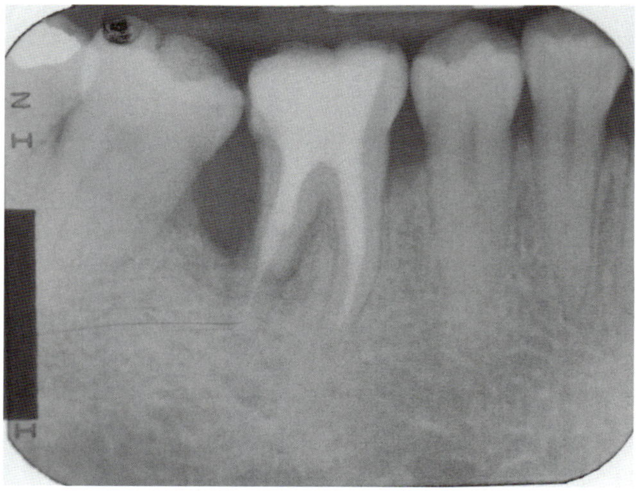

Fig 11.19 Case 4 post root canal treatment.

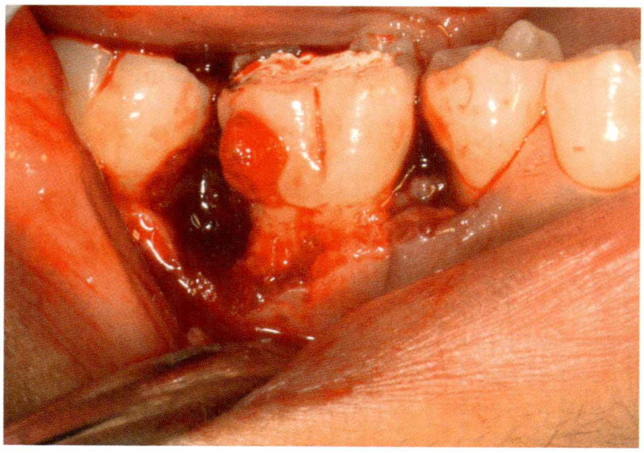

Fig 11.20 Case 4 after the full-thickness mucoperiosteal flap is raised to visualize the extent of bone loss and the furcation area.

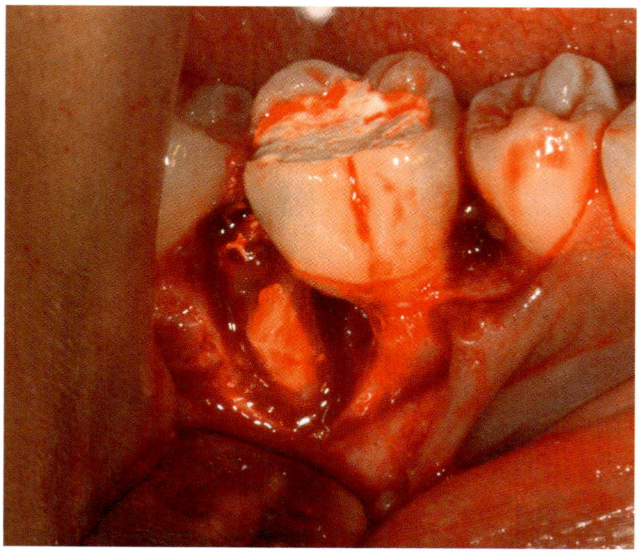

Fig 11.21 Resection through the distal root.

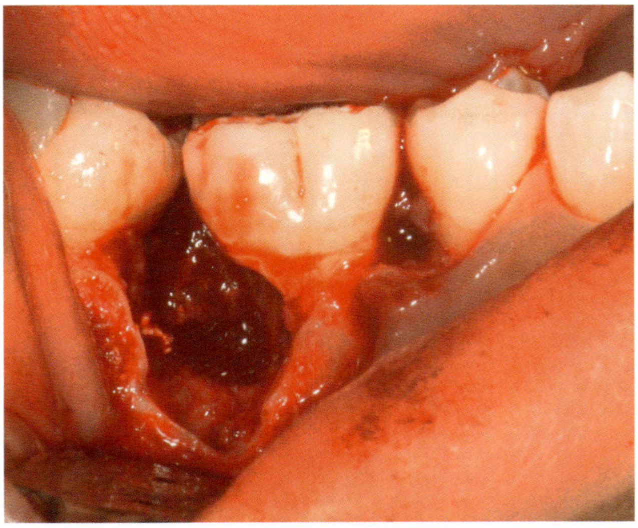

Fig 11.22 The root has been elevated, and the edges of the root trunk have been finished to avoid any ledges.

A full-thickness mucoperiosteal flap was raised buccally and lingually to provide maximum visualization of the distal root and furcation area (Figure 11.20). An oblique cut was made with a bur, starting from just below the contact point to the furcation, and the distal root was elevated (Figure 11.21). To allow future access for plaque control and debridement, it is important to ensure that no ledges are left in the furcation area (Figure 11.22). The root canal entrance on the severed root trunk was sealed with glass ionomer cement. The tooth was restored with a full-coverage gold crown to protect the remaining tooth structure (Figure 11.23).

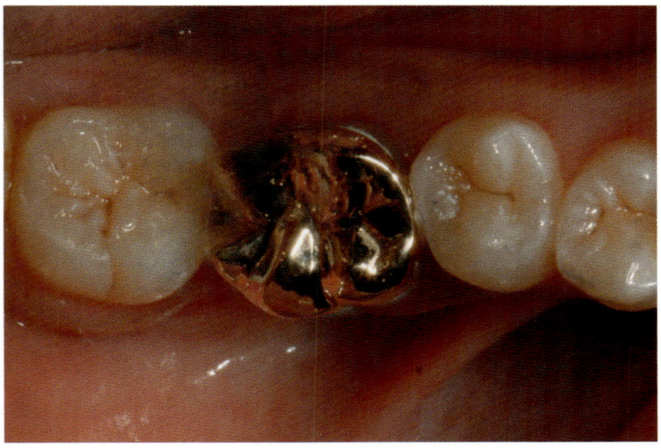

Fig 11.23 The final restoration.

Summary

There are a number of clinical situations in which treatment decisions need to take into account how to best address the biological, functional, and aesthetic requirements. When choosing which technique to use, careful consideration needs to be given to the thickness of the attached gingiva, whether access to alveolar bone crest is essential, and the planned future restoration.

Chapter 12

Periodontal regeneration

Introduction

"Lesson one" for any student of periodontology usually describes periodontitis as occurring when gingivitis spreads to the deeper periodontal tissues, causing irreversible loss of marginal alveolar bone and periodontal ligament and also apical migration of the junctional epithelium. Thus, periodontitis is considered to cause irreversible tissue loss, and it is not surprising that for many years one of the major challenges in periodontal research has been to devise and implement methods to regenerate the tissues that are lost due to the disease process.

A number of different techniques are now in use for promoting periodontal regeneration (also sometimes referred to as "new attachment therapies"). In this chapter, these techniques are outlined, their clinical indications are described, the outcomes that can be achieved by these methods and the factors that may influence outcomes are discussed, and a brief review of possible future developments is considered. It should be stated at the outset that success with periodontal regenerative therapies is dependent on the skill and the experience of the operator, and consequently these procedures are normally considered as within the realm of the trained periodontal specialist. The general dentist, however, should be aware of the methods used and their possible applications, but it is not the intention of the discussion here to give a comprehensive description of the detailed techniques used during regenerative procedures.

Overview of regenerative therapies

Periodontal regeneration can be defined as the regeneration of periodontal tissues to replace those lost due to disease, resulting in the formation of new bone, cementum, and functionally orientated periodontal ligament. Because these criteria can only be confirmed definitively by histological examination, in clinical use their outcome is assessed by increased gain in clinical attachment level and increased bone height, either by radiographic evaluation or sometimes, particularly in studies, by direct "bone sounding" using a probe under local anaesthesia. All of the techniques have (to a greater or lesser extent) been evaluated for histological evidence of actual regeneration, mainly in animal models of periodontal regeneration.

There are three main types of regenerative therapy:

- Barrier membranes (guided tissue regeneration)
- Graft materials
- Biologically active materials that stimulate the periodontal tissues to regenerate

Guided tissue regeneration

Guided tissue regeneration (GTR) is the use of barrier membranes to exclude the superficial gingival tissues from a healing periodontal surgical wound and thus promote wound repopulation by cells of the periodontal ligament which are able to regenerate the periodontium. The basic technique involves the placement of a thin membrane overlying the periodontal defect under the gingival flap during periodontal surgery. The membrane is secured in place, usually with an internal suture, and the flap is repositioned and sutured over the membrane (Figures 12.1 and 12.2). Originally, membranes made of expanded PTFE fibres (GORE-TEX) were used. This material is very biocompatible, but the main disadvantage of its use is that a second surgical procedure is required 6 weeks after membrane placement in order to remove the material. Consequently, a range of resorbable membrane materials have been developed that are used in a similar way but do not require re-entry surgery at a later date. These include membranes of polylactate/polyglycolate polymers (similar to the material used for resorbable sutures) and membranes made from collagen obtained from animals, typically of bovine source.

Graft materials

A wide range of graft materials have been described for placement in periodontal defects to promote periodontal regeneration. The types of graft are summarized in Table 12.1. The biological principle behind their use is that they act as a three-dimensional scaffold within the surgical defect to promote the in-growth of periodontal ligament and bone cells, ultimately resulting in resorption of the graft and replacement with healthy bone. In addition, theoretically, some of these materials have bioactive properties such as the presence of growth factors within the matrix that may further promote regeneration. However, the significance or superiority of this potential activity has not been convincingly demonstrated over and above the "osteoconductive" activity of the graft as a scaffold material. Histological studies of graft materials suggest that in some cases they are not completely resorbed but become merely encapsulated by fibrous tissue. Thus, there is debate about whether the radiographic appearance of bone regeneration seen with these methods is actually always equivalent to true periodontal regeneration. Nevertheless, the clinical improvements seen with grafting materials are similar to those of other regenerative techniques.

The surgical procedure used is similar to that used with GTR, except that rather than covering the defect with a membrane during surgery, the defect is packed with the graft material before suturing the flap (illustrated in Case 1).

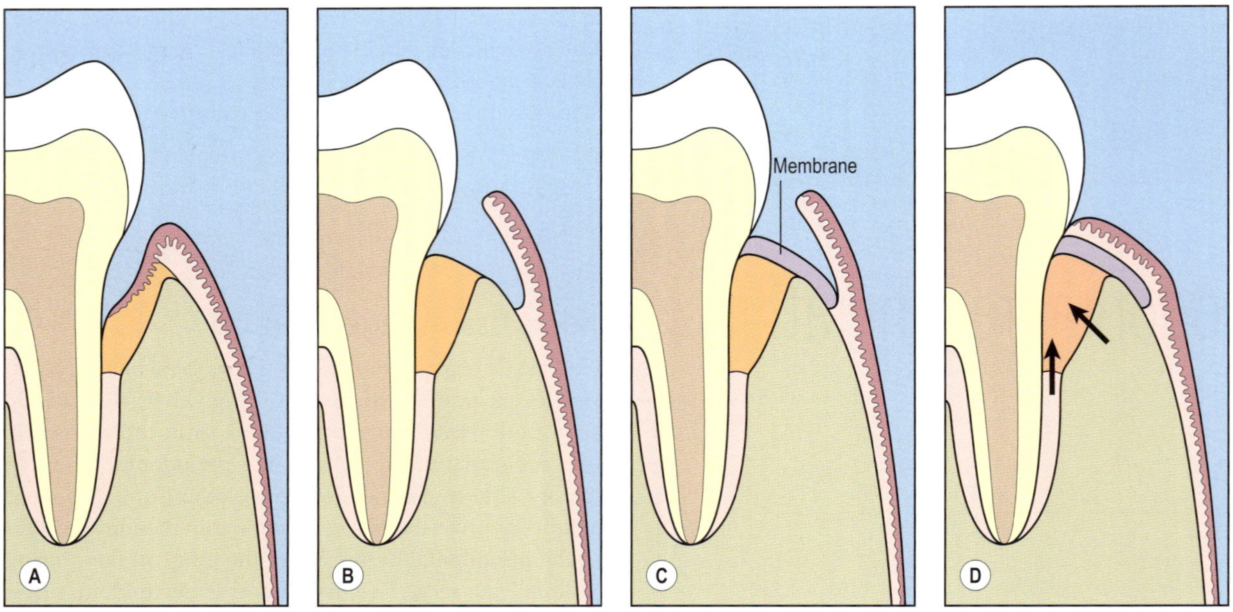

Fig 12.1 Diagram of the principles of guided tissue regeneration. (A) Pocket formation and infrabony defect. (B) Flap raised surgically, and granulation tissue from infrabony defect removed. (C) Membrane placed over defect. (D) Flap replaced and sutured. Membrane forms a barrier to exclude gingival tissues from surgically debrided defect and promotes wound repopulation by cells migrating from the periodontal ligament and bone (arrows).

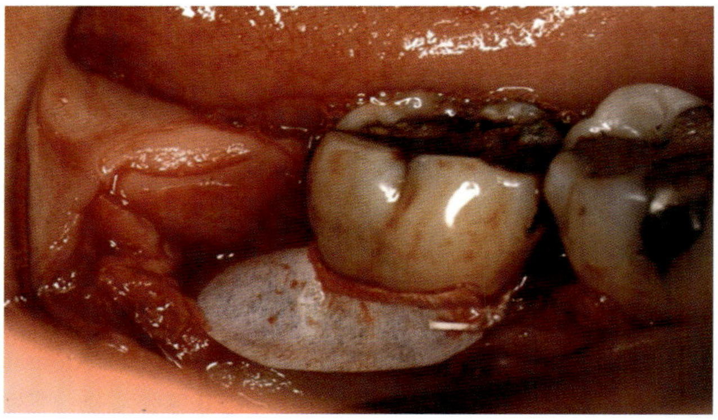

Fig 12.2 Membrane placed in defect during GTR surgery.

Table 12.1 Types of graft material for periodontal regeneration

Type	Description	Additional comments
Autografts	Autogenous bone harvested from a donor site from the same patient and placed in the periodontal defect	Bone harvesting from donor site (e.g., mental region of mandible, tuberosity of maxilla, iliac crest) is associated with considerable increased patient morbidity
Allografts	Graft preparation taken from human (cadaveric) bone; commercially available from "bone banks"; include irradiated cancellous bone, demineralized freeze-dried bone matrix	Theoretical risk of disease transmission (e.g., viral or prion disease), although considerable care is taken in preparation to minimize the risk. Acceptability of cadaveric bone may be an issue with some patients
Xenografts	Graft preparation taken from animal-derived bone; include acellular bovine bone matrix products	Theoretical risk of disease transmission (e.g., viral or prion disease), although because the product is deproteinized, this is considered to be very minimal. Considerable care is taken in preparation to minimize any theoretical risk. Acceptability of a bovine graft material may be an issue with some patients
Alloplasts	Synthetic bone substitute materials	A range of materials, including "bioactive" silica-based glass granules, hydroxyapatite, and β-tricalcium phosphates

Biologically active materials

The main biologically active-based material used for periodontal regeneration is a preparation of porcine enamel matrix derived from developing teeth. The commercially available product Emdogain consists of the enamel matrix derivative (EMD) preparation in a propylene glycol alginate carrier, and overall it has the consistency of a very fluid gel. The enamel matrix derivative contains a number of proteins, including the enamel matrix protein amelogenin, which is believed to be responsible for the preparation's activity.

The action of EMD is based on the observation that during root formation of the tooth, Hertwig's epithelial root sheath cells express enamel matrix proteins, and it is thought that these may be involved in inducing the formation of cementum. Therefore, it is postulated that addition of EMD to periodontal defects will promote new cementum formation and periodontal regeneration. In fact, the precise biological mechanisms of action of EMDs in periodontal regeneration are not fully understood, but it has been shown that they can induce periodontal cell proliferation and bone formation *in vitro*. Clinical and histological studies of EMD certainly have demonstrated their ability to promote regeneration. As discussed previously, the surgical procedure involves debriding the defect. Prior to application of the EMD material, the root surface is conditioned with EDTA to promote adherence of the EMD to the root surface, and the material is then applied to the defect with a syringe and blunt cannula prior to flap replacement and suturing.

In addition to the use of EMD for regeneration, a collagen-based cell binding peptide (Pepgen) has been reported for use in promoting periodontal regeneration, and there is much interest in the use of other biologically active molecules, notably growth factors (which are a group of growth-promoting cytokines), as regenerative treatments. One commercial preparation consists of recombinant human platelet-derived growth factor (PDGF) with a β-tricalcium phosphate graft material as a carrier. PDGF is mitogenic and angiogenic, and it is an important regulator of wound healing physiologically. In the United States and some other countries, this product is classified as a "medical device" and is commercially available. In Europe, the product has been classified as a "pharmaceutical product" and is not currently licensed for use in periodontal applications. The one clinical trial of this material from the United States suggests that it can improve clinical outcomes compared with the graft material alone, particularly in promoting increased bone growth.

Applications of regenerative therapies

Despite the array of different techniques available, regenerative therapies are only of use in specific, fairly limited, circumstances. Regenerative techniques are only indicated where used in isolated infrabony defects or in class II furcation defects. The likely success of these procedures is dependent on how enclosed the defect is; thus, they can be useful in two-wall or three-wall vertical bony defects but are less successful in one-wall defects. The techniques do not have any effect on bone height or clinical attachment level on horizontal defects. In fact, some limited "spontaneous" regeneration is sometimes seen in enclosed defects even in the absence of a specific regenerative technique being used (Figure 12.3).

Clinical studies do not appear to show any consistent advantage of one regenerative technique over another in terms of outcomes (with the possible exception from one study of the use of PDGF, in which PDGF + β-tricalcium phosphate gave superior results to β-tricalcium phosphate alone). GTR techniques are particularly surgically demanding, whereas alloplastic materials and Emdogain are technically much more straightforward to use, but all demand a high degree of surgical skill in managing the tissues and achieving primary closure. In addition, there is little evidence to support the use of combined techniques (e.g., EMD + GTR and EMD + graft) to improve outcomes compared with single techniques alone.

Case 1

A 50-year-old man presented with a history of periodontal problems and with recent discomfort from the lower right region. He was medically healthy and a nonsmoker. On examination, there was a deep suppurating pocket at LR6 distally, and the radiograph showed a deep two-walled infrabony defect in this area (Figure 12.4). The tooth was heavily restored but vital. After completion of initial treatment, LR6 was scheduled for regenerative surgery using an allograft material of irradiated allogenic human bone particles (Figure 12.5). Healing was uneventful, and at review after 7 months there was marked pocket depth reduction and complete infill of the bony defect seen radiographically (Figure 12.6).

The outcome in this case is nearly the maximum possible to achieve with regenerative techniques because it has resulted in apparent complete bony infill of the defect combined with pocket depth reduction and only slight, if any, recession. As noted previously, with mineralized graft materials, one cannot be absolutely certain that the radiographic changes seen are the result of true periodontal regeneration or whether some of the radiographic improvement is the result of persisting bone graft material. However, whichever is the case, the clinical improvements achieved have been highly successful in managing a pocket that was close to resulting in a perio/endo lesion and compromising the

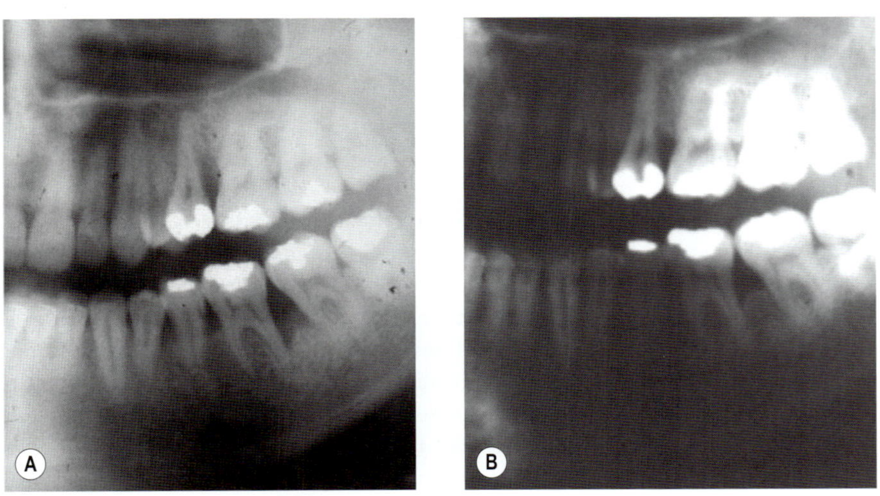

Fig 12.3 "Spontaneous" regeneration. Detail of rotational tomograms of a 36-year-old man with localized periodontitis particularly affecting the UL5 distally, the LL6 distally, and the LL7 mesially. The patient was treated with oral hygiene instruction and root surface debridement followed by 3-monthly maintenance visits. (A) The pretreatment view. (B) The view 1 year postoperatively. Although the quality of the radiographs is rather poor and not directly equivalent, there appears to have been significant gain in bone height on all three of these defects, most markedly on UL5. In addition, in the postoperative radiograph, a well-formed lamina dura is seen at these sites, which is considered to be indicative of good bony healing.

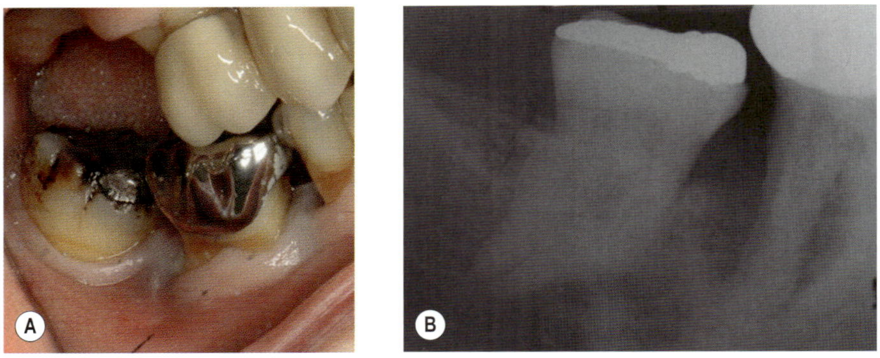

Fig 12.4 Clinical presentation of Case 1. Suppuration of deep pocket at LR6 clinically, and radiographically there is a deep infrabony pocket that extends apically to approximately 80% or more of the root surface.

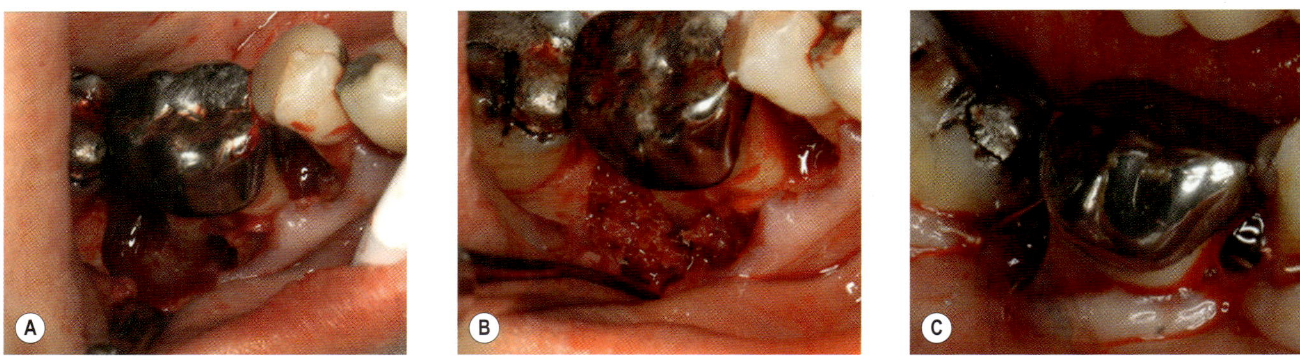

Fig 12.5 Regenerative surgical treatment of LR6. (A) Flap is raised to access the deep infrabony pocket distally and that extends buccally to the furcation region. (B) Defect packed with allograft material. (C) Flap is replaced and carefully sutured to obtain primary closure and good wound stability.

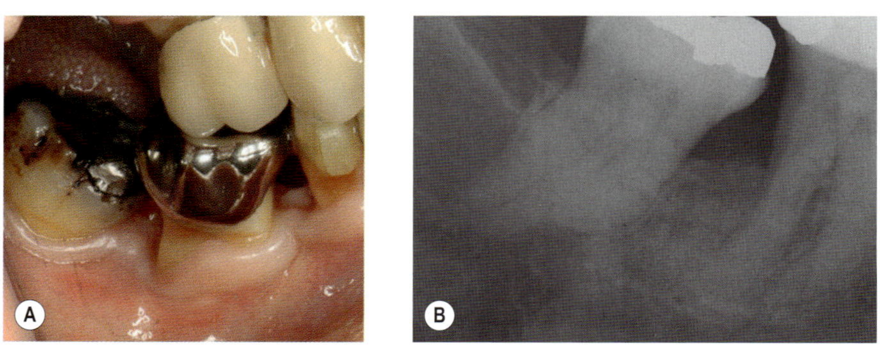

Fig 12.6 (A) Clinical appearance and (B) radiographic outcome 7 months postoperatively. The tissues are uninflamed, and there has been complete bony infill of the infrabony defect.

tooth permanently. It is interesting to note the extent of the bone loss seen when the flap was raised compared to the radiographic appearance. It is common during any surgery to find that bone loss is far more extensive than that anticipated from the radiograph, and this should be considered when planning cases for regenerative surgery.

Two additional cases showing radiographic outcomes of regenerative surgery, in these cases treated with EMD, are shown in Figures 12.7 and 12.8.

Outcomes of periodontal regenerative treatments

Although the results of regenerative treatments shown here are very favourable, the many clinical trials of these different treatments demonstrate that regeneration can be a highly variable and unpredictable outcome. Systematic reviews that collectively analyse the results of different studies of these techniques suggest that the average benefit of such a procedure compared with a conventional flap surgery technique is less than 2 mm of additional clinical attachment level gain. Obviously, the average result is not a very good indication of an expected outcome in an individual case because the average includes many excellent results far superior to this but also others for which little or no benefit has been shown. The outcome of these procedures may depend on a number of factors, some of which are listed in Table 12.2.

It must again be emphasized that in addition to a degree of unpredictability of these procedures, they have only limited applications, do not address the issue of more horizontal patterns of bone loss, and do not

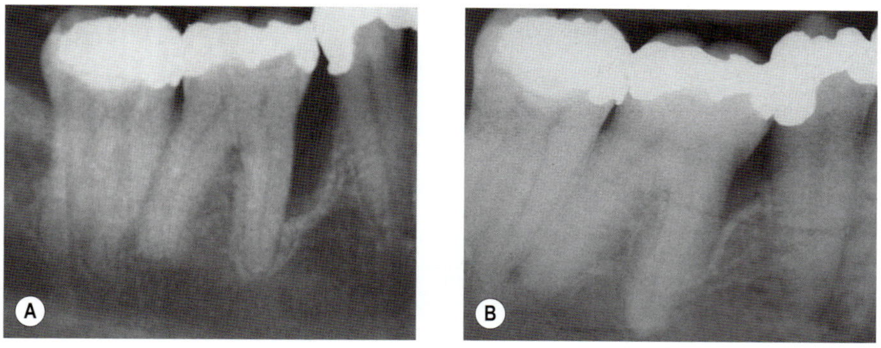

Fig 12.7 Radiographic appearance of outcome of surgery with EMD on infrabony defect on mesial of LL6 in a 47-year-old woman. Marked but incomplete bone fill of defect is seen 2 years after surgery. It was associated with pocket reduction from 9 to 3 mm.

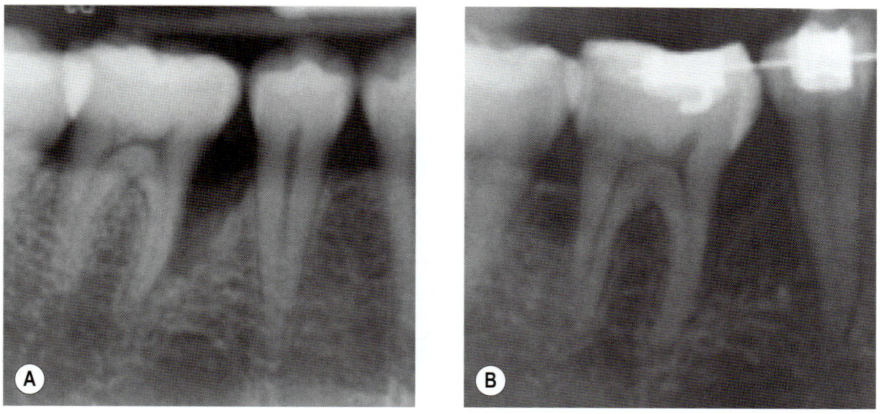

Fig 12.8 Radiographic appearance of outcome of surgery with EMD on infrabony defect on mesial of LL6 in a 24-year-old woman with localized aggressive periodontitis. Incomplete bone fill of defect is seen 1 year after surgery. Pocket reduction from 8 mm initially to 4 mm is seen. (Postoperatively, the patient was also receiving orthodontic treatment for alignment of incisors.)

Table 12.2 Favourable and unfavourable factors affecting outcomes of regenerative techniques

Favourable	Unfavourable
Maintenance of good plaque control	Smoking
Shape of defect—the more enclosed it is (e.g., three-walled, very deep enclosed defect), the better the outcome	Shape of defect—shallow or wide infrabony defects, one-walled defects, grade III furcation lesions
Experience of the operator	
Achieving complete primary closure of flap	Exposure of membrane/graft to oral cavity during healing
Stable, immobile wound (this has led to development of the use of single or minimally invasive flaps for regeneration)	Tooth mobility; failure to maintain space within defect, for example, because of membrane collapsing

allow reconstruction of soft tissue profiles of the dental papillae.

Future developments

Because of the current limitations of regenerative treatments, extensive research continues to be conducted with the goal of improving these techniques. The main areas under investigation include the following:

- The use of growth factors to stimulate regeneration
- The development of new biomaterials for use either as grafts or as membranes
- The use of periodontal ligament stem cell reimplantation following isolation and expansion in the laboratory

As some of these treatments become available for clinical use, it will be particularly important for them to be evaluated fully by randomized trials to determine what really works and what does not.

Chapter 13

Local and systemic antimicrobial agents

Introduction

Given the microbial aetiology of periodontal diseases, it is not surprising that many different antimicrobial agents have been used in the management of periodontal disease. These agents include a range of antiseptics used for chemical plaque control and antibiotics that are used mainly as adjunctive treatments for periodontal pocketing. This chapter describes the use of both antiseptic agents and antibiotics, with particular emphasis on consideration of when antibiotics may be indicated and their potential effects.

As a microbial biofilm, mature dental plaque is inherently somewhat resistant to antimicrobial agents because they are unable to effectively penetrate deep within the plaque. Consequently, chemical plaque control agents tend to be more effective in preventing or inhibiting plaque growth rather than eliminating established plaque; similarly, antibiotic agents are used in combination with mechanical debridement of the biofilm.

Antiseptic agents and chemical plaque control

A wide range of antiseptic agents have been used in toothpastes, dental gels, and mouthwashes. Many of these are listed in Table 13.1. Products containing these agents are used for a variety of applications, including plaque control, oral and throat infections, and mucosal ulceration. All of these agents are effective at killing bacteria in laboratory conditions, and in general, bacterial resistance to them does not develop. However, only some of them have been shown to have significant inhibitory effects on dental plaque. The effectiveness of these agents depends particularly on their ability to persist in the oral cavity and remain active over a period of time, which is referred to as their "substantivity."

Chlorhexidine

Chlorhexidine digluconate is the most effective of all the antiseptic agents used for controlling plaque. Studies demonstrate that it is able to completely inhibit plaque growth when starting from a clean tooth. Chlorhexidine is strongly cationic and thus binds to teeth and oral mucosal surfaces, and it remains active for many hours. This excellent substantivity accounts for its high efficacy. It is mainly used as a mouthwash (0.2% w/v), but it has also been produced as a 1% dental gel, in the form of sprays, and in a toothpaste. However, it is not suitable for use in most toothpaste formulations because the detergents present inactivate the chlorhexidine. Thus, as a mouthwash, ideally it is best used after toothbrushing and thorough rinsing.

Chlorhexidine is safe for long-term use, but its main side effect is that it causes extrinsic staining, which can be troublesome and extensive, particularly if used for long periods. Therefore, it tends to be used for short periods of time from a few days to a few weeks for specific purposes rather than as a long-term adjunct to plaque control. The staining that it causes is the result of its cationic, binding properties. Occasionally, chlorhexidine can cause hypersensitivity reactions resulting in salivary gland swelling or mucositis, but these reactions are very rare.

For controlling plaque, chlorhexidine is indicated for use when normal plaque control measures cannot be carried out or as an adjunct for plaque control for short periods of time. Thus, it is used for preventing plaque post-surgery, following trauma, during intermaxillary fixation, and sometimes when people are unable to carry out adequate manual brushing. It is also useful as an adjunct to mechanical plaque control measures when there is severe inflammation, to try to speed up the resolution of gingival inflammation. Inflammation actually promotes plaque accumulation, so resolving the inflammation by plaque control measures is much more difficult than preventing recurrence of inflammation once it is under control. Another example of when it may be useful as an adjunctive treatment is shown in Figure 13.1. Finally, the use of chlorhexidine preoperatively has been suggested as a way of reducing the oral flora and minimizing risk of bacteraemia.

Overall, chlorhexidine is an extremely useful and effective plaque control agent. However, it is not a substitute for proper periodontal management, including effective regular home care procedures. Its effects are also mainly limited to the supragingival flora, and there is little evidence that irrigation of pockets with it is useful.

Other antiseptic agents and plaque control

As shown in Table 13.1, a number of other antiseptics are available for routine use in oral care products to inhibit plaque, including triclosan, zinc ions, sanguinarine, and essential oils. Triclosan is widely used in toothpastes and in some mouthwashes as an antiplaque agent. In some preparations, it is formulated with a Gantrez copolymer to improve its substantivity, and in others it is used in combination with zinc ions, which enhance the antibacterial activity. In clinical studies under well-controlled conditions, these products can reduce plaque and gingivitis by approximately 30%. Essential oil mouthwashes have similar effects on plaque and gingivitis. Sanguinarine is a plant extract that also has some antiplaque effects, and it is available in toothpaste and mouthwash preparations.

Table 13.1 Antiseptic agents used in oral care products

Agent	Details and preparations	Evidence of effects on plaque inhibition?
Chlorhexidine digluconate	Bisbiguanide; in mouthwash, gels, sprays, and toothpaste	Yes
Triclosan	Chlorinated bisphenol; in toothpaste and mouthwash	Yes
Zinc ions	As zinc citrate; in toothpaste, usually with triclosan	Yes
Essential oils	Oils of thymol, menthol, eucalyptol; in mouthwash	Yes
Sanguinarine	Quaternary ammonium compound from plant extract; in toothpaste	Yes
Povidone iodine	As mouthwash	Minimal
Cetylpyridium chloride	Quaternary ammonium compound; in mouthwash	Minimal
Hexetidine	In mouthwash	Minimal

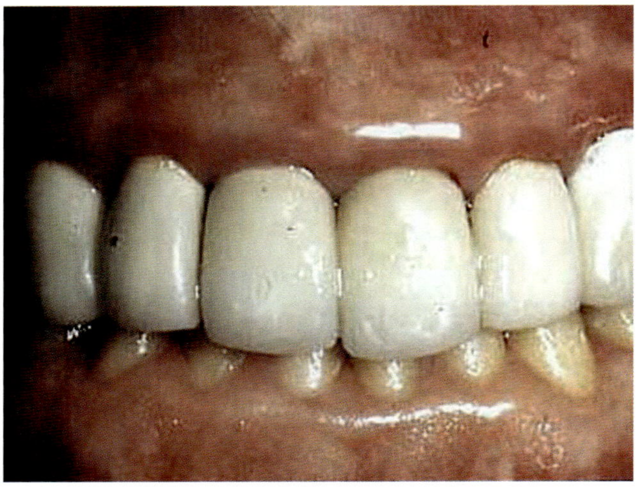

Fig 13.1 Catch-22? Severe gingival inflammation associated with poorly fitting margins of upper anterior crowns. The inflammation is unlikely to resolve while the margins are still there, but one cannot successfully remake the crowns until the inflammation has resolved. In this case, the crowns can be removed and replaced with well-fitting laboratory-made acrylic temporary crowns. To assist the gingival resolution, adjunctive use of chlorhexidine together with good plaque control measures would be appropriate.

Although these products are in widespread use, it is difficult to measure their effects on a population basis. Due to the size of their effect, it is unlikely that one will see a marked clinical change in a patient when switching to one of these products, which is not to say that they may not be having significant effects on plaque and gingivitis. On an epidemiological scale, it is interesting to speculate about the effect of a 30% reduction in plaque on the prevalence of periodontal disease.

Other antiplaque agents

In addition to antiseptics, a number of other ways of inhibiting plaque formation have been proposed, including using enzymes in toothpastes that activate salivary antibacterial mechanisms and using chemical ingredients that inhibit formation of the acquired pellicle and thus inhibit bacterial colonization and plaque growth. This latter action particularly seems to be, at least in theory, an attractive way of inhibiting plaque, but there are no products currently available that act in this way.

Systemic antimicrobial agents

The widespread use and misuse of antibiotics in medicine and dentistry has resulted in a major increase in multiple resistant organisms, to such an extent that for some serious infectious diseases it is sometimes difficult to find an effective antibiotic drug. In addition, although many of these drugs are safe in the majority of cases, they all have the risk of unwanted adverse effects. Thus, the decision to use antibiotics in the management of periodontal disease should not be taken lightly, and in the vast majority of cases, periodontal diseases can be (and should be) managed without prescribing antibiotics.

However, it is undoubtedly the case that occasionally antibiotic use can have a major positive impact on the management of periodontal diseases, and in these cases its use can be justified on the basis of the major improvements that can be obtained in clinical outcomes of managing what are usually very severe and difficult periodontal problems. As stated at the beginning of this chapter, antibiotics should only be used as adjunctive treatments to mechanical debridement to ensure proper disruption of the plaque biofilm. Without this, antibiotics on their own tend to be very ineffective or only give very short-term benefits at best.

Acute conditions

Necrotizing periodontal diseases (acute necrotizing ulcerative gingivitis and necrotizing periodontitis) respond very well to a short course of antibiotics, which rapidly alleviates the symptoms and resolves the underlying destructive lesions. These are usually treated with metronidazole 200 mg TDS for 3 days, or where this may be contraindicated, then amoxicillin 500 mg TDS for 5 days may be used. This should be combined with gentle debridement, oral hygiene instruction, and follow-up appointments.

Acute lateral periodontal abscesses result in an acute flare-up in a periodontal pocket. Because they are superficial, they are often much less severe than periapical abscesses of endodontic origin and do not require antibiotic treatment. They should be managed initially by drainage achieved by debridement of the pocket, and they should be followed up for further periodontal management of the pocket. Because of their superficial nature, periodontal abscesses only extremely rarely show any systemic signs such as pyrexia or local spread of infection, but if either of these is present, antibiotic treatment is appropriate.

Treatment of periodontal pocketing

Systematic reviews of studies that have investigated the use of adjunctive antibiotics in the treatment of periodontitis show increased pocket depth reductions compared to mechanical therapy alone in both chronic and aggressive periodontitis. A number of studies have focused on severe disease groups, including generalized and localized aggressive periodontitis, and on patients who have responded poorly or who appear to be resistant to conventional periodontal treatments. Some have suggested that antibiotic use should be based on microbial testing, but this is difficult, expensive, and of uncertain benefit given the very wide array of bacterial species present in plaque. In particular, the presence of *Aggregatibacter actinomycetemcomitans* has been proposed as an indication for adjunctive antimicrobials because this facultative organism is strongly associated with severe disease and is difficult to eliminate by mechanical debridement alone compared to, for example, *Porphyromonas gingivalis*, which is much more readily eliminated by effective disruption of the biofilm because it is an obligate anaerobe and much more fastidious about its environmental requirements for survival.

Nevertheless, the decision to prescribe adjunctive antimicrobials is in most cases an empirical one, for cases of aggressive periodontitis and chronic periodontitis that is unresponsive to conventional treatment (sometimes referred to as "refractory periodontitis"). Given the complexity of these cases, it has been argued that this decision is best taken by an experienced periodontal specialist.

A number of different antibiotic regimes have been utilized for such cases, and these are listed in Table 13.2. There is no evidence of the superiority of one regime compared to others. Tetracyclines (oxytetracycline and doxycycline) inhibit matrix metalloproteinase activity and are anti-inflammatory in addition to their direct antibacterial activities, although the therapeutic advantage of this is not known. In addition, long-term sub-antimicrobial dose doxycycline (20 mg BD for up to 9 months) has also been tested and is licensed for use in periodontitis. However, its specific indications are not certain, and there is at least a theoretical risk of inducing bacterial resistance, although this has not been demonstrated. Whichever antibiotic regime is chosen, patients should have all quadrants of root surface debridement (RSD) completed and start taking the antibiotics at the completion of mechanical therapy.

Table 13.2 Antibiotic regimes for adjunctive periodontal treatment

Regime	Dosage	Comments
Amoxicillin (500 mg) + metronidazole (200 mg)	TDS for 7 days	Widely used combination; main side effects include penicillin hypersensitivity and "antabuse" reaction of metronidazole with alcohol
Oxytetracycline	250 mg QDS for 21 days	Broad-spectrum bacteriostatic; also has anti-inflammatory properties; compliance difficult
Doxycycline	100 mg OD for 14 days	Same family and similar properties as tetracycline; easier compliance
Amoxicillin and clavulanic acid	375 mg TDS for 14 days	Same as amoxicillin; β-lactamase resistant
Azithromycin	500 mg OD for 3 days	Concentrated in inflamed sites/neutrophils; remains at active concentrations for up to 14 days; may have anti-inflammatory properties; easy compliance

Finally, there is no evidence to support the use of antibiotics routinely after periodontal surgery.

Case 1

A 37-year-old man was referred to the periodontist for severe periodontal disease. He complained of some tooth mobility and some discomfort in the lower right region, but otherwise he had few symptoms. He was medically fit and had never smoked. He had been a regular attender and brushed his teeth twice daily with an electric toothbrush. He had been using interdental brushes on the advice of his dentist. There was no family history of gum problems.

On examination, the gingivae looked largely uninflamed and plaque control was good (Figure 13.2). No calculus deposits were noted. However, a 6-point probing chart showed localized deep pocketing, and radiographs showed severe vertical bony defects in a number of areas and a perio/endo lesion affecting LR7 (Figure 13.3).

A diagnosis of generalized aggressive periodontitis was made. The patient received a course of nonsurgical periodontal therapy that reinforced his (already good) oral hygiene, and full-mouth RSD was carried out under local anaesthesia over two visits. The LR7 was extracted during treatment. On the second visit, he was given a prescription for doxycycline 100 mg once daily for 2 weeks and scheduled for reassessment 6 weeks later. He was subsequently unable to attend the review appointment, and he was eventually seen for reassessment 3 months after completing the treatment. At reassessment, the patient reported no

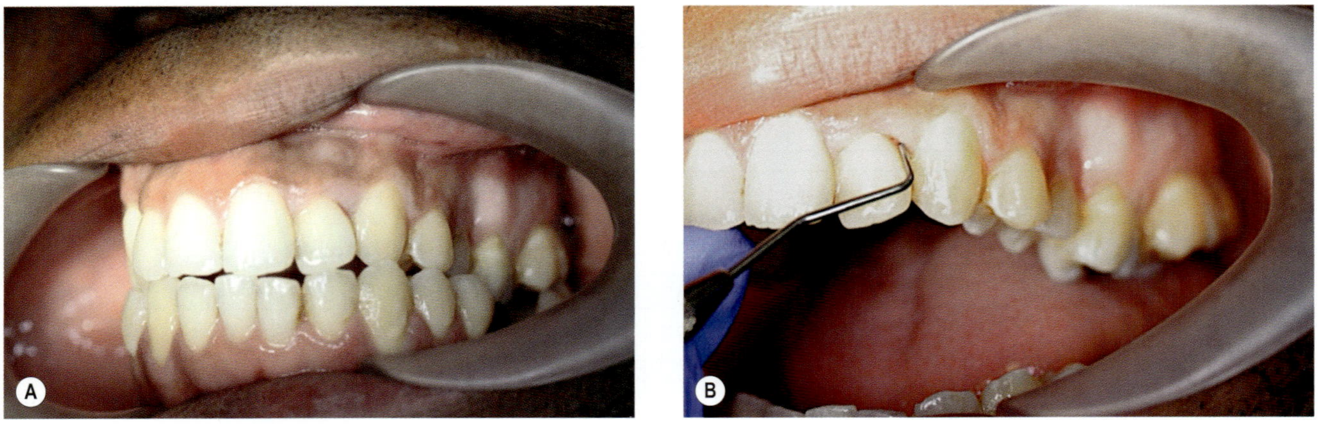

Fig 13.2 Clinical appearance of Case 1 at presentation. The gingivae look largely healthy and plaque control was good, but many localized deep pockets were evident on probing.

problems, and a 6-point pocket chart showed very marked pocket depth reduction in all sites except for LR6 mesially (Figure 13.4). The LR6 was planned for further assessment (including a periapical radiograph of the apparently two-walled infrabony defect) to consider surgical treatment in this region and particularly to assess the suitability of the defect for a regenerative surgical procedure.

This case is typical of those that might be considered immediately for adjunctive antibiotic therapy. First, he had a clear diagnosis of aggressive periodontitis, with the absence of significant calculus deposits, and his plaque control was good. In cases in which there are obvious local factors, particularly subgingival calculus, it is appropriate to carry out an initial course of treatment without antibiotics to determine initial response to treatment. In the final analysis, the cutoff point for those to be prescribed antibiotics during the first round of treatment is an empirical judgement and will vary among clinicians.

Although the average additional benefit of adjunctive antibiotics over RSD alone in clinical studies is relatively modest, such dramatic improvements as seen here are frequently seen in cases in which there is little inflammation and minimal deposits at presentation.

Case 2

This is the clinical Case 1 described in Chapter 9. The patient was a 39-year-old woman who, on presentation, was initially treated with nonsurgical and surgical treatments and responded well to this management. After 6 months of maintenance, she attended complaining of new bleeding gums but could not attribute the change in her periodontal condition to anything in particular. She remained in good health and was a nonsmoker. On examination, her plaque control remained good (plaque score of 18%), but the gingivae looked slightly inflamed and the pocket chart showed a severe and generalized relapse in pockets that in many cases were at least as deep as they were prior to initial therapy (Figure 13.5). A new radiograph was taken, which showed clear signs of significant disease progression, particularly at LR7 and UR6 (Figure 13.6).

The main significant feature here is the generalized nature of the disease recurrence, which is not the result of smoking, apparently not the result of poor compliance, and not due to specific failures of, for example, a surgical procedure. Based on the discussion in Chapter 9, she is now a nonresponding patient. There were no signs of other explanations for this recurrence, and there were no other risk factors or signs of type 2 diabetes. She is demonstrably a highly disease-susceptible patient and thus was treated with an additional round of RSD under local anaesthesia during two visits together with a course of azithromycin 500 mg once daily for 3 days. She was followed up at 6 weeks and 3 months after completing this new course of treatment and reported that the gums rapidly felt much better again. The new chart taken at 3 months showed marked improvements in all sites, although the pocketing and severe bone loss with furcation involvement at LR7 remain a concern (Figure 13.7). Whether she will show further tendencies to such dramatic recurrences remains to be seen.

Although the patient's most recent outcome is impressive, the question in this case is whether as good a response would have been achieved without the use of adjunctive antibiotics.

This patient is perhaps not the typical "nonresponding patient" because she initially showed an excellent response to treatment but subsequently relapsed quickly. A more typical "nonresponding patient" who might be considered for adjunctive antibiotics could be defined as someone with a failure to respond to treatment in deep sites throughout

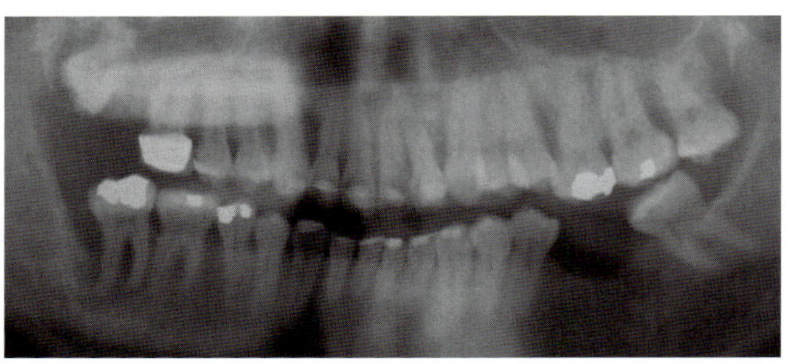

Fig 13.3 Rotational tomogram of Case 1 at presentation. Multiple infrabony pockets are evident, and there is a perio/endo lesion on LR7. Note also arch wire/composite splints fitted to the upper and lower anterior regions.

		8	7	6	5	4	3	2	1	1	2	3	4	5	6	7	8
Post treatment	B			2 2 3	2 1 3	2 2 1	2 1 4	5 2 2	2 1 2	2 1 2	3 3 5	3 2 3	3 2 4	3 3 3	4 2 4	5 3 5	4 2 3
Initial diagnosis	B			3 2 3	3 2 4	3 2 6	10 5 9	6 2 3	2 2 2	2 1 5	3 9 10	3 2 4	3 2 3	3 12 7	3 2 3	2 2 6	3 2 3
Initial diagnosis	P			3 2 3	4 2 2	3 2 3	9 2 5	6 3 3	3 2 4	3 3 7	2 1 10	4 3 4	1 3 3	14 10	2 2 2	5 2 6	4 4 4
Post treatment	P			2 2 3	2 3 3	2 2 2	4 2 3	3 2 2	2 1 2	2 1 2	2 1 2	2 2 3	3 1 2	2 1 2	2 1 2	2 1 3	3 2 3

		8	7	6	5	4	3	2	1	1	2	3	4	5	6	7	8
Post treatment	L			2 3 7	4 2 3	3 2 4	2 2 2	2 1 2	1 1 2	2 1 2	2 1 2	2 1 3	2 1 2	2 1 2		2 2 2	
Initial diagnosis	L		9 3 9	5 2 8	4 3 3	4 3 5	4 2 3	3 2 3	2 1 2	1 1 1	1 1 3	2 1 3	2 1 2	2 1 4		2 1 3	
Initial diagnosis	B		10 4 4	3 2 6	4 2 3	2 2 5	3 1 2	2 1 2	2 2 3	2 1 2	1 1 2	2 1 3	2 2 2	1 1 2		1 2 3	
Post treatment	B			3 2 7	3 1 2	2 1 4	3 3 2	2 1 2	1 1 1	1 1 2	2 1 2	1 1 2	2 1 2	2 1 2		2 4 4	

Fig 13.4 Pocket chart of Case 1 taken at initial diagnosis and 3 months after completion of nonsurgical treatment combined with adjunctive doxycycline. Note the dramatic improvement in all deep sites with the exception of LR6 mesially.

	8	7	6	5	4	3	2	1	1	2	3	4	5	6	7	8
12/12 POST SURGERY		888	989	766	423	212	426	754	423	212	111	223	212	736	744	
6/12 POST SURGERY		412	333	212	333	222	324	422	323	212	212	212	233	333	323	
PRESENTATION	433	524	747	523	323	333	347	633	455	434	333	423	423	635	444	334
	8	7	6	5	4	3	2	1	1	2	3	4	5	6	7	8
PRESENTATION	433	521	744	522	322	331	344	634	452	431	322	522	522	744	555	331
6/12 POST SURGERY		333	422	212	222	212	323	422	322	322	222	333	322	313	222	
12/12 POST SURGERY		999	747	622	432	222	257	666	555	311	222	333	313	646	557	

	8	7	6	5	4	3	2	1	1	2	3	4	5	6	7	8
12/12 POST SURGERY		7710	646	337	326	323	222	211	111	212	222	312	223	822	524	
POST INITIAL THERAPY	422	335	624	224	333	111	111	111	111	111	112	212	222	635	544	335
PRESENTATION	433	226	535	335	333	212	112	212	211	111	212	222	333	736	534	445
	8	7	6	5	4	3	2	1	1	2	3	4	5	6	7	8
PRESENTATION	522	335	726	534	322	212	212	111	111	112	112	312	313	635	745	333
6/12 POST SURGERY		222	322	233	212	111	111	111	111	112	112	222	222	333	344	
12/12 POST SURGERY		8810	836	446	323	212	111	111	112	212	211	223	233	722	525	

Fig 13.5 Pocket chart of Case 2 at initial presentation, 6 months following completion of active therapy, and a further 6 months later, showing serious generalized recurrence of disease.

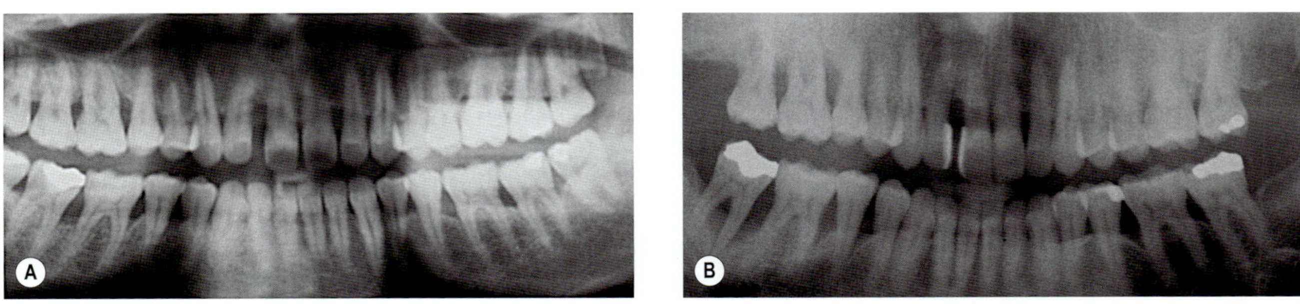

Fig 13.6 Rotational tomograms of Case 2 taken at initial presentation (A) and at diagnosis of disease recurrence (B). Note marked progression of disease particularly at LR7 and UR6.

	8	7	6	5	4	3	2	1	1	2	3	4	5	6	7	8
AFTER AB THERAPY		644	555	324	422	211	313	422	212	112	211	323	222	423	335	
AT RELAPSE		888	989	766	423	212	426	754	423	212	111	223	212	736	744	
	8	7	6	5	4	3	2	1	1	2	3	4	5	6	7	8
AT RELAPSE		999	747	622	432	222	257	666	555	311	222	333	313	646	557	
AFTER AB THERAPY		633	544	332	211	111	133	443	322	111	212	213	213	444	533	

	8	7	6	5	4	3	2	1	1	2	3	4	5	6	7	8
AFTER AB THERAPY		666	433	222	322	222	211	111	111	112	211	222	322	433	333	
AT RELAPSE		7710	646	337	326	323	222	211	111	212	222	312	223	822	524	
	8	7	6	5	4	3	2	1	1	2	3	4	5	6	7	8
AT RELAPSE		8810	836	446	323	212	111	111	112	212	211	223	233	722	525	
AFTER AB THERAPY		467	445	333	332	112	211	211	111	112	111	122	214	332	425	

Fig 13.7 Pocket chart of Case 2 at relapse (12 months after surgery completed) and 3 months after completion of new round of RSD with adjunctive antibiotics.

the mouth, despite good compliance, thorough debridement, and a nonsmoker who is medically healthy.

Overall, antibiotics can be a very useful adjunctive treatment in a small number of carefully selected cases, as illustrated here. The dramatic improvements illustrated here are not uncommon in these cases. However, such improvements are not typically seen in patients with less severe disease.

Locally delivered antimicrobial agents

A number of antimicrobial agents have been produced and tested that are designed to introduce antimicrobial agents locally into a periodontal pocket. A key factor in the design and utility of such products is the ability to sustain bacteriocidal concentrations of the agent for a sufficient amount of time to be effective using a delivery vehicle that provides for slow release of the agent. Antimicrobials that have been prepared in this way include doxycycline, minocycline (a synthetic tetracycline), metronidazole, and chlorhexidine. Delivery vehicles vary from simple gels, which are syringed into a pocket and from which the material slowly leaches out, to gelatin inserts and impregnated fibres, which are packed into the pocket, and thixotropic gels with improved slow-release drug kinetics. Some of the potential advantages and disadvantages of locally delivered antimicrobials compared with systemic agents are listed in Table 13.3. In clinical studies comparing RSD with RSD together with locally delivered antimicrobials, the antimicrobial treatment results in slightly superior pocket depth reductions and increased elimination of bacteria of the "red complex." However, the evidence for their use is rather weak and gives little indication of when it would be appropriate to use them clinically. This is probably partly due to a dilemma between commercial and clinical interests. Commercial companies would like their products to be used as often as possible (and therefore will pay for studies that show their general efficacy), whereas clinicians would like to use them as little as possible but would like to know if they are particularly useful in specific applications or circumstances. As with other antimicrobial treatments, they should never be used as substitute for thorough mechanical debridement.

Table 13.3 Potential advantages and disadvantages of locally applied antimicrobial agents compared with systemic agents

Advantages	Disadvantages
Treatment directed at specific sites	Expensive and needs to be applied professionally
Very high therapeutic concentrations achievable	Lack of general effect (e.g., anti-inflammatory effects in tissues, possible benefit of treating shallow sites)
No issues with drug compliance	May encourage bacterial resistance (due to suboptimal doses present close to treated sites, with chlorhexidine being the exception)
Little or no circulating drug—minimal side effects	Relative lack of evidence base for efficacy or indications for use

Chapter 14

Gingival recession

Introduction

Gingival recession is defined as the apical migration of the gingival margin below the cementoenamel junction, resulting in exposure of the root surface. It can be localized or generalized and is a common problem that can be caused by periodontal disease, periodontal treatment, or chronic trauma in otherwise periodontally healthy patients. Recession can sometimes be self-limiting and cause few problems, but it can also result in a range of problems for patients and represents a difficult challenge to manage.

The principles of management of gingival recession include the following:

- Assessment of the aetiology of the condition
- Identification of the patient's concerns about the condition
- Removal of any aetiological factors when possible
- Monitoring the stability of the recession
- Management of any sequelae of the condition, such as dentine sensitivity
- In some cases, correction of the gingival recession is indicated

Assessment

In assessing gingival recession, a careful history of the condition needs to be taken followed by clinical examination to assess the extent and severity of the condition and to identify the aetiology. A list of the aetiological factors of recession is shown in Table 14.1. A key factor in most cases of recession is the associated anatomical factors that predispose to the condition. The major determinant of many cases of recession is the thickness of the gingivae, which is referred to as the gingival biotype. Recession mainly occurs where there is a thin gingival biotype and where the gingiva is thin because of its position, such as the labial gingivae of the lower incisor regions or labial gingivae of the upper canine teeth. In some cases, the biotype is sufficiently thin that developmentally there is no labial alveolar bone, known as a dehiscence. In these cases, gingival recession can develop rapidly in the presence of chronic minor trauma, such as toothbrushing and possibly even from the minor trauma from everyday masticatory loads. Where a tooth is malpositioned, such as proclined or rotated, this can again result in the absence of overlying alveolar bone because the tooth root is now outside the envelope of the alveolar bone.

Anatomical factors of the soft tissues may also play a major role in the aetiology of recession. These are particularly related to the presence of frenal attachments, especially in the lower labial mucosa. A high frenal attachment may extend close to the gingival margin of the tooth, and there may also be an associated lack of attached gingiva, such that the forces during, for example, mastication are directly transmitted to the gingival margin and promote recession. In addition, high frenal attachments may also impair adequate plaque control in the region, resulting in localized periodontal disease that manifests as recession.

Gingival recession defects can be classified according to Miller's classification, which grades the severity of defects according to whether the recession extends to the mucogingival junction and whether it has resulted in interproximal attachment loss and recession of the interdental papilla (Table 14.2). Miller's classification is particularly applied to defects when being considered for corrective surgery, with those classed as I or II considered amenable to surgical intervention and those classed as III or "IV" considered not amenable.

By itself, gingival recession may often be localized, self-limiting, and harmless. However, in many cases, there are important sequelae associated with the condition, and it is important to assess these when deciding on the management of recession. A list of problems associated with gingival recession is shown in Table 14.3. Patients with localized recession associated with chronic minor trauma such as toothbrushing typically have very clean, healthy mouths and no associated periodontal disease, but they often are concerned that the condition is indicative of generalized periodontal disease and worry about the risk of eventual tooth loss. In these cases, patients need to be carefully reassured that the condition is not indicative of periodontitis and that tooth loss is actually a very rare consequence of progressive recession in these cases. The assessment and management of gingival recession is illustrated in the cases presented next.

Case 1

A 46-year-old man presented complaining of generalized gingival recession. He had been aware of the recession for a number of years but believed that it had become noticeably worse in the past 12 months. He had persisting tooth sensitivity to cold stimuli but was not concerned about the appearance of the recession because he believed that his lips concealed the recession. He was also concerned about the risk of tooth loss in the long term. He was medically fit and well and a nonsmoker.

He was brushing his teeth four times a day with a hard toothbrush. He had a low-sugar diet and drank approximately 1 L of orange juice every day. He had previously used a toothpaste for sensitive teeth but was not currently using this.

Table 14.1 Aetiological factors in gingival recession

Aetiological factor	Specific examples	Comments
Chronic trauma	Particularly vigorous toothbrushing; also habitual trauma such as picking at gums and from tongue studs; direct trauma to gingivae from opposing teeth due to malocclusion	Usually gingivae healthy and uninflamed; seen particularly where there are associated anatomical factors such as thin gingival biotype
Gingival biotype	Thickness of the gingivae varies considerably between patients and at different sites in the mouth; bony dehiscences	Typically affecting labial surfaces of lower incisors and upper canines
Malocclusion	Proclination or rotation of teeth, resulting in root surfaces outside the bony envelope of the jaws, creating bony dehiscences	Similar effect to thin gingival biotype
Frenal attachments/ lack of attached gingivae	Typically labially on lower anterior teeth	Frenal pulls may directly enhance recession but also may impair plaque control
Periodontal disease	Although attachment loss in periodontitis usually causes pocketing, where predisposing anatomical factors present it may result in recession instead	Gingivae inflamed and plaque accumulation evident
Smoking	Smoking reported to increase gingival recession	
Periodontal treatment	All types of periodontal treatment can result in some recession; most marked in pocket elimination surgery (apically positioned flaps) in which recession is a deliberate outcome	Widespread and generalized with loss or recession of interdental papillae; determined by the amount of underlying bone loss
Overeruption of teeth	Due to tooth wear or lack of opposing teeth	

Table 14.2 Miller's classification of gingival recession defects

Class I: Defect that does not extend to mucogingival junction
Class II: Defect that extends to the mucogingival junction, but with no interproximal attachment loss
Class III: Recession that includes loss of attachment interproximally
Class IV: Severe recession involving extensive interproximal attachment loss

Table 14.3 Problems associated with gingival recession

Progression of recession—ultimately endodontic involvement and tooth loss
Dentine sensitivity
Risk of root caries
Tooth surface loss—erosion and abrasion of root surfaces
Poor aesthetics

The clinical appearance at presentation is shown in Figure 14.1. The main feature of note is the marked labial recession seen in both upper and lower incisor teeth. The interdental tissues were unaffected. The recession defects were classified as Miller class I because they do not extend to the mucogingival junction and do not involve the interdental tissues. Some tooth surface loss of the exposed root surfaces

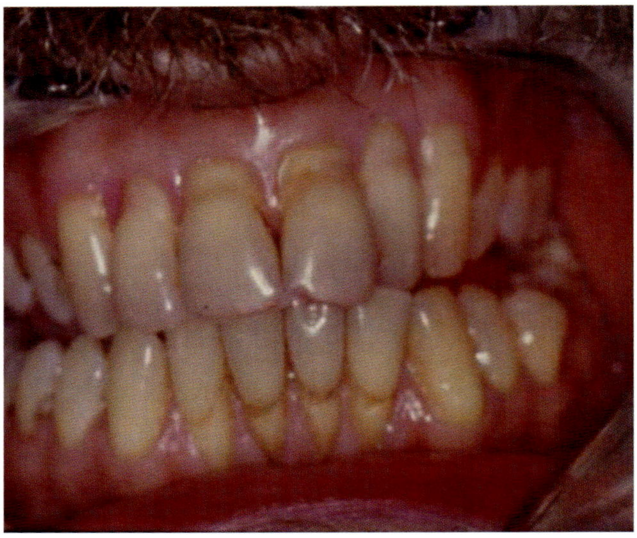

Fig 14.1 Generalized gingival recession in Case 1. Gingivae are uninflamed, and plaque control is good. There is thin gingival biotype and signs of tooth erosion and toothbrush abrasion.

was evident. The appearance of this was consistent with a combination of abrasion and erosion arising from the toothbrushing and the high acidic dietary intake. The patient had excellent plaque control, and there was no gingival bleeding or other signs of periodontal disease elsewhere. A full chart of the recession was made. He was asked to demonstrate his toothbrushing method, which consisted of a vigorous scrubbing action with his hard manual toothbrush. The clinical examination noted the thin gingival biotype on the anterior teeth.

Overall, the recession was diagnosed as being due to the vigorous toothbrushing and the presence of thin gingival biotype. The patient was reassured that the recession was not indicative of poor periodontal health or neglect and that this recession was not likely to result in tooth loss. Given that the patient's main complaint was sensitivity, he was not concerned about appearance, and the considerable difficulty that would be posed by trying to correct the recession surgically, it was agreed to manage the case conservatively.

First, alginate impressions were taken and study casts were prepared and given to the patient to use as an accurate record of the existing recession to monitor future progression. Study models are a much more accurate method of recording the amount of recession for future reference than relying on charting methods. In addition, in this case study, models would also allow monitoring of the tooth surface loss to ensure that this was not progressing. Second, a softer manual toothbrush was recommended and the patient given careful instructions in the Bass technique to carry out toothbrushing. This was followed up to check that the method was implemented and that the patient's plaque control remained effective. As an alternative, an electric toothbrush might also have been considered.

The patient was given dietary advice to reduce his intake of acidic food and drink (1) to help manage the sensitivity and (2) to reduce the risk of further erosive tooth surface loss. Fluoride varnish was applied to the exposed root surfaces and the patient prescribed a daily fluoride mouthwash to help manage the sensitivity. At a review appointment 4 weeks later, the sensitivity was gone and it was recommended that the patient stop using the fluoride mouthwash but regularly use a toothpaste formulated for management of sensitive teeth. It was not considered that the extent of tooth surface loss warranted restorations, but occasionally glass ionomer cement restorations may be placed if the wear is severe.

At a review appointment 1 year later, it was demonstrated that there had been no further progression in the recession, and the patient remained symptom free and without any periodontal problems.

Many, but not all, patients with recession complain of sensitivity. There are a wide range of treatments for sensitivity that act mainly by blocking the exposed dentinal tubules or may desensitize the odontoblast tubular processes. Sensitivity is often a transient phenomenon that is readily managed by the use of sensitive toothpaste, but where the symptoms are more intractable, particular note should be taken of the diet history. Regular high intake of acidic food and drinks is an important aetiological factor in sensitivity because it results in re-exposure of the patent dentinal tubules. In some cases, it is necessary to try a range of different treatments before successfully controlling the symptoms. A list of treatments for dentine sensitivity is given in Table 14.4.

Many cases of gingival recession, such as shown here, can be managed conservatively and do not require corrective surgery.

Case 2

A 28-year-old woman was referred to a periodontist and complained of gum recession on a lower tooth along with sensitivity of this tooth and generalized bleeding gums. She was medically fit and a nonsmoker. She reported that the recession had been getting slowly worse during the past 5 years. She attended the dentist regularly, brushed her teeth twice daily, and used dental floss intermittently. She was particularly concerned about the progression of recession and risk of losing the tooth.

On examination, there was generalized gingivitis with a plaque score of 65%, but no attachment loss was noted. The clinical appearance of the recession at presentation is shown in Figure 14.2, along with a periapical radiograph of the area. The gingivae are swollen and inflamed, and there is an isolated labial recession defect on the LR1 that extends to the mucogingival junction but does not involve the interproximal region. Plaque accumulation at the gingival margin of LR1 was prominent. There is generalized crowding of the lower anterior teeth, with the LR1 labially placed. In addition, there is a high frenal attachment at the midline, mesial to the LR1 that extends coronally above the apical extent of the recession defect.

The diagnosis was generalized gingivitis and a Miller class II recession defect of LR1 associated with periodontal disease, a high frenal attachment, and crowding resulting in the labial position of the tooth. It was noted that the defect was potentially amenable to surgical correction and that the tooth would benefit from surgical excision of the high frenal attachment to facilitate plaque control in the region and to eliminate any frenal pull that may be increasing the risk of

Table 14.4 Treatments for dentine sensitivity

Treatment	Comments
Diet analysis and avoidance of acidic foods and drinks	Important treatment for managing intractable sensitivity; useful as an adjunct to other treatments
Toothpastes to encourage blocking of dentine tubules	Usually contain strontium chloride or arginine. High-fluoride-containing (5000 ppm) toothpastes also of value (available by prescription in the United Kingdom)
Toothpastes to desensitize odontoblast processes	Contain potassium nitrate
Fluoride varnish	Applied professionally; works instantly but effects tend to wear off in a few days
Fluoride mouthwash	Daily fluoride mouthwash (0.05% w/w) often very effective
Resin sealants	Can be effective if retained well
Glass ionomer restorations	Useful where there is marked tooth surface loss
Surgical correction of recession	Relies on achieving complete coverage of recession defect and therefore not a very reliable method for managing sensitivity; not a primary indication for corrective surgery of recession defects

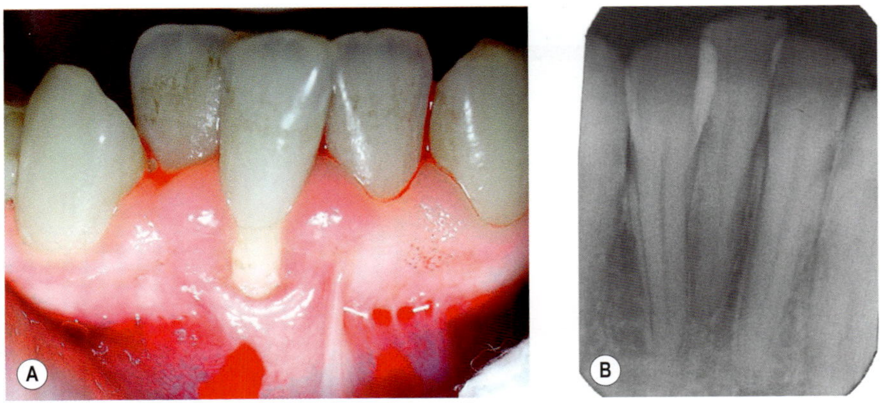

Fig 14.2 (A) Clinical presentation in Case 2. Localized Miller class II recession defect of LR1 associated with periodontal disease, high frenal attachment, and labial position of the tooth. Plaque accumulation is visible at the gingival margin of the recession. (B) Radiograph shows normal interproximal bone levels.

further recession. It was considered that there was a risk of further recession given the apical extent of the defect and the position of the tooth, which meant that the overlying labial gingival was particularly thin.

The treatment initially was planned to manage the generalized gingivitis (and thus eliminate the primary aetiological factor of the recession) before deciding on a definitive treatment for the recession defect, and in particular to consider surgical correction.

During two visits, the patient was given oral hygiene instruction and scaling was performed to remove all calculus deposits. A review visit was held 6 weeks after completion of initial treatment. At the review visit, the gingivitis had largely resolved and the plaque score had reduced to 16%. The possible future treatment options were discussed in full with the patient. It was explained that there was a significant risk of further progression of the recession if no further treatment was carried out. A frenectomy (to remove the frenal attachment) was advised to improve accessibility for plaque control and eliminate the frenal pull on the tissue. The option of further surgical treatment to correct the defect was also discussed in detail, and after consideration the patient expressed her wish to proceed with this.

The patient was then planned for surgical treatment. A first surgical procedure was carried out to excise the frenum, and the patient was allowed to heal. In many cases, this procedure can be carried out simultaneously with the gingival grafting procedure, but in this case it was considered that the grafting would be easier if the frenum was removed prior to the main surgical procedure. After healing, the patient was then scheduled for a connective tissue graft procedure, together with coronal positioning of the flap over the graft to cover the root surface defect (Figure 14.3). A connective tissue graft is a graft of connective tissue that is taken from the subepithelial tissue of the hard palate. The defect is first exposed by raising a split-thickness flap over the area to leave the fibrous periosteum intact, thus providing a vascular bed to accept the graft. The graft is then sutured into place over the defect and covered (or partially covered) with the flap by coronally advancing it over the graft.

The patient experienced marked postoperative pain, particularly from the graft donor site in the hard palate, but healing was otherwise uneventful. Plaque control in the area was managed by chlorhexidine mouthwash until healing was complete and the patient able to carry out normal plaque-control procedures.

The appearance of the site 6 months postoperatively is shown in Figure 14.4. The site shows excellent healing, with full coverage of the root surface and a good band of attached gingivae that was largely indistinguishable from the surrounding area. The patient reported that she had no problems and was very pleased with the final outcome.

◇ *Surgical procedures for treating recession defects*

As seen here, surgical correction of Miller class I and II defects can be extremely successful and predictable when carried out by experienced hands. This type of mucogingival surgery is mainly in the realm of the experienced periodontist who has undergone extensive postgraduate training, has experience in managing such defects, and is likely to carry out sufficient numbers of such procedures to remain properly skilled at them. Thus, for the undergraduate and the general dentist, it is mainly important to be familiar with the possibilities of these procedures, and have a working knowledge of what is involved, rather than being competent in carrying them out.

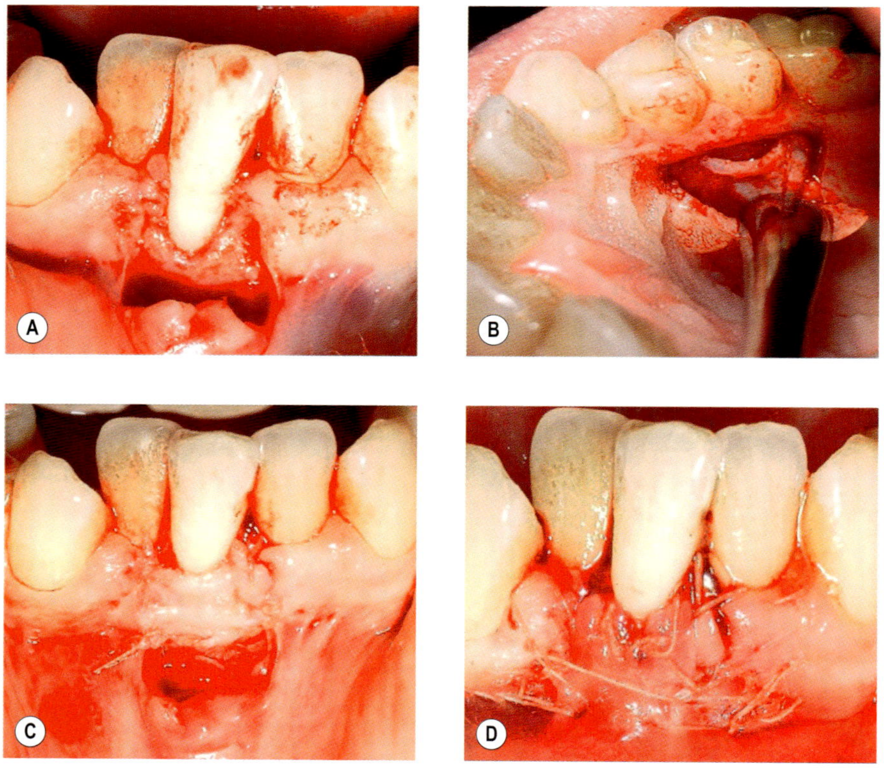

Fig 14.3 Connective tissue graft procedure. (A) Split-thickness flap raised over defect. (B) Harvesting connective tissue graft. The palatal epithelium is elevated and the graft dissected out from the subepithelial tissue. (C) Graft sutured in place over defect with resorbable sutures. (D) Wound closed by coronally advancing the split-thickness flap and sutured in place.

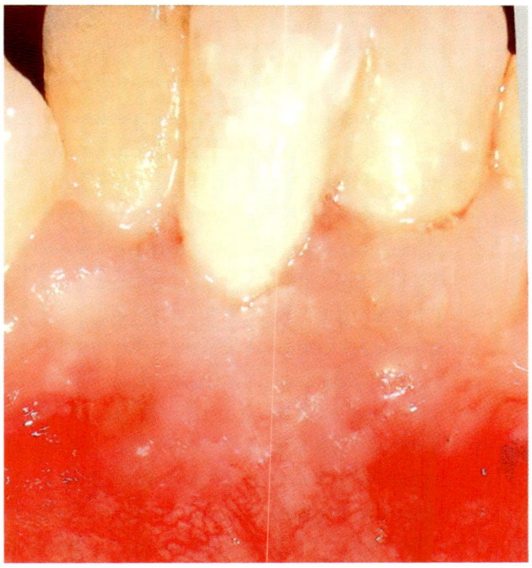

Fig 14.4 Follow-up of connective tissue graft 6 months postoperatively. There is full coverage of the previous recession defect and good levels of attached gingivae.

The main indications for corrective mucogingival surgery are to prevent risk of future progression and for aesthetic reasons. There may also be benefits for managing dentine sensitivity, but there are probably better ways of managing sensitivity, as discussed previously, particularly because managing sensitivity by corrective surgery is dependent on achieving complete coverage of root surfaces.

A variety of different surgical techniques have been described for the management of gingival recession defects. In general, use of connective tissue grafts, or the use of commercially available acellular dermal grafts, is the preferred method for obtaining full root surface coverage. Some of these methods are summarized in Table 14.5. However, a range of modifications to these techniques have been described.

Recession following periodontal treatment

In general, the management of postoperative recession following periodontal treatment represents an entirely different and more demanding challenge to the cases of recession described previously. All types of periodontal treatment will potentially cause generalized recession, and this is much more widespread than that determined by the local anatomy of the gingivae. Following periodontal treatment, the amount of recession occurring will be partly dictated by the gingival biotype but most particularly by the extent of the underlying bone loss that has occurred during the disease process. In general, surgical periodontal treatment will tend to cause the most recession immediately postoperatively, particularly where pocket elimination (apically positioned flap) procedures have been used because these deliberately create gingival recession to eliminate pocketing. However, the evidence suggests that in the medium to long term (3–5 years +), the amount of recession occurring with all types of periodontal treatment will tend to converge. Because the recession seen following periodontal treatment tends to particularly involve the interproximal tissues (i.e., Miller class IV recession defects), this is usually not amenable to surgical correction and represents a major cause of distress for many patients (Figure 14.5).

Table 14.5 Surgical techniques used for the management of gingival recession defects

Technique	Comments
Frenectomy	Removes the aetiological factor but does not correct existing defect; simple to perform
Free gingival graft	Graft harvested from palatal gingiva, which includes palatal epithelium; increases attached gingiva and provides increased gingival thickness to stabilize risk of future recession
Connective tissue graft	Subepithelial graft harvested from palate; allows epithelialization of grafted site by adjacent tissue or coronally advanced flap; superior to free gingival graft for obtaining root coverage
Acellular dermal graft	Commercially available processed graft material obtained from human skin graft donors, which has similar effects as connective tissue graft but avoids morbidity and trauma associated with normal graft harvesting; recent surgical development that requires further evaluation
Laterally positioned flap	Pedicle graft that preserves the blood supply of the tissue; difficult to control full coverage and risk of recession in adjacent donor site
Coronally positioned flap	Useful in conjunction with connective tissue graft or following free gingival graft to provide sufficient extra tissue to allow coronal advancement; pedicle flap that preserves blood supply

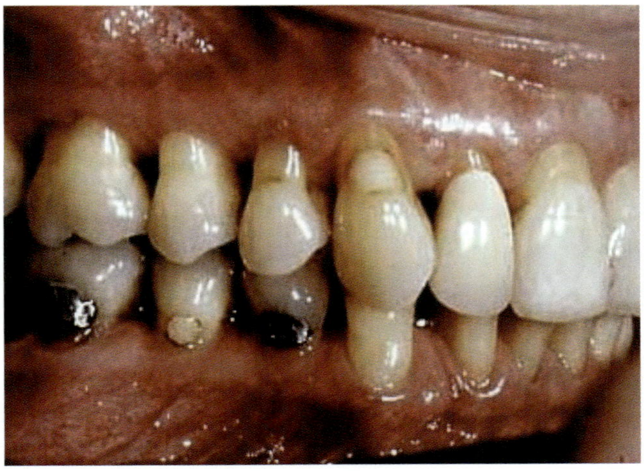

Fig 14.5 Generalized recession in a patient who has had periodontal treatment. There is marked recession involving the interproximal regions, resulting in the appearance of spaces between the teeth due to recession of interdental papillae, so-called "black triangle disease."

Case 3

A 31-year-old woman with severe periodontal pocketing was referred to a periodontist. She complained of progressive looseness of her teeth and had recently lost two lower teeth due to mobility, had previously lost her upper posterior teeth, and had been provided with an acrylic upper partial denture to replace these teeth. Her plaque control was good, and minimal calculus deposits were noted. There was severe generalized attachment loss, particularly of the remaining upper teeth.

She was diagnosed as having generalized aggressive periodontitis and was treated with a course of nonsurgical periodontal therapy of root surface debridement in all quadrants under local anaesthesia together with an adjunctive course of doxycycline 100 mg daily for 2 weeks.

At review, she demonstrated a dramatic reduction in all pocket depths, and the tissues looked uninflamed. However, there had been severe gingival recession, particularly of the upper anterior teeth, which deeply concerned the patient. The clinical and radiographic features are shown in Figure 14.6.

The options for managing this recession are extremely limited. Surgical intervention did not offer any solution to this problem. The options for treatment were either provision of a removable labial gingival veneer or extraction of the teeth and replacement with a larger upper partial denture. After discussion, it was agreed to construct an acrylic labial gingival veneer to replace the missing gingival tissues prosthetically. This is a nondestructive solution, and thus it was believed that the worst-case scenario was that the patient would not be able to wear the veneer and other options for management would have to be considered.

A primary alginate upper impression was taken, from which a labially approaching special tray was constructed to fit the buccal gingivae extending to the first molar teeth. During the second visit, a mould of the upper palatal teeth was made to block out the undercuts though the interdental papillae, and this was liberally coated with Vaseline (to prevent bonding to the subsequent impression) and inserted *in situ* to prevent impression material becoming engaged in the palatal undercuts. The special tray was then used to take an impression of the labial upper gingivae in medium body addition silicone impression material. During the next visit, the labial gingival veneer was fitted (Figure 14.7).

The patient was delighted with the improvement achieved and at follow-up reported that she now wore the veneer at all times and had completely become accustomed to it.

An additional case of the construction of an acrylic gingival veneer is shown in Figure 14.8. In this case, the patient had had marked gingival bleeding associated with the crowns present on the upper anterior teeth. Following periodontal treatment, the recession that occurs resulted in very unsightly exposure of the now supragingival crown margins. In this case, the use of a gingival veneer was a much better option, and much more effective, than the highly destructive option of remaking the crowns.

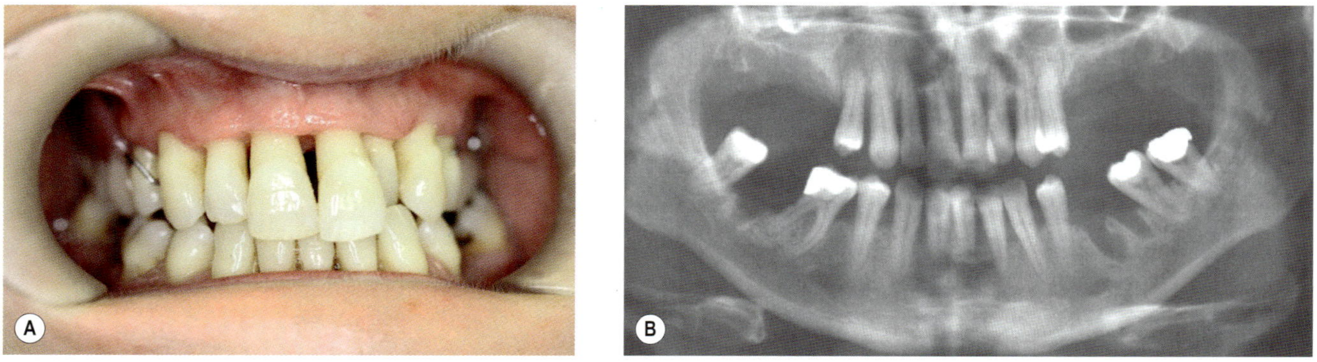

Fig 14.6 (A) Clinical and (B) radiographic features of Case 3. There has been dramatic recession following resolution of the very deep pockets affecting particularly the upper anterior teeth.

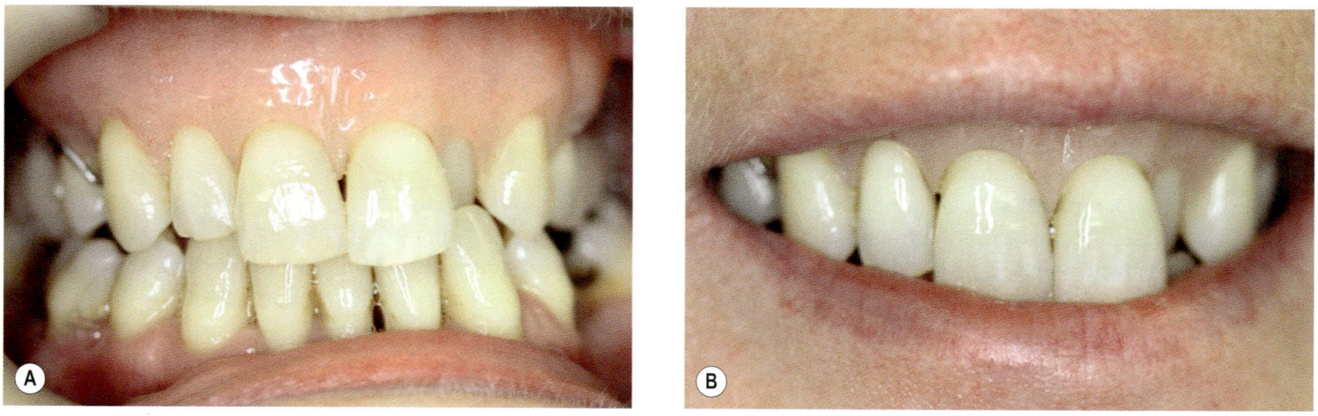

Fig 14.7 Acrylic gingival veneer to hide the gross gingival recession resulting from periodontal treatment. (The contour of the anterior teeth has also been slightly adjusted with composite and slight incisal grinding to improve the appearance of the incisors.)

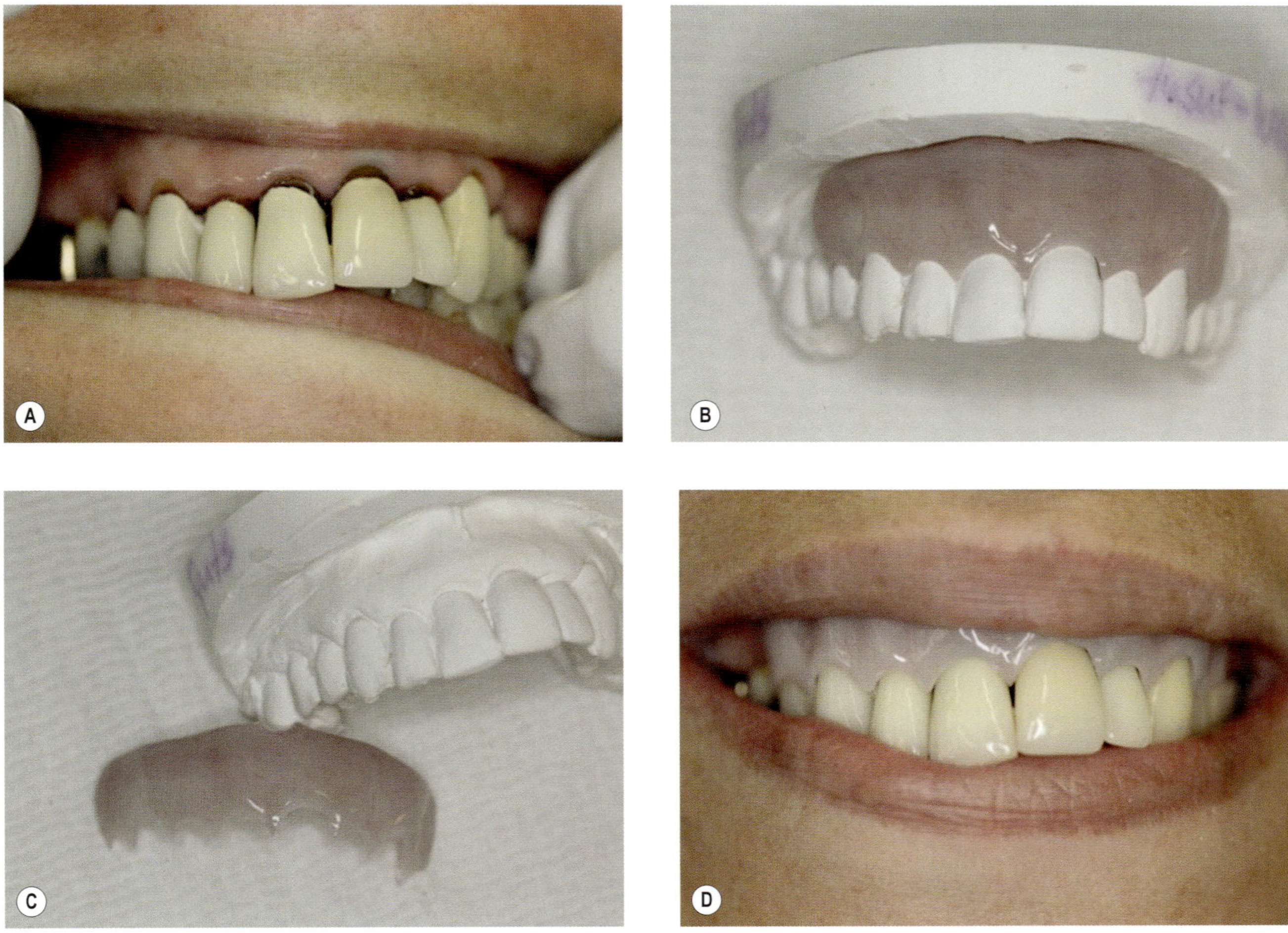

Fig 14.8 Gingival veneer constructed to conceal unsightly crown margins exposed by gingival recession after periodontal treatment.

The management of postoperative gingival recession, particularly in the anterior region, remains a major challenge that we do not seem to be near solving using biological methods. Gingival veneers can be made in acrylic, as shown here, or in a silicone material that is softer and has some flexibility, although there is no clear guide on the superiority of one compared to the other beyond individual clinician preference. The use of removable gingival veneers does not seem like a modern solution to this difficult problem, but they are remarkably popular with patients, probably because the gain in appearance, confidence, etc., considerably outweighs the inconvenience of wearing these prostheses.

Chapter 15

Postoperative care and periodontal maintenance therapy

Introduction

Active periodontal treatment should have a clear endpoint as its objective. It is important that an active diagnostic decision is taken to determine the satisfactory outcome of this treatment rather than simply enter a cycle of constant repetition of, for example, further courses of nonsurgical or surgical treatments. As discussed in Chapter 9, the ideal outcomes of active therapy include the achievement of a satisfactory level of plaque control, elimination of gingival inflammation, control or removal of associated risk factors, and the reduction in pocket depths to less than 5 mm. These outcomes are based on many studies that demonstrate that these are associated with the ability to maintain good periodontal health in the future.

Occasionally, it may be judged that achievement of these objectives may be compromised—for example, when compliance continues to be poor or if the patient continues to smoke. In these circumstances, it may be necessary to accept less than perfect outcomes and to arrange supportive periodontal therapy to try to reduce the risk of further disease in the future.

On completion of active periodontal treatment, two very important challenges remain for the clinician: (1) the management of any consequences of periodontal disease and (2) preventing the risk of recurrence of disease in the future. The aims of this chapter are to consider the management of some of the unwanted consequences of periodontal disease, to emphasize the crucial importance of establishing a maintenance programme for the patient, and to describe the requirements for a successful maintenance programme.

Managing the consequences of periodontal disease

Because periodontal disease causes tissue destruction that is largely irreversible, even following successful treatment, it causes a range of unwanted sequelae that can sometimes be more challenging to the clinician than the actual control of the disease per se. These sequelae are often the major concern of affected patients, and although it is important for the patient to understand the primary requirement of managing the periodontal disease, the clinician needs to take careful note of the patient's concerns and to agree on a plan to address these.

The common consequences of periodontal disease that patients may complain about and that may require further management are listed in Table 15.1. The management of recession and dentine sensitivity are also discussed in Chapter 14.

A full discussion of the restoration of the periodontally compromised dentition is beyond the scope of this book. However, the cases presented here illustrate some of the issues that may arise and some management options available. In all cases, the management of the periodontal disease is the essential prequel to being able to address these problems, and as with all periodontal treatment, active maintenance programmes are required for long-term success.

Case 1

A 27-year-old man attended for review following previous treatment for severe localized periodontitis that had particularly affected the incisor teeth. He reported no problems with his gums, but he was deeply upset about the appearance of his upper anterior teeth, which had always been imbricated, but this appearance was now exacerbated by recent additional drifting and by gingival recession.

On examination, it was noted that he had responded extremely well to the previous periodontal treatment and there were no persisting pockets greater than 4 mm, no gingival bleeding, and plaque control was good. The upper anterior teeth showed marked crowding and imbrication, with UR2 retroclined and UL2 proclined, together with unevenness of the central incisors. The patient had an anterior open bite, and none of the teeth exhibited any increased mobility (Figure 15.1).

The teeth were carefully assessed, and although it was considered that following periodontal treatment their prognosis was good, the options for improving the aesthetics were limited. Because of the imbrication, there was loss of space overall for the upper incisors. Orthodontic treatment was not considered a suitable option in this case because of lack of space and the severely compromised periodontium of the teeth. Therefore, it was agreed that the only suitable solution would involve extraction of some or all of the teeth.

To assess further, study models were made and a range of options explored by diagnostic wax-ups, including extraction of upper lateral incisors and replacement with single pontic cantilevered resin-bonded bridges. However, because of the lack of space and the irregularity of the central incisors, it was agreed with the patient that extraction of all four incisors would give by far the best aesthetic result, recognizing that the central incisors would be made slightly narrower mesiodistally to allow for an even matching of the teeth. Consequently, the incisors were extracted and initially replaced with an immediate acrylic partial denture and finally replaced by a resin-bonded bridge using the UR3 and UL3 as abutments (Figure 15.1).

Extraction of the incisors was a major issue for the patient, but ultimately he was delighted with the outcome. Sometimes extraction of teeth is the right treatment not because they have existing disease but, rather, for overall aesthetics. In this case, the use of the upper canine teeth as abutments for the bridge was readily considered because these teeth were largely unaffected by the severe periodontal disease seen on the incisors and also because the occlusal loading on the bridge was relatively low, given the anterior open bite.

More generally, the decision regarding the use of periodontally compromised teeth as abutments for fixed or removable prostheses requires careful assessment. First, it is imperative that such teeth have been successfully treated for periodontal disease, but in these circumstances studies convincingly show that increasing occlusal load on teeth by using them as abutments will not result in renewed attachment loss provided that they are well maintained in a plaque-free state. However, the increased occlusal load on an already compromised tooth can further increase tooth mobility. Thus, when determining whether to use a periodontally compromised tooth as an abutment, consideration has to be made regarding the magnitude of the likely increased occlusal load to which it will be subjected, if it is possible to spread the load over a number of abutment teeth, and in the most extreme cases, whether to incorporate "cross-arch bracing" to prevent mobility of prostheses.

Table 15.1 Patient-centred unwanted consequences of periodontal disease

Consequence	Comments
Poor aesthetics	Due to recession, loss of interdental papillae ("black triangle disease"), tooth drifting and spacing, etc.
Dentine sensitivity	Due to root surface exposure from recession
Risk of root caries	Due to root surface exposure/dietary sugar intake
Tooth mobility	Resulting in compromised function/discomfort
Tooth loss	May require tooth replacement
Oral malodour (halitosis)	Periodontal disease is most common cause of oral malodour; should improve with active periodontal treatment; tongue brushing and mouthwashes may also help
Gingival swelling and bleeding	Should be addressed during active periodontal treatment phase

Case 2

A 46-year-old woman with generalized severe chronic periodontitis that had been successfully treated complained of marked mobility, particularly of UL1, and some spacing of the upper incisors. She has good plaque control but is a smoker of approximately 10 cigarettes a day. She is committed to trying (again) to quit smoking.

On examination, the UL1 showed grade 2 mobility and the UR1 grade 1 mobility. The patient reports the UL1 is uncomfortable, particularly on eating, and thus affects her masticatory function. She is always concerned about "catching" the UL1 during function and making it even more mobile.

The mobility was managed by the use of a fibreglass-reinforced composite splint applied to the incisors, and the contour and spacing of the teeth improved by composite buildups (Figure 15.2). She was given careful instruction in how to keep the area clean using interdental brushes, and further maintenance visits were arranged.

Acid-etch bonded composite materials are very useful in managing some spacing and drifting and are the basis for most types of splinting methods. Although using

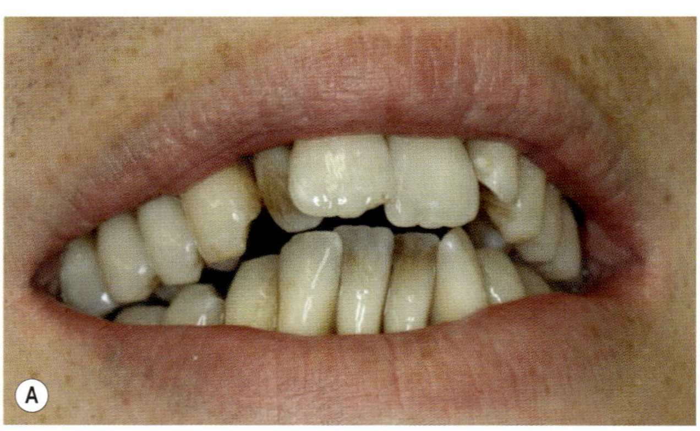

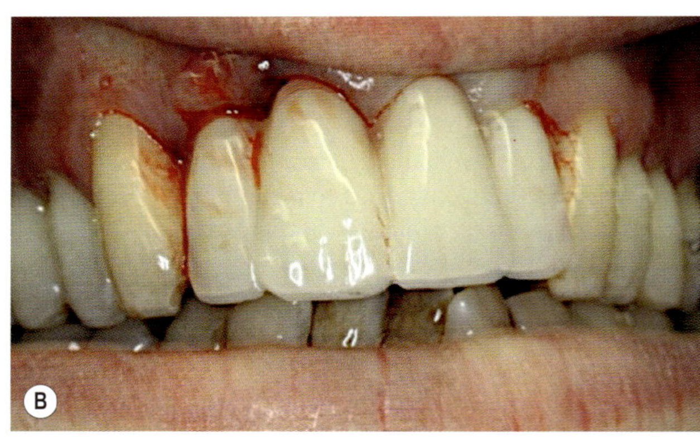

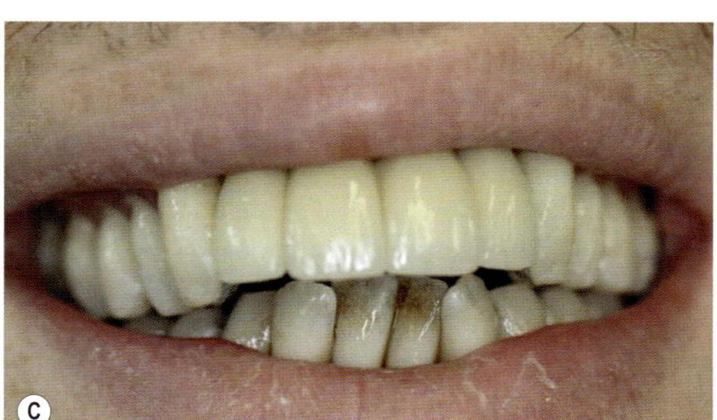

Fig 15.1 Case 1 (A) at presentation and (B) at extractions and fitting of immediate acrylic partial denture. (C) Teeth replaced with resin-bonded bridge with abutments at UL3 and UR3.

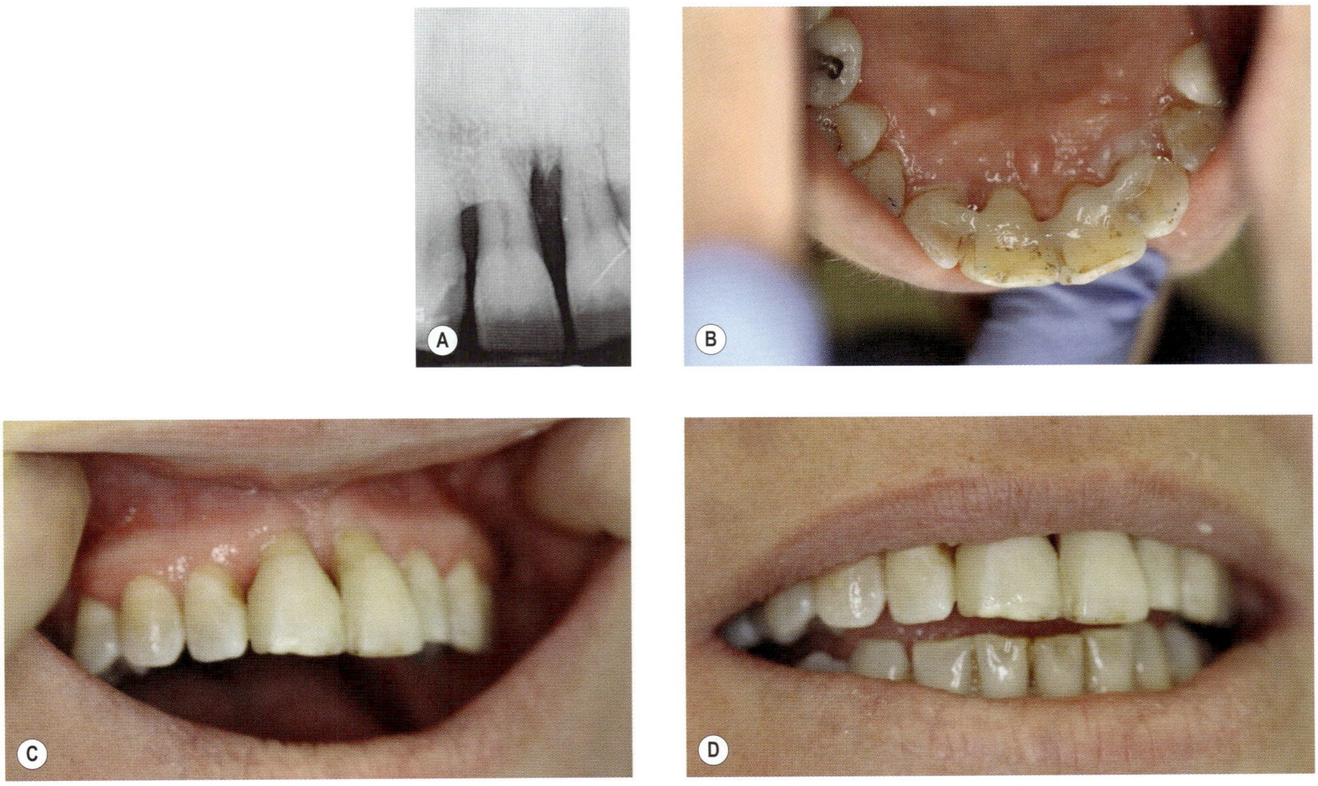

Fig 15.2 Case 2. (A) Radiograph of upper central incisors showing severe bone loss, particularly at UL1. (B) Fibreglass-reinforced splint placed on incisors. The splint has had to be placed quite apically to avoid occlusal interferences, and it requires very careful maintenance because of the increased risk of plaque accumulation. (C and D) Labial view of splinted teeth. Composite buildups have been placed as part of the splint to improve contours of teeth, particularly at UR1 distal and UL1 mesial.

composites to manage spacing is inevitably a bit of a compromise, they are nondestructive, relatively quick to place, and can be aesthetically excellent when carefully carried out.

Mobile teeth are a common consequence of periodontal disease. The mobility of a tooth is ultimately dependent on the amount of occlusal loading placed on a tooth and thus will be determined by

- the amount of periodontal attachment loss; and
- the relative or actual increase in occlusal load due to
  - normal occlusal loads in a compromised periodontium;
  - excessive occlusal loads due to occlusal interferences and dysharmonies; and
  - parafunction.

In assessing tooth mobility, it is important to assess the patient's functional occlusion for occlusal dysharmonies and for parafunctional habits. Where detected, occlusal adjustment and occlusal splints may be indicated. When carrying out occlusal adjustment in these cases, it is usual to accept and preserve the current occlusion and adjust individual occlusal dysharmonies by (1) eliminating occlusal interferences in intercuspal position (to eliminate premature contacts) and establishing centric stops and (2) adjusting dysharmonies in lateral and protrusive movements while preserving centric stops. It is not difficult to destabilize patients' occlusal function by inexperienced hands; thus, patients requiring extensive occlusal adjustment will benefit from expert input from an appropriate specialist.

Permanent splinting can be very effective in stabilizing teeth following periodontal treatment, which can dramatically improve patient comfort and function. The main indications for provision of permanent splinting are

- to immobilize mobile teeth that are causing discomfort or affecting function for a patient;
- to immobilize teeth where there is progressive increase in mobility; and
- to prevent further movement of teeth, including drifting, overeruption, or relapse of orthodontically treated teeth.

For splinting to be successful, it is essential that the periodontal disease is managed first and that it is recognized that a splint will make it more difficult to maintain plaque control around teeth. A wide range of different methods of splinting have been described throughout the years, many of which are listed in Table 15.2. In the case described here, a fibreglass-reinforced composite splint was used. These fibres are treated so that they form a chemical bond with the composite, providing enormous strength and adaptability for a wide variety of applications. Thus, the main risk of failure is at the actual bond between the composite and the tooth, which if well carried out is usually very reliable. The adaptability of a fibre-reinforced type of splint is also demonstrated in Case 3. Two other splint types—arch wire splints and composite splints—are shown in Figures 15.3 and 15.4. Without any mechanical reinforcement, composite is too brittle and fractures too readily to be used reliably as a permanent splinting method, but it is potentially useful for short-term splinting.

Table 15.2 Methods of providing permanent splinting

Method	Comments
Fibreglass-reinforced composite	Chemical bond between fibre and composite; very strong and adaptable; can incorporate composite buildups; debonding can sometimes occur at bonding between composite and tooth
Arch wire and composite	Effective and simple; less adaptable and more obtrusive than fibreglass; debonding can sometimes occur at bonding between composite and tooth, or of composite material retaining the arch wire
Resin retained bridge/splint	Adapted from "Maryland style" bridges; debonding occurs frequently and is troublesome
Composite	Too weak to be regarded as permanent splinting; material is brittle and fractures easily
Linked crowns	Very effective if replacing existing restorations; otherwise, extremely destructive of healthy tooth tissues

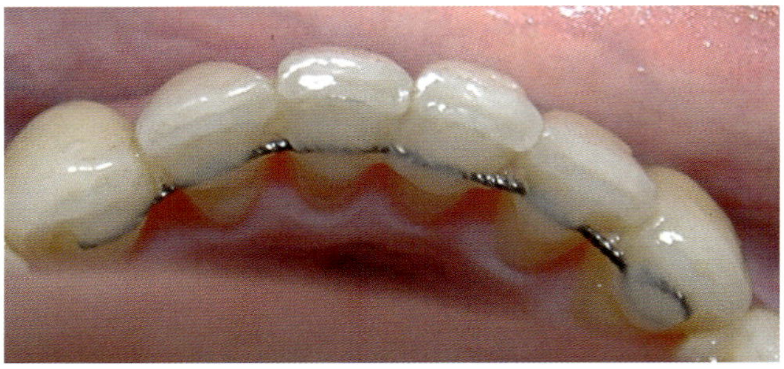

Fig 15.3 Example of arch wire splint. Wire is prebent on a model in the laboratory and retained with composite resins. These splints are used widely as orthodontic retainers but are also effective in other situations.

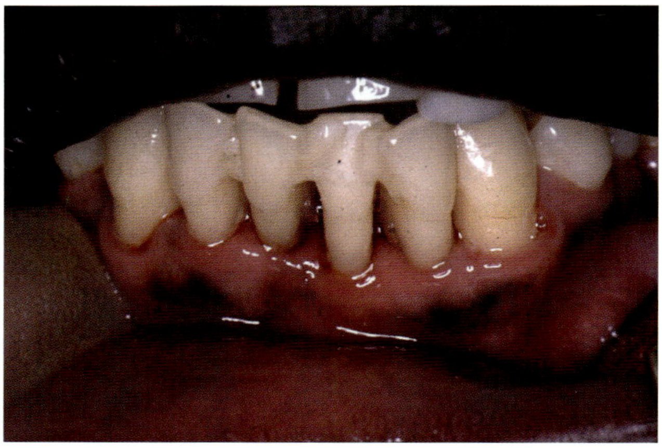

Fig 15.4 Composite resin splint. This is useful as a temporary splint because it can be placed relatively quickly, but when not reinforced the material is too brittle to use successfully for permanent splinting.

Case 3

A 62-year-old man was referred to the periodontist by the patient's physician for investigation and management of his gum problems. The patient suffered from metastatic renal cell carcinoma and was currently being treated with bevacizumab. He was also initially taking amlodipine, but this was stopped early in his periodontal treatment.

Bevacizumab is an inhibitor of the receptor for vascular endothelial growth factor and is currently being trialled for the management of a number of specific advanced-stage carcinomas. Although its effects on the periodontal tissues are not fully reported, it is known that the drug impairs wound healing and increases the risk of bleeding.

The patient had rather poor plaque control and was smoking "a few" small cigars daily. Periodontal examination showed an unusual, almost greyish, irregular inflamed appearance of the gingival tissues. There was generalized chronic periodontitis, and the patient believed that his periodontal condition had deteriorated rapidly during his recent illness and its treatment. During initial periodontal therapy, the patient attended with an acute flare-up of UL1, which had suddenly become very mobile, painful, and was suppurating.

The patient required extraction of the UL1 as soon as possible, particularly in view of his medical history, and it was believed that provision of an immediate partial denture would not be helpful for his rapidly changing periodontal condition and perhaps would represent a further minor indignity for the patient because he was undergoing extensive hospital interventions. Therefore, the tooth was extracted during this visit and a fibreglass splint placed palatally on the upper anterior teeth. The root of the extracted UL1 was cut off *ex vivo* with an air turbine and long tapered diamond bur, and the crown of the tooth was bonded to the splint to act as an immediate bridge pontic, with a small portion of the coronal root remaining to preserve tooth height to the extraction socket (Figure 15.5). The socket healed uneventfully, and the patient had no further problems with this area 1 year following extraction.

Periodontal maintenance therapy

As previously emphasized, successful periodontal therapy depends on a number of factors, notably

- correct diagnosis;
- adequate plaque control;
- management of modifiable risk factors;
- subgingival debridement (which may be by both nonsurgical and surgical methods); and
- long-term maintenance.

Periodontal maintenance therapy, also referred to as supportive periodontal therapy, is therefore one of the most important determinants of successful periodontal therapy.

One of the major risk markers for future periodontal disease is past disease experience. Therefore, the periodontal patient who has been successfully treated will still be at risk from further breakdown and attachment loss. The key to preventing this is maintaining adequate plaque control, which can be achieved through the patient's own efforts at home, regular professional cleaning of plaque deposits and plaque retention factors, continued management of any other modifiable risk factors, and early detection and professional intervention where there are signs of disease recurrence.

A totally clean tooth is recolonized by bacteria almost as soon as cleaning has finished, resulting in the formation of

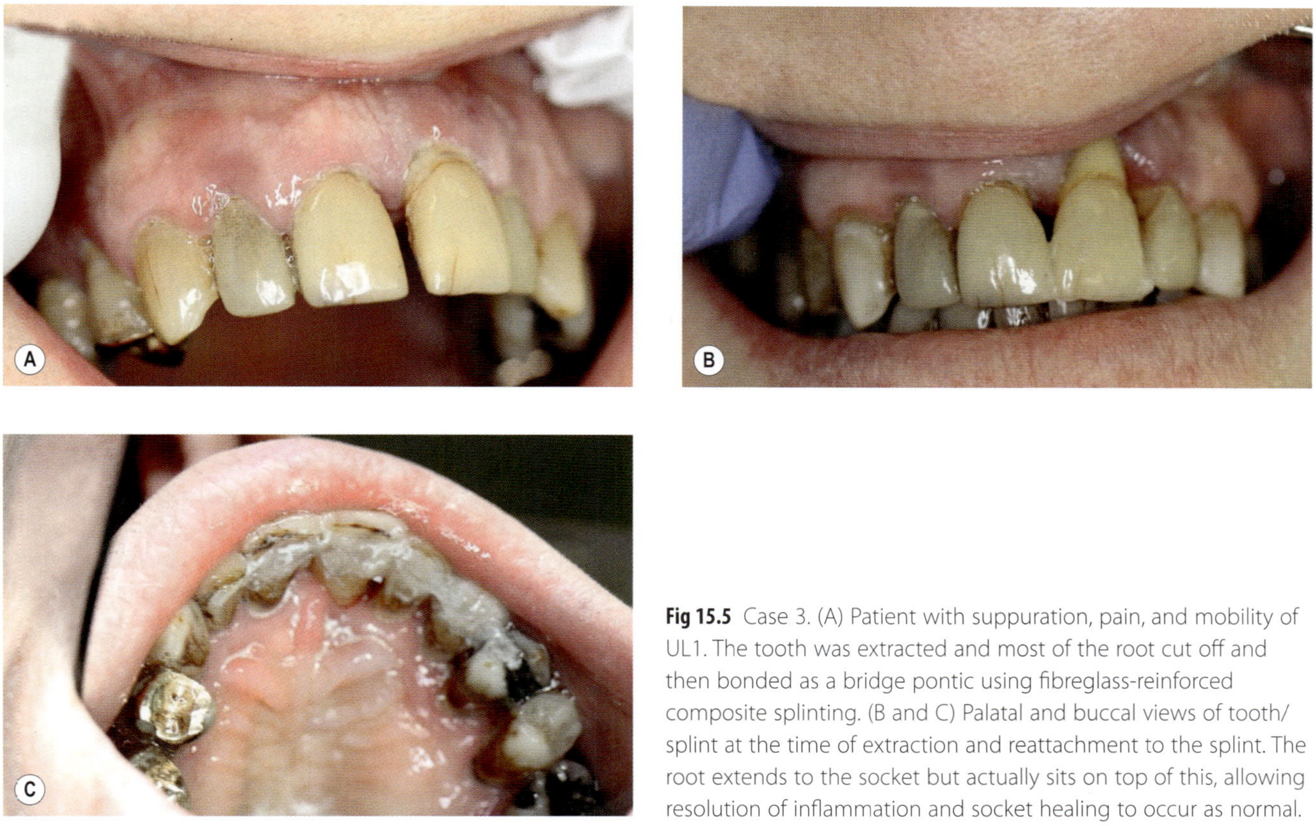

Fig 15.5 Case 3. (A) Patient with suppuration, pain, and mobility of UL1. The tooth was extracted and most of the root cut off and then bonded as a bridge pontic using fibreglass-reinforced composite splinting. (B and C) Palatal and buccal views of tooth/splint at the time of extraction and reattachment to the splint. The root extends to the socket but actually sits on top of this, allowing resolution of inflammation and socket healing to occur as normal.

a new plaque biofilm. If this is allowed to mature, this new plaque may begin the whole process of periodontal breakdown anew. Regular disruption of this biofilm will obviously prevent this from happening. The patient is able to do this supragingivally, and evidence suggests that adequate supragingival plaque control will also reduce subgingival plaque formation and maturation in shallow pockets that are less than 5 mm in depth. However, subgingival plaque control is most effectively carried out by professional cleaning, which empirically is typically carried out every 3 months in a maintenance regime, although this interval must be based on the individual's needs.

During approximately the past 40 years, a considerable periodontal literature has established the importance of periodontal maintenance as a major determinant of long-term success. This is demonstrated by seminal studies by Axelsson and Lindhe and others, whose work demonstrated that periodontal maintenance could prevent future disease, whereas those who did not have a planned maintenance programme were much more likely to show disease reoccurrence and future progression of disease.

It is tempting to think that once sufficient improvement in plaque control by a patient is achieved, it is likely to be sustained because the patient will see the benefits he or she has gained from this. However, many patients will, in time, slip in their oral hygiene and will need re-motivating through the discussions and demonstrations that were described in Chapter 7. When re-motivating patients, it is particularly helpful if they have had a successful outcome so far that they can be reminded of and also be reminded of the effects of neglecting their oral hygiene. Thus, it is likely that one of the major benefits of a regular maintenance programme is simply that continuing to emphasize the importance of good plaque control reinforces the need for this with patients, who might otherwise think that they are "cured" of their condition. Furthermore, the objective measurement of plaque and bleeding by using indices or scores is a potentially powerful motivational and educational tool when discussed with a patient. It is also recognized that patients can perform excellent oral hygiene on the day of their visit and have 0% plaque. However, the bleeding score will reveal more about how they have been doing with their plaque control in the weeks before their visit.

Evidence for the value of repeated instrumentation of affected sites as a way of preventing future disease is lacking, but this is well accepted as an important part of maintenance care and is biologically sensible. The opportunity to detect early signs of recurrence of disease and implement early interventions to prevent progression is also considered an important part of maintenance therapy.

Recently, the basis for maintenance therapy has emphasized the importance of continuous risk assessment, which involves decisions made on a patient basis, tooth basis, and site basis recognizing that each patient's needs and susceptibilities may differ. The concepts of risk assessment both at the patient level and at the tooth level were described indepth in previous chapters. It is of note, however, that studies have suggested that during a maintenance phase of treatment, the presence of persisting bleeding on probing of approximately 30% of sites may be a useful negative prognostic indicator and is suggestive of the need for further intervention.

A typical maintenance visit may involve the following:

- Asking the patient to report any problems or complaints experienced since the last visit

- Checking plaque control and gingivitis (by debris and bleeding indices or plaque and bleeding distribution)
- Checking pocket depths, especially sites of previous deep pocketing, at each visit and carrying out a full pocket chart regularly (e.g., yearly)
- Reinforcing oral hygiene instruction
- Removal of calculus and other secondary factors
- Planning further intervention for sites showing signs of recurrence of disease or signs of new disease

The interval between maintenance visits is usually approximately 3 months. Intervals can be varied for individuals on the basis of their assessed risk of future disease, particularly in the long term. For example, for a patient who persistently shows excellent maintenance of periodontal health, lack of gingival bleeding, and no signs of deterioration in plaque control, a longer recall interval may be reasonably prescribed. However, for a patient who shows repeated signs of deteriorating plaque control, or who has other risk factors such as persisting smoking or a contributory systemic factor such as diabetes, it may be necessary to keep the recall interval at 3 months or even ideally to shorten the interval between appointments.

Providing continued maintenance and support to periodontal patients is an area in which the dentist and the hygienist can work very closely together, sharing the responsibility for this care. In addition, this may also be shared between a specialist periodontist, the general dentist, and the hygienist. Indeed, in most practices, the hygienist carries out most of this therapy, although findings, particularly negative ones, should always be reported and discussed and a mutual way forward for the patient decided upon. Because the final responsibility for diagnostic decisions remains with the dentists, they should ensure that they reassess patients at regular intervals (e.g., yearly), when full 6-point probing charts can be retaken.

Overall, the published data indicate that periodontal treatment is extremely successful in preventing future disease progression and tooth loss, particularly when an adequate long-term maintenance programme is implemented.

Case 4

A 68-year-old woman visited a dental hygienist at a periodontal department for a routine maintenance visit. She had no complaints or problems. Review of her patient records showed that she had been a regular attender at the department for 23 years. She had initially presented (at age 45 years) following referral by her general dentist with a diagnosis of severe periodontitis. Her dentist told her that she was likely to lose many or all of her teeth. She complained of tooth mobility of some of the lower teeth, particularly on the right side. The original radiograph taken at that time is shown in Figure 15.6A. At that time, there was severe bone loss noted in the upper right molar region and the lower anterior teeth, with severe angular defects of approximately 80% and bone loss at LR543 and LL35.

A course of nonsurgical periodontal therapy was carried out at the time of initial presentation. Good pocket depth reductions were noted, and the patient was then put on a maintenance programme that originally set at 3-month intervals but more recently had been extended to 6-month intervals. At the time of the original treatment, a "Rochette"-style splint had been fitted to LR54321 to manage the mobility in this region.

The presentation at the review appointment 23 years later is shown in Figures 15.6B and 15.7. The patient had excellent plaque control and no gingival bleeding or deep pockets, and severe gingival recession occurring throughout the years since initial treatment had been noted. There were no significant changes in bone levels on any of the teeth compared with the previous radiograph (taken 23 years ago). The patient was not troubled by the aesthetics of the recession because this was largely concealed by her lip lines, and she was delighted that she had retained all the teeth that were present at the start of treatment, particularly given the original prognosis that had been offered for the survival of her teeth.

This case is unusual not because of the spectacular outcome of simple treatment and careful maintenance in a case of severe periodontitis; the published data support this as a common or normal achievable outcome of periodontal treatment in many patients. It is unusual because it is rare to be able to document such cases because patients rarely continue to have maintenance therapy at the same site for so many years.

A number of other interesting observations can be made from the case. First, the severe recession that has occurred is unfortunately the normal long-term outcome of treatment when the underlying bone has been so severely affected. In this case, the patient was not concerned about the aesthetics

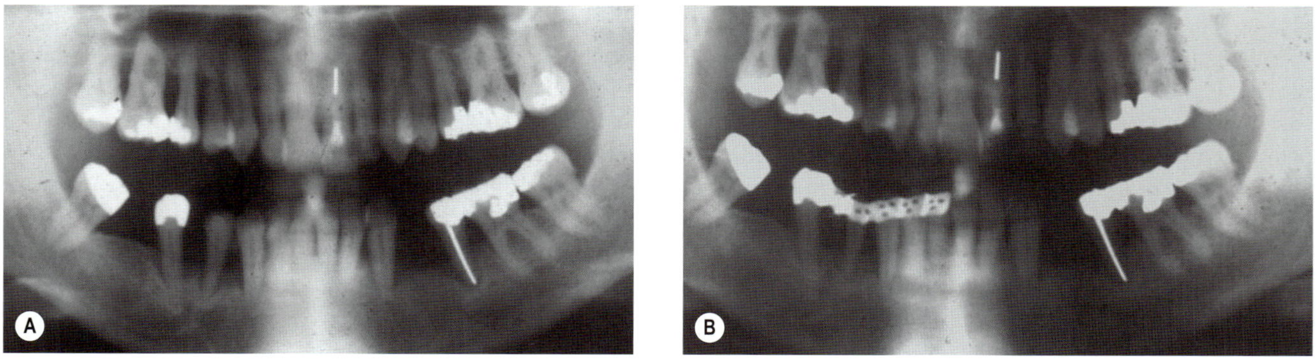

Fig 15.6 Rotational tomogram radiographs of Case 4. (A) At initial presentation. (B) At routine maintenance visit 23 years later. Note the absence of significant changes in bone levels between visits.

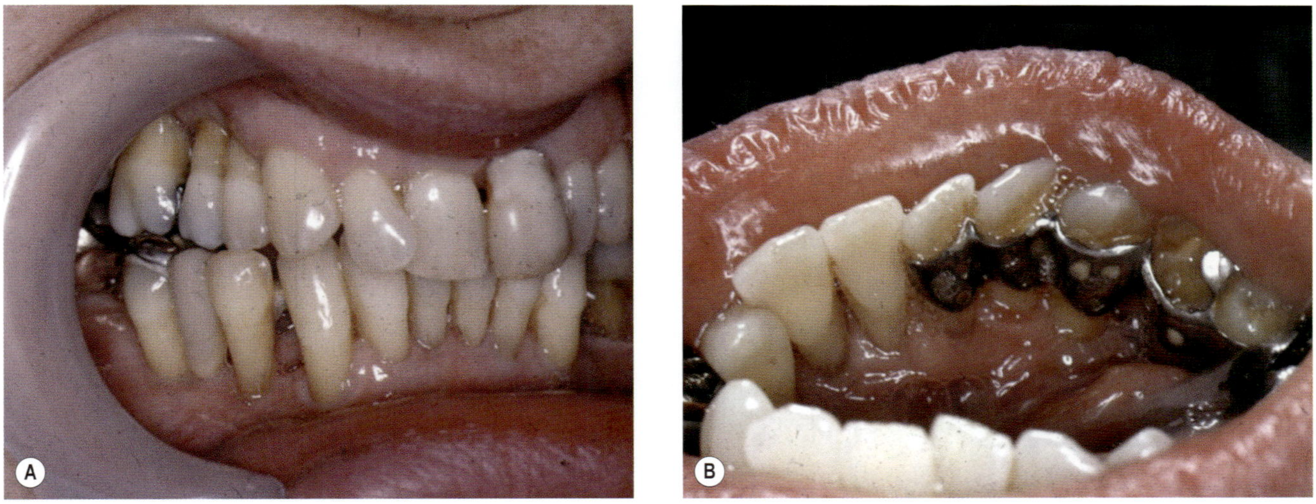

Fig 15.7 Clinical appearance of Case 4 at visit 23 years after initial therapy. Note the healthy periodontal tissues, severe recession and Rochette splint on LR teeth.

of this because it did not show very much during normal function and there was no associated sensitivity of root caries. The patient also considered that retention of her teeth was a much more important outcome than the negative effects of the recession. Second, the provision of the splint had successfully managed the functional impairment caused by the mobility of LR45 particularly. The type of splint used is a Rochette splint, which was the earliest type of metal/resin-bonded splint and depends entirely on mechanical retention between the composite and the metal to prevent failure. Consequently, failure of these splints in the medium term was probably the norm, whereas some of the approaches used today are much less likely to fail. In this case, the remarkable survival of the splint may be the result of the additional retention features incorporated, including a buccal occlusal clasp on the LR5 and the rest seat on LR4. Nevertheless, the survival of this splint for this period of time is unusual. In addition, as can be seen, the bulk of the metal used in this type of splint is a perfect plaque trap for interdental plaque formation. Again, because of the patient's high compliance and dexterity with plaque control measures, further disease has been prevented.

Summary

Managing the consequences of periodontal disease presents many major challenges and may require a range of techniques and specialist expertise. When carefully executed, periodontal therapy is usually extremely effective but crucially requires an adequate maintenance plan tailored to individual patient risk and needs.

Section 3

Introduction to dental implantology

Chapter 16

Indications for dental implant treatment

Patients often present with a desire to replace missing teeth or are faced with the need to have teeth extracted for a variety of reasons (Figures 16.1 and 16.2). Replacement of teeth with fixed implant restorations or the use of implants to support and retain removable dentures are evidence-based treatment options with the potential for very high success rates. Often, alveolar bone and soft tissue also require replacement, so implant treatment frequently involves replacement of alveolar tissues using both biological and prosthetic means.

This chapter discusses indications for dental implants by considering the factors shown in Table 16.1.

Why does the patient wish to replace missing teeth?

To improve aesthetics?

The wish to replace missing teeth is often understandably driven by a desire to smile with confidence and conform to socially accepted norms of appearance.

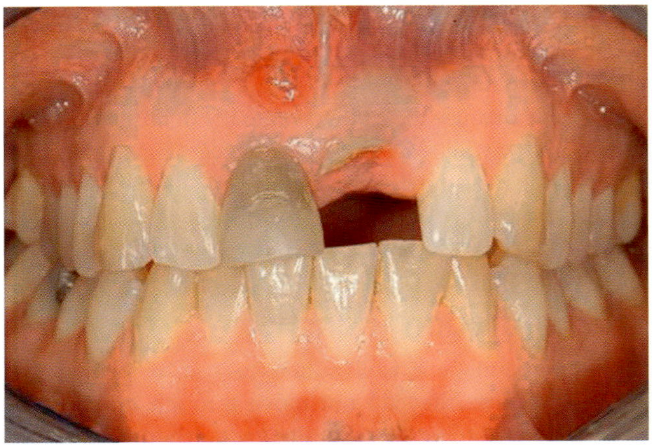

Fig 16.1 Both of the central incisors have suffered irreparable damage as a result of trauma. Periradicular infection at the upper right central incisor is manifest as a fluctuant swelling on the buccal mucosa.

To improve masticatory function?

Because teeth perform keys roles in mastication of food, their absence often causes compromise in chewing function and may also indirectly affect nutritional status by influencing food choices.

To improve speech function?

The presence of teeth and alveolar structures is critical in production of certain speech sounds. Their absence can affect speech intelligibility (how an individual is able to communicate through speech).

To enable wind instrument playing?

Some wind instruments require anterior teeth to be present to enable the appropriate embrasure to be formed around the mouthpiece of the instrument.

To regain what has been lost?

Loss of a body part (e.g., a tooth) may be associated with a deep-seated desire to replace what is missing, irrespective of the role played by the anatomical part.

What are the prosthodontic advantages of implant treatment?

To avoid tooth preparation and possible sequelae

Removal of tooth structure, the inevitable exposure of cut tooth surface to bacteria in saliva, and other procedures involved in attaching bridge retainers to teeth are associated

Table 16.1 Indications for dental implant treatment

- Why does the patient wish to replace missing teeth?
- What are the prosthodontic advantages of implant treatment?
- What is the problem with an existing fixed restoration or the natural teeth?
- Is there a denture-related problem the patient wishes to solve?
- Does the cause of missing or failing teeth have any influence on indication for implants?
- Does the timing of tooth loss have any influence on indication for implants?
- What are the main drawbacks of implant treatment?
- Are there contraindications to implant treatment?

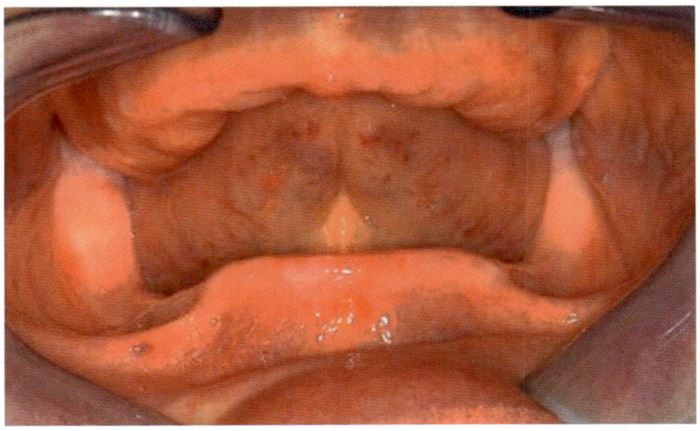

Fig 16.2 An edentulous patient with loose, uncomfortable dentures who wishes to discuss the possibility of using dental implants to improve the situation.

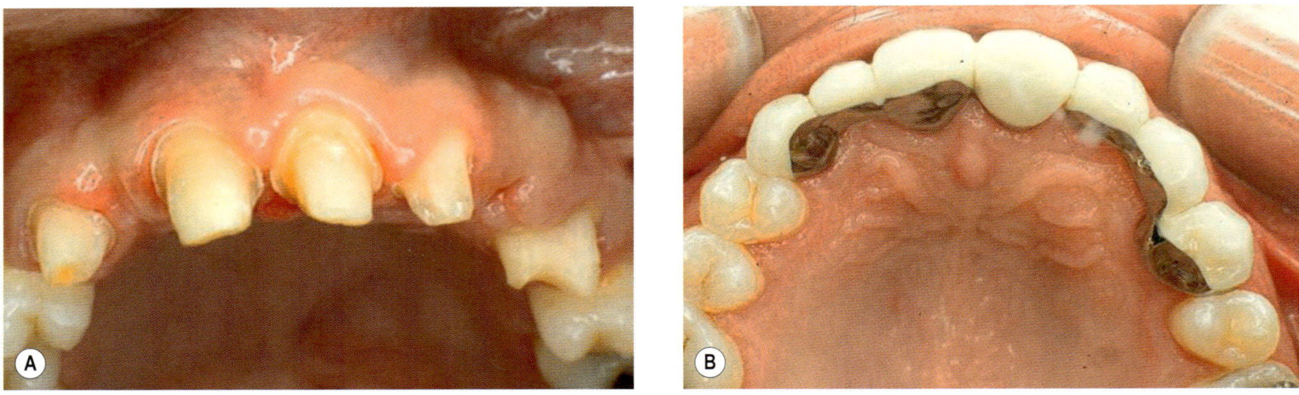

Fig 16.3 Developmental hypodontia treated with bridges utilizing full-coverage retainers necessitating removal of substantial amounts of tooth structure. The upper left central incisor carried a preexisting crown.

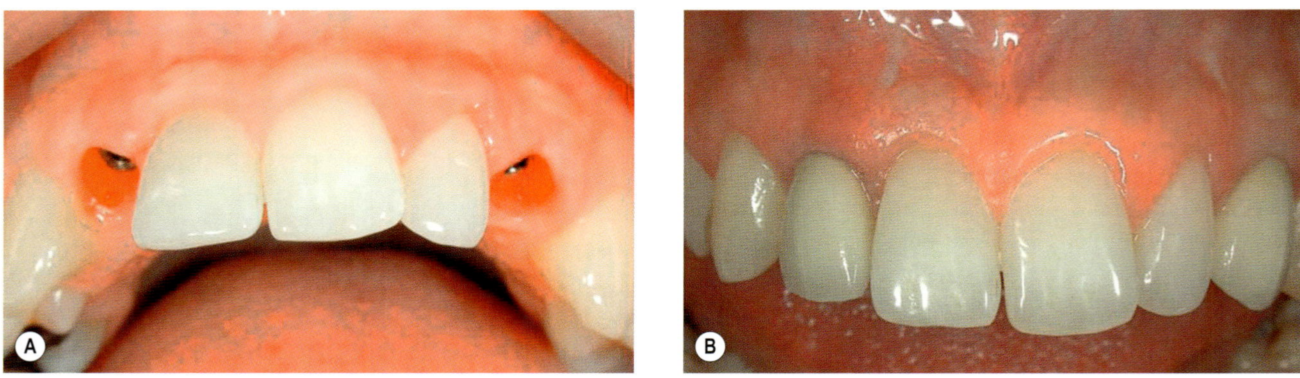

Fig 16.4 Developmental hypodontia treated with dental implants without the need to prepare intact teeth to attach bridge retainers.

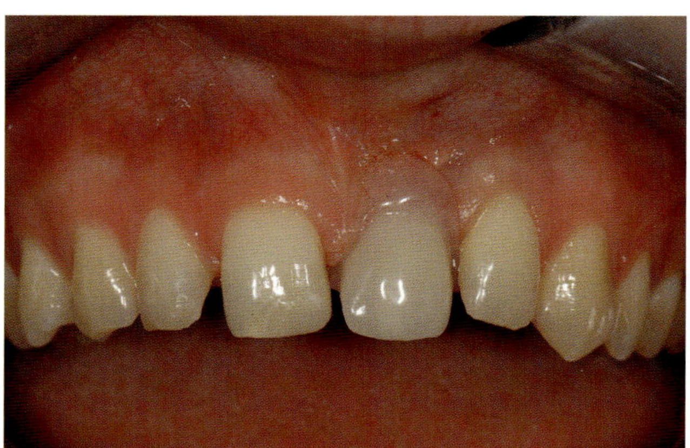

Fig 16.5 This patient, who has a missing upper left central incisor that was replaced with a removable denture, wants to maintain the interdental spaces. A dental implant avoids the need for a connector, which would be difficult to hide from view, attaching a bridge pontic to abutment(s).

with a risk of pulp necrosis and the need for either extraction or endodontic treatment (Figures 16.3 and 16.4).

No need for connectors between pontic and abutment teeth

Implants are ideally suited to restoring missing teeth where there are interdental spaces, particularly in the aesthetic zone (Figure 16.5).

Avoids mechanical risks of conventional bridges

The longer the span of a fixed bridge, the higher the risk of mechanical complications such as superstructure fracture or decementation of a retainer. It follows that the longer the edentulous space, the more likely it is that implants are indicated as fixed tooth replacements.

The deep complete overbite—No need to accommodate a denture connector

When the mandibular incisors contact the palatal mucosa in the intercuspal position, it is difficult to provide a removable denture because the connection to the denture tooth will often produce an occlusal interference (Figure 16.6). A dental implant as the definitive replacement can circumvent this occlusal difficulty.

Concurrent use of an implant as an orthodontic anchor

Dental implants are well suited to use as orthodontic anchors because they do not move through the alveolus when subjected to low-level prolonged (orthodontic) forces. The prosthodontic advantage lies in the ability to use a provisional restoration on an implant as a guide to orthodontic alignment and ultimately to replace the provisional restoration with a definitive one (Figure 16.7).

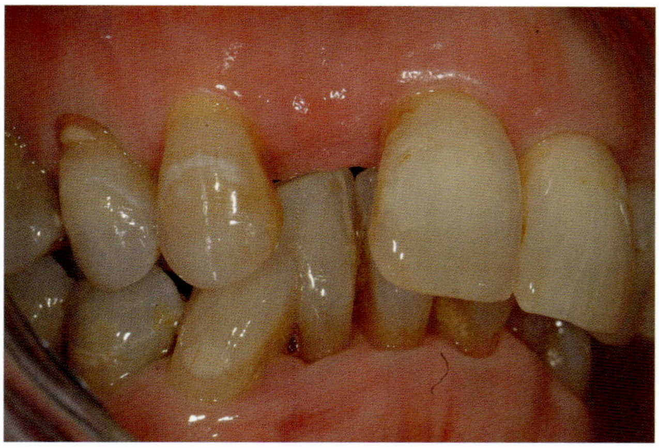

Fig 16.6 In occlusion, the deep complete overbite means that there is no space to accommodate a connector between a denture tooth and the major connector.

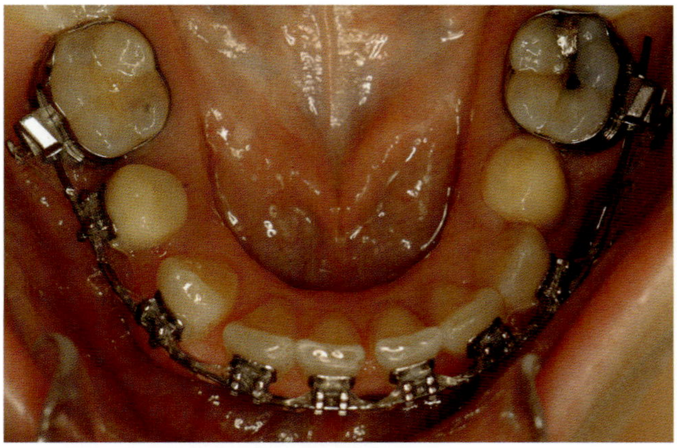

Fig 16.7 Four premolars have been replaced with two implants carrying provisional restorations. The right premolar is being used as an orthodontic anchor. Both implant crowns act as guides to appropriate tooth positioning within the arch.

Linking implant restorations together

Linking natural teeth together for whatever reason is a concern because of the potential for differential tooth movement causing failure at the tooth–restoration interface that can be difficult both to diagnose and to manage. Because implants have negligible differential movement, linking them together is prosthodontically acceptable (Figure 16.8). A practical advantage of linking implant restorations together is that it reduces the number of interdental contacts that may require adjustment in order to achieve accurate fit. Linking also provides the opportunity to share occlusal loads between a number of implants.

Retrievability of the restoration

It is common for an implant restoration to be attached to the underlying implant in a way that allows it to be retrieved. This can allow for repair, replacement, or inspection if necessary (Figure 16.9).

Denture retention and support

Removable dentures can be significantly enhanced by implants, which provide both support and retention (Figure 16.10). This is a particular advantage for a complete denture in the edentulous mandible. Recording the jaw relations can also be facilitated by incorporating attachments into the registration appliances.

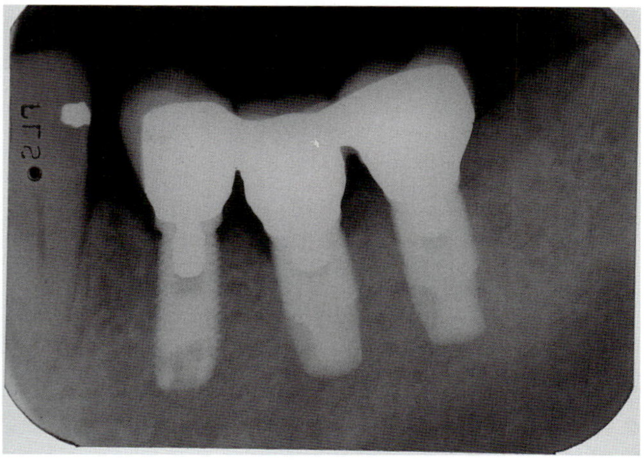

Fig 16.8 Implants in the posterior mandible linked by the restoration in order to help distribute occlusal loads.

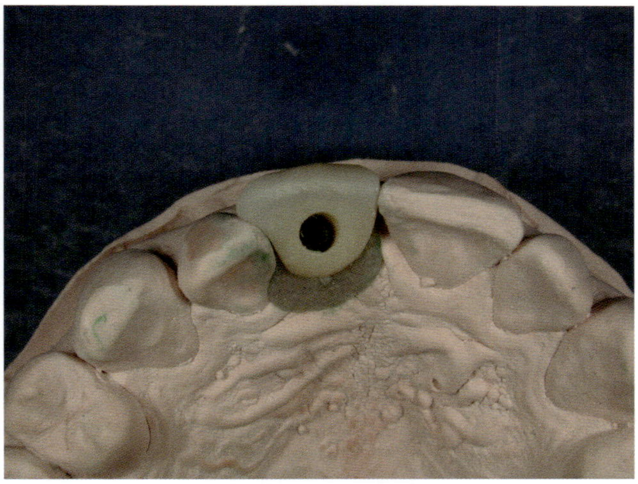

Fig 16.9 The upper right central incisor is replaced by a restoration screwed directly to an implant. The screw access hole is not visible from the front.

To take advantage of machined fitting parts

One of the challenges of conventional crown and bridge dentistry is the need to capture accurate impressions of tooth preparations and adjacent gingival margins. Implant dentistry allows for the easy use of machined components to facilitate the impression stages of construction (Figure 16.11).

What is the problem with an existing fixed restoration or the natural teeth?

Problematic bridgework

Both conventional and minimal preparation adhesive bridges may fail for a number of reasons, including failure of the cement lute. It may be possible to restore the abutment teeth and improve their prognosis by leaving them as single units, replacing the missing teeth with implant restorations.

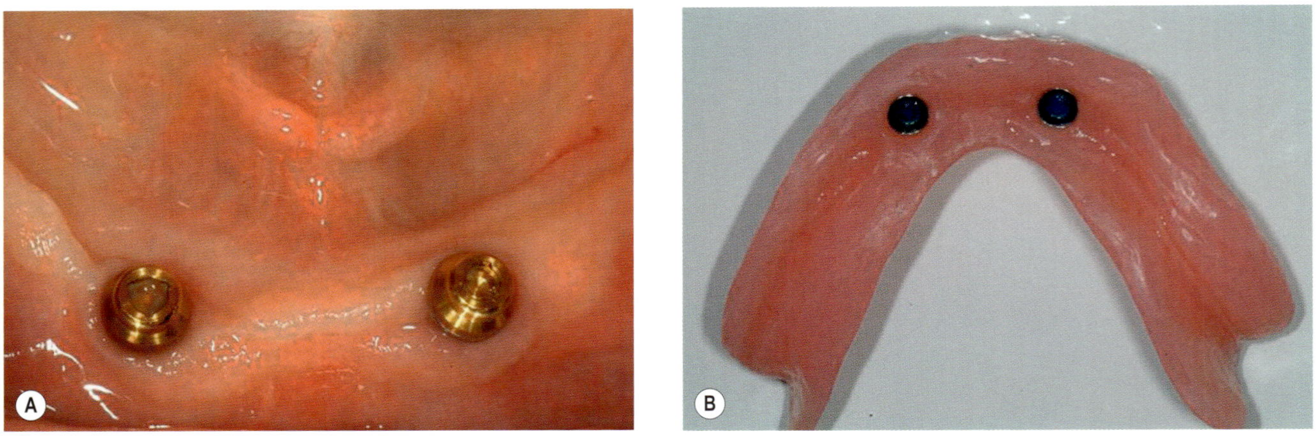

Fig 16.10 An overdenture using implants for both support and retention.

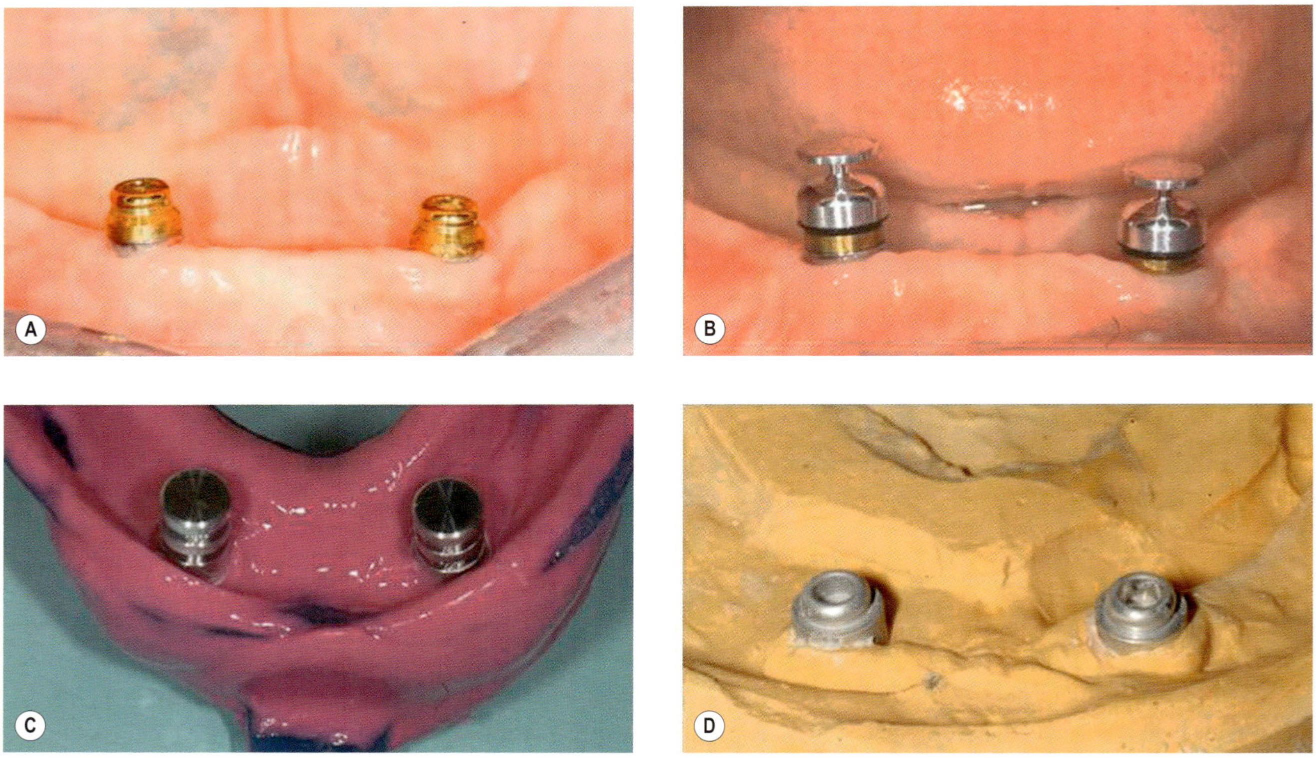

Fig 16.11 Transfer impression copings used to generate a working cast containing abutment replicas for an edentulous patient in preparation for a mandibular overdenture.

Metallic retainers have the potential to significantly alter the shade of abutment teeth, particularly if they are thin. This problem is circumvented by using implants (Figure 16.12).

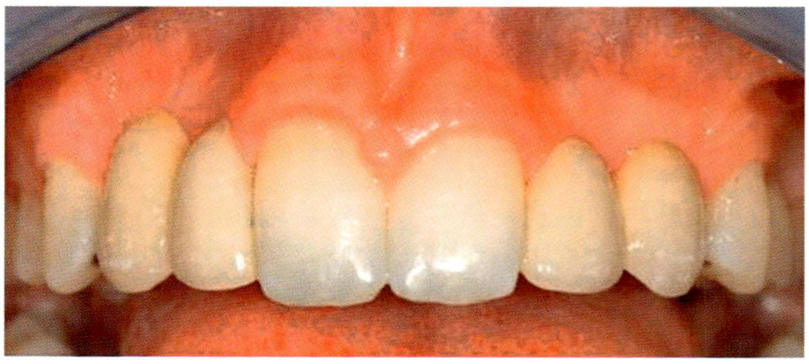

Fig 16.12 The grey discoloration at the central incisors due to adhesive bridge retainers attached to their palatal aspects would be avoided by the use of dental implants.

Periodontal disease

Periodontal disease may manifest as tooth hypermobility and migration causing discomfort, aesthetic problems, and occlusal difficulties. Alone or in combination, the latter can complicate the design of fixed and removable restorations. It may be appropriate to remove such teeth when providing dental implants. It is also important to consider the risk of future peri-implant infection arising from pathologic bacteria in the remaining periodontium and disease susceptibility of the individual. Unfortunately, periodontal disease causes loss of alveolar bone, which can severely compromise the volume of bone available for optimal implant placement (see Chapter 18).

Unrestorable teeth

Apart from replacement of missing teeth, decisions are often required about teeth that are badly affected by caries, pulp/periapical disease, root resorption, and mechanical failure. There are many factors to take into account when making what can be difficult decisions about the predictability of restoring teeth compared with extraction and replacement with implants.

Is there a denture-related problem the patient wishes to solve?

Improved removable denture

By helping to support and retain removable dentures, a number of denture-related problems can be overcome, such as a tendency for loose dentures to stimulate a gag reflex or dentures that are loose and painful because they move in function. Implants give the potential to construct dentures without the need for visible clasps or palatal coverage (Figure 16.13).

Fixed restoration instead of removable denture?

It is not difficult to appreciate the desire patients may have to avoid a removable denture altogether (Figure 16.14). Not only is there the potential for improved function but also ageing-related perceptions of removable dentures may be avoided.

Unfortunately, the pattern of alveolar resorption in the maxilla can make it difficult to construct fixed implant restorations that match the aesthetic and phonetic qualities of removable dentures. Multiple implants and the possible need for bone grafts also make this style of restoration expensive.

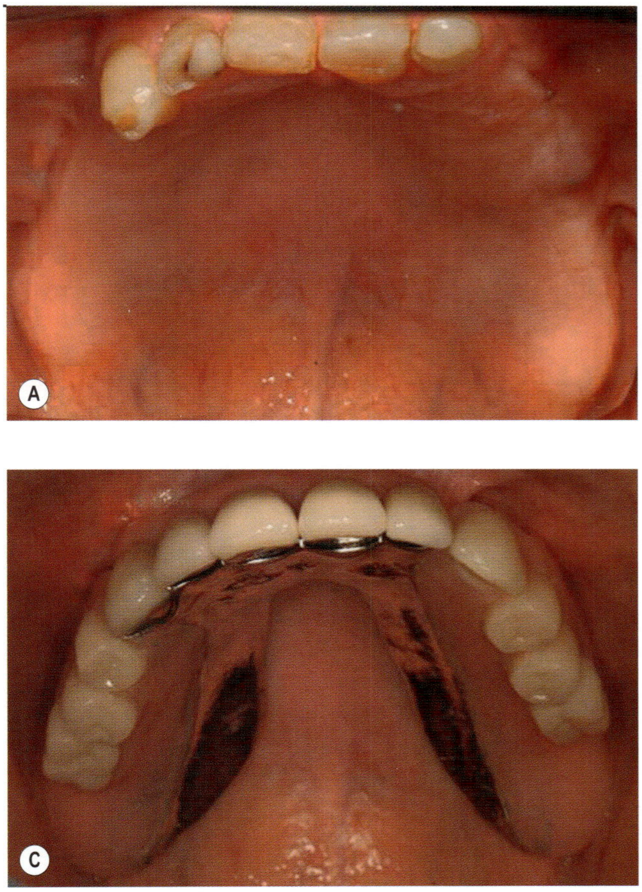

Fig 16.13 A bar-retained implant overdenture in conjunction with maxillary anterior crowns.

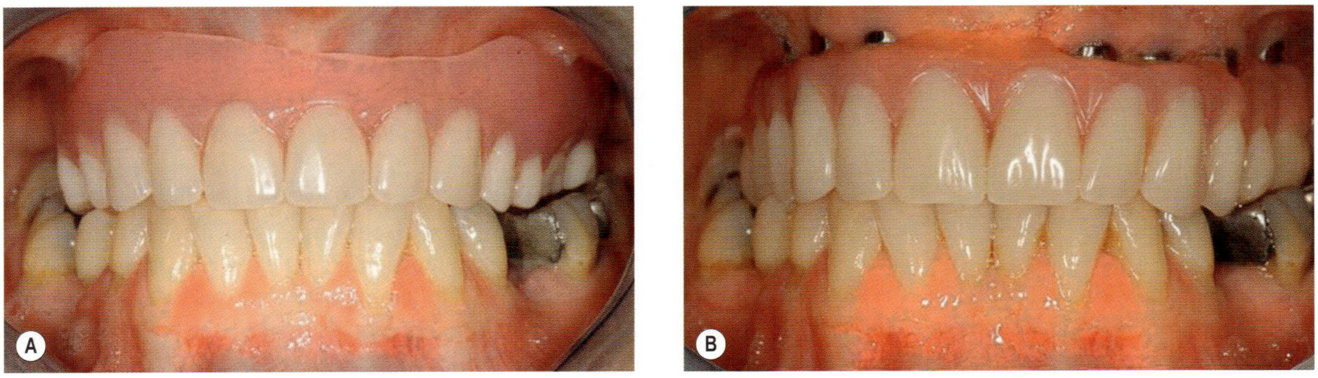

Fig 16.14 A fixed implant restoration (B) to replace a removable denture (A) in a patient with an edentate maxilla.

Does the cause of missing or failing teeth have any influence on the indication for implants?

In some situations, the cause of tooth loss may have a particular bearing on planning, treatment, and success of implant restorations. Pertinent factors are discussed in the following sections.

If the patient is involved with medicolegal proceedings related to the loss of teeth, there may be an expectation that damage payments will fund implants. All parties must be fully aware of the circumstances and claim status.

Periodontal disease

Loss of alveolar bone, complications due to further tooth loss, and the risk of future peri-implant disease pose challenges and limitations for this group of patients.

Congenital/developmental absence

Failure of development of permanent teeth (and supporting tissues) can result in inadequate alveolar volume for dental implants. Malposition and malformation of the permanent teeth that do develop pose additional challenges. These patients may benefit from specialist multidisciplinary management (Figure 16.15).

Patients in this category may also present at a young age when dental implants may not be advisable. Once integrated, implants will not migrate with the growing alveolus as healthy teeth do, so they can become malpositioned by the time craniofacial growth slows.

Ectopic teeth that fail to erupt can pose an obstruction to implant positioning. Removal of ectopic teeth to allow implant insertion may result in an alveolar defect that can complicate implant placement.

Caries

Planning for implants is more straightforward if the oral environment is stable. If caries is ongoing, it may mean that further tooth loss will occur with deleterious consequences for a long-term plan involving implants.

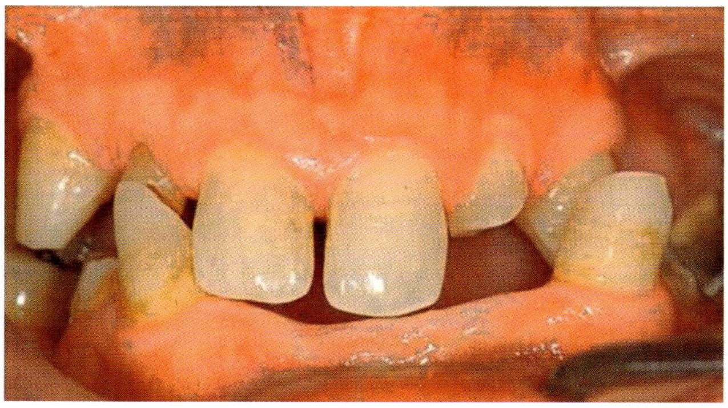

Fig 16.15 Failure of teeth to develop makes implant provision for this patient challenging for several reasons.

Related to treatment for head and neck cancer

Compromised teeth may need to be extracted when radiotherapy is to be used to treat head and neck cancer. Side effects of radiotherapy, such as oral dryness and poor-quality mucosa, can significantly affect the success of mucosa-borne removable dentures, making implant-supported restorations a helpful option. However, there is a risk of precipitating osteoradionecrosis if implants are placed in irradiated alveolar bone.

Tumour excision may involve dentoalveolar structures leaving a range of anatomical defects that may be amenable to restoration with fixed or removable prostheses (Figure 16.16). The need for ongoing tumour surveillance must be borne in mind when designing restorations for these patients.

Trauma

Young adults who have lost individual or small numbers of teeth as a result of trauma frequently present seeking replacement with implants. Implants may be particularly desirable if adjacent teeth are intact and would require significant irreversible adjustment to fashion them into bridge abutments. More extensive trauma may be accompanied by loss of alveolar or even basal bone (Figure 16.17). Resulting defects may require bone and soft tissue grafts to create sufficient alveolus to provide support and aesthetic frame for implants. There will be a limit to what is feasible and realistic in each case. It is important to consider whether lifestyles that pose a risk of traumatic damage to the teeth could likewise leave implant restorations at risk of damage.

Root resorption

Teeth that undergo replacement root resorption during alveolar development may produce alveolar deficiency because a possible effect of tooth ankylosis is to inhibit local alveolar growth (Figure 16.18). The result may be a challenging vertical and horizontal alveolar volume deficiency. If replacement root resorption takes place after growth has ceased, then there is the potential for more bone to remain for an implant than would be the case after extraction of a nonresorbed root.

Periradicular infection

Residual periradicular infection has the potential to cause infection at an implant inserted in the vicinity (see Figure 16.1). Implant insertion immediately after extraction of a tooth with periradicular infection is likely to carry a greater risk than insertion at a later date when there has been a chance for residual infection to be resolved.

Periradicular infection is commonly associated with inflammatory bone resorption (Figure 16.19). Teeth that have been subjected to root surgery will also either have had periapical bone removed for surgical access or be associated with pathologic inflammatory bone resorption. Residual periradicular bone defects clearly have the potential to complicate implant insertion.

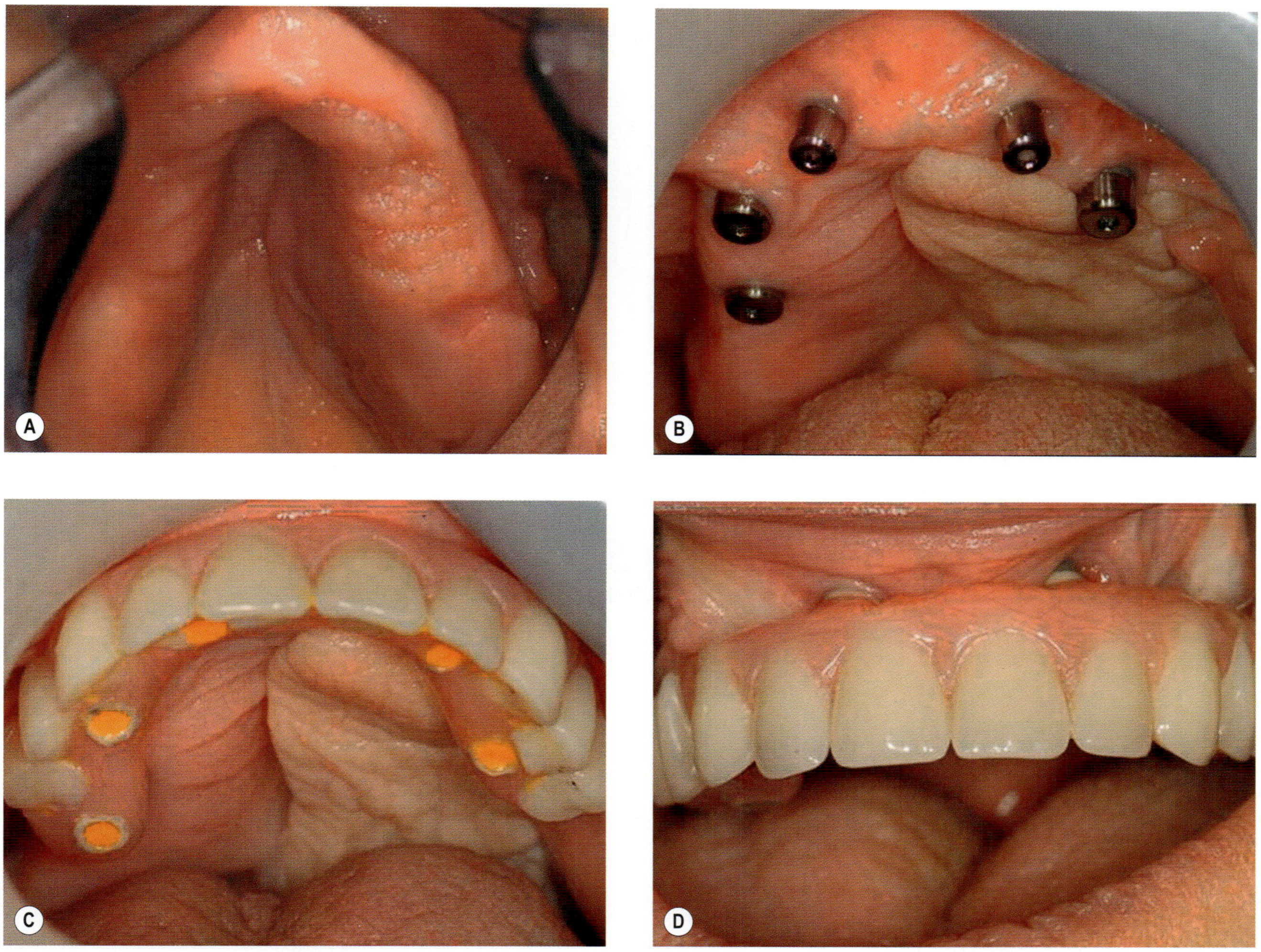

Fig 16.16 A fixed implant bridge for a patient with a malignant tumour of the left posterior maxillary alveolus. At presentation (A), note the enlarged left maxillary alveolus. The tumour has been excised and the defect reconstructed using a vascularized composite fibular graft that has subsequently had implants inserted (B). An acrylic bridge is in place with silicone material used for provisional screw access hole closure (C and D). This patient did not receive radiotherapy.

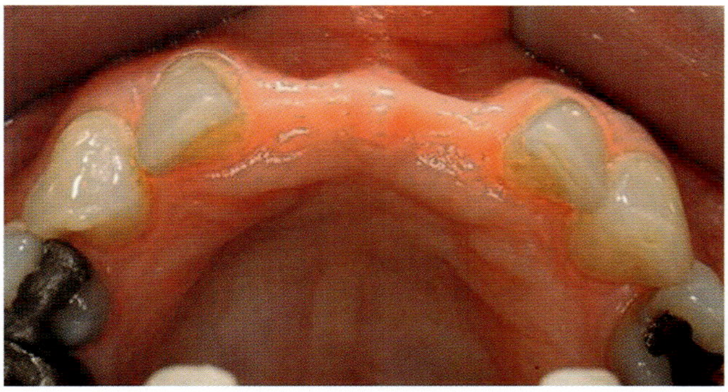

Fig 16.17 Alveolar loss is evident after healing in a patient whose maxillary central incisors have been lost as a result of trauma.

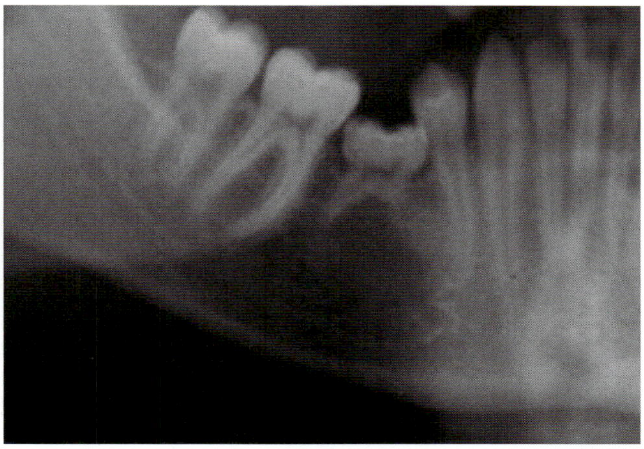

Fig 16.18 A mandibular second deciduous molar without a successor undergoing replacement resorption. It has inhibited local alveolar growth and gives the appearance of having become secondarily impacted as the adjacent teeth have tilted.

Does the timing of tooth loss have any influence on indication for implants?

Resorption of bundle bone around a tooth root and further localized alveolar remodelling begins when a tooth is lost. There may be a window of opportunity of up to 3 months following extraction or traumatic avulsion of teeth during which implant insertion can be more straightforward than if the alveolus is left to remodel for longer with likely loss of bone volume. Delaying may run the risk that implantation is not feasible without preliminary bone grafting to augment the alveolus (Figure 16.20).

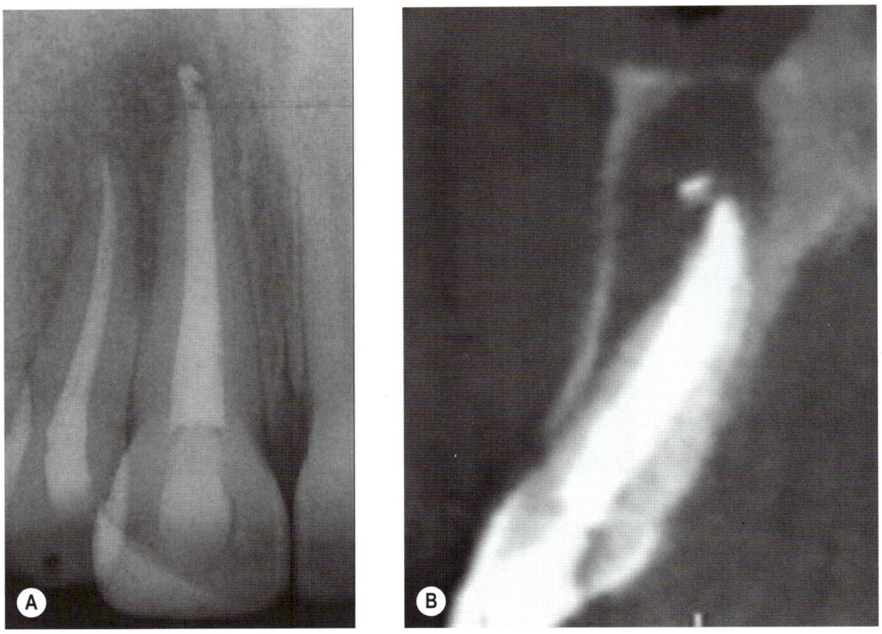

Fig 16.19 The cross section from a cone beam computed tomography scan (B) shows obvious periradicular bone loss at a root-treated maxillary right central incisor. The bone loss is much less easily seen on the periapical radiograph (A). Courtesy of Dr John Whitworth, Senior Lecturer, School of Dental Sciences, Newcastle University.

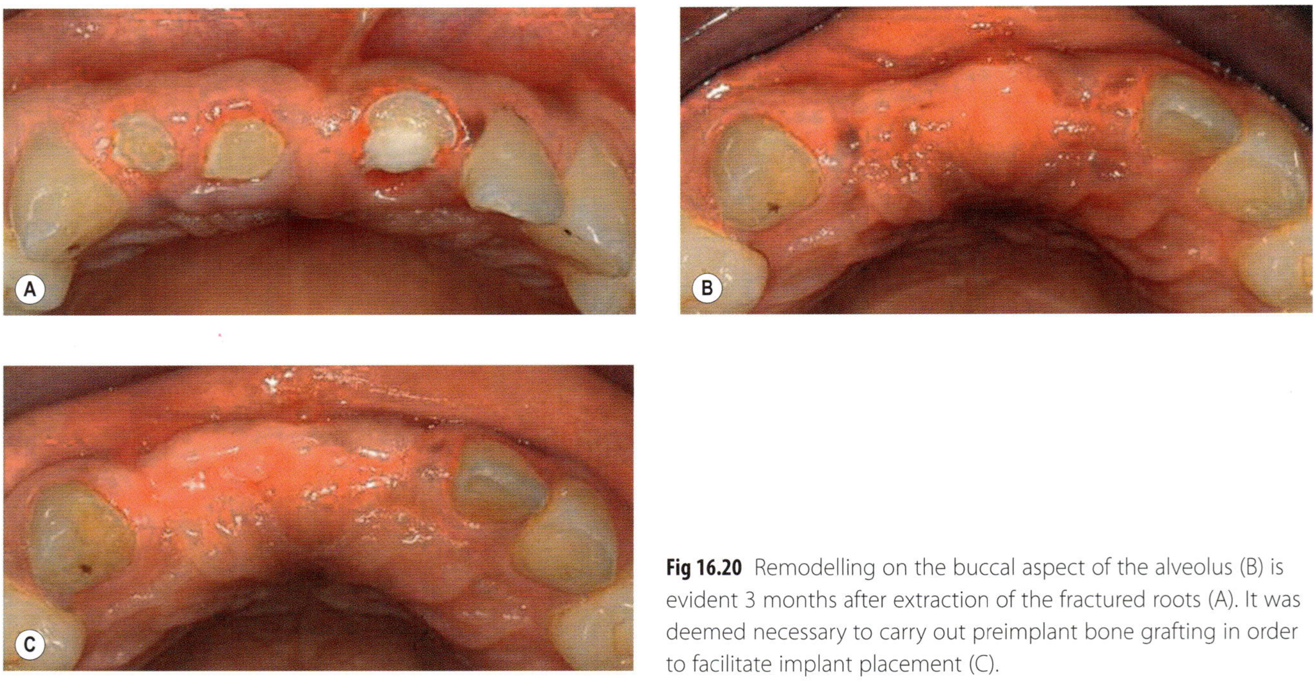

Fig 16.20 Remodelling on the buccal aspect of the alveolus (B) is evident 3 months after extraction of the fractured roots (A). It was deemed necessary to carry out preimplant bone grafting in order to facilitate implant placement (C).

What are the main drawbacks of implant treatment?

The need for surgery

Provision of implants involves some level of surgical intervention, which may be seen as a drawback. The extent of surgery, the risk of damage to neighbouring structures, the likelihood of postoperative side effects and complications, and patient responses will vary greatly depending on numerous patient- and operator-related factors (see Chapter 17).

Cost and duration of treatment

Implant treatment tends to be more expensive than non-implant alternatives. It is also common for treatments to extend over several months or longer because of the need to wait for hard and soft tissue healing.

Lack of implant product standardization

Because there are hundreds of ever-evolving implant systems in use worldwide, patients may have difficulty locating a dentist who is willing and able to maintain and perhaps refurbish or repair restorations made with an unfamiliar implant system. Although not inevitable, mechanical and biological complications do occur, particularly for implant overdentures.

Possible need for a tooth-free period

There are occasions when a patient may not be able to have tooth replacement for short periods (days) during stages of treatment: typically, immediately following surgery to provide bone grafts or place implants. It may also be necessary for a patient to use a removable denture for a period of time during treatment even when fixed implant restorations are the ultimate objective.

Difficulty achieving aesthetic perfection and easy access for oral hygiene

Unless patient expectations are managed effectively, there is a risk of patient dissatisfaction with the aesthetic outcome of implant treatment. The main challenge in this respect is in relation to achieving a perfectly natural-looking gingival frame around an implant restoration in the anterior maxilla (often referred to as the aesthetic zone).

Despite best efforts, the form of an implant superstructure may not be conducive to regular easy access for oral hygiene by the patient. In addition, what may be possible to clean when the patient has good dexterity and eyesight at the outset may prove impossible to clean if these faculties deteriorate with age or illness.

Are there contraindications to implant treatment?

To answer this question, a comprehensive patient assessment is required. Most contraindications are relative. See Chapter 17 for a detailed discussion.

Chapter 17

Assessing the patient for implant placement

A patient presents having lost the upper right central incisor as a result of trauma (Figure 17.1). What are the general factors to consider in relation to replacing the missing tooth with a dental implant?

This chapter discusses the general factors in the assessment of patients for treatment with dental implants (Table 17.1). Chapter 18 examines treatment planning for specific situations.

What are the patient's expectations and can they be safely met?

The goal of assessment is to provide the information required to formulate a detailed individually tailored treatment plan that is likely to safely meet the realistic expectations of the patient. Both implant and nonimplant options for tooth replacement should be considered and presented to the patient. All treatment options must be evaluated and discussed in light of the general oral and systemic health of the patient. To make these decisions, it is necessary to undertake a thorough assessment that involves taking a detailed history, performing a thorough examination, and carrying out or requesting and then interpreting the results of appropriate investigations.

Does the treating team have the ability to meet the expectations of the patient?

◇ *What training has been undertaken?*

Implant dentistry is usually introduced during undergraduate dental training but often only in theory with little or no practical experience. This situation is changing as implant dentistry becomes more commonplace. Where regulation of dentistry exists, implant dentistry is regarded as an area of practice that requires additional appropriate postgraduate training both for the dentist and for the other members of the dental team.

◇ *Is the appropriate equipment available and are the practice premises suitable to carry out implant dentistry?*

In addition to the high standards required for an effective, safe general dental practice, there are a number of additional requirements in order to undertake implant dentistry. For example, it is necessary to have the appropriate product-specific instruments such as screwdrivers available. If surgical implant dentistry is being carried out, additional instruments and equipment are required, such as a speed-reducing motor control unit, effective suction (with backup equipment to manage any malfunctions), and a range of implants and matched drills. The room used for operating must have effective lighting; enough space for layout of sterile instruments; and facility for proper surgical scrub, gowning, and gloving procedures. The ability to obtain detailed images of the jaw anatomy may require that computed tomography (CT) be used. CT should be easily accessible either in the practice or through a local referral. Intravenous sedation is a useful patient management adjunct in implant dentistry, and its use according to published standards requires dedicated equipment, premises, and training.

Is the patient able to give valid informed consent?

In order for the patient to make a decision about whether to proceed with implant treatment (or not), a number of key aspects of care need to be made clear, and these must be documented in the patient's record. To assist this process, written information with images and/or accredited website addresses about implants are helpful, along with a detailed costed treatment plan and terms and conditions. Patients should also be informed about what the evidence base reveals about likely success rates of similar treatment carried out under similar conditions and by dentists with comparable levels of experience.

◇ *What are the time-scales for the completion of treatment?*

Implant treatments tend to take longer than conventional dentistry. Patients need to be made aware of the likely number, frequency, and duration of appointments. They need to be advised that some treatments require periods of extended healing to allow for tissue maturation. Patients need this kind of information to plan how treatment can fit with occupational and lifestyle commitments.

◇ *Will the patient be able to attend for maintenance?*

Prosthesis designs with a high anticipated maintenance requirement need to be planned with consideration of whether there is access to the appropriate level of dental follow-up care.

◇ *Can the patient afford the treatment and maintenance?*

Implant treatment is often costly. A clear statement of total changes, invoicing arrangements, and any fees for possible unexpected events is essential at the outset. In addition, financial arrangements and responsibilities for ongoing follow-up and maintenance as well as any warranty period must be made transparent. Some types of implant restoration, such as removable overdentures, predictably require ongoing adjustment or replacement of parts; patients need to understand this and the likely cost before committing to treatment.

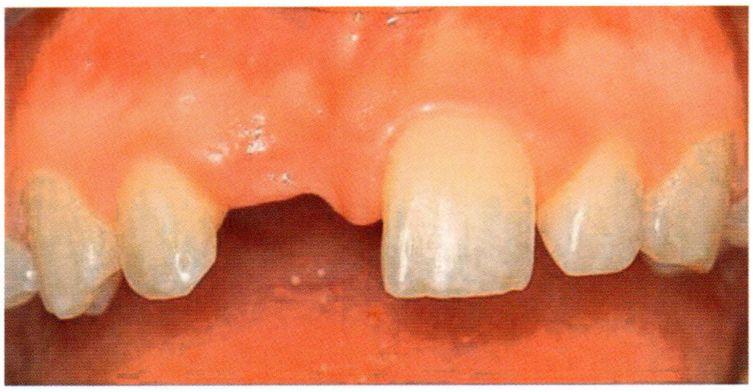

Fig 17.1 A patient presents with loss of a central incisor as a result of trauma.

Table 17.1 Questions that need to be addressed in a general assessment for possible implant treatment

- What are the patient's expectations and can they be safely met?
- Is it possible to communicate effectively to obtain a reliable history?
- Are there any pre-existing general factors that might compromise the establishment of bone and soft tissue integration?
- Will it be possible to access the oral cavity to perform the required diagnostic, surgical, and prosthodontic procedures with acceptable risk?
- Is the patient likely to tolerate surgery, anaesthetic, and anxiety management techniques with acceptable risk?
- Is there a risk from ionizing radiation in pregnancy?
- Is there any risk of compromised wound healing due to underlying medical conditions or the effect of current or past therapies?
- Is the oral environment stable and disease-free?
- Is the patient's age relevant?
- Are there any lifestyles or habits that might influence treatment options or that might pose a risk to implant restoration longevity?

◈ *Might there be periods during treatment without tooth replacement and how might teeth be replaced temporarily?*

Although it is sometimes possible to restore implants with dental restorations at the time of implant placement, it is frequently necessary to use other means of tooth replacement for a period following extraction, bone grafting, or implant placement. The motivation for seeking implant treatment is often to avoid or do away with a removable denture, so patients need to be fully informed about any need to use removable prosthesis during treatment. This information is particularly pertinent for patients with no removable denture experience who aspire to make the transition from a failing dentition to fixed implant restorations. There are also circumstances in which the patient may be advised not to use any form of tooth replacement. This is typically for short periods following preparatory grafting or implant placement, with consequent aesthetic and functional compromise.

◈ *What side effects from surgery are to be expected, and what are the more unusual but significant risks?*

The side effects experienced after dental implant surgery are highly dependent on the details of the surgery and the tolerance and healing capacity of the patient. The perception of pain, for example, is not solely related to the degree of physical trauma but also the result of complex subjective and objective interactions. However, patients should be warned to expect some pain and swelling. Additional warnings about

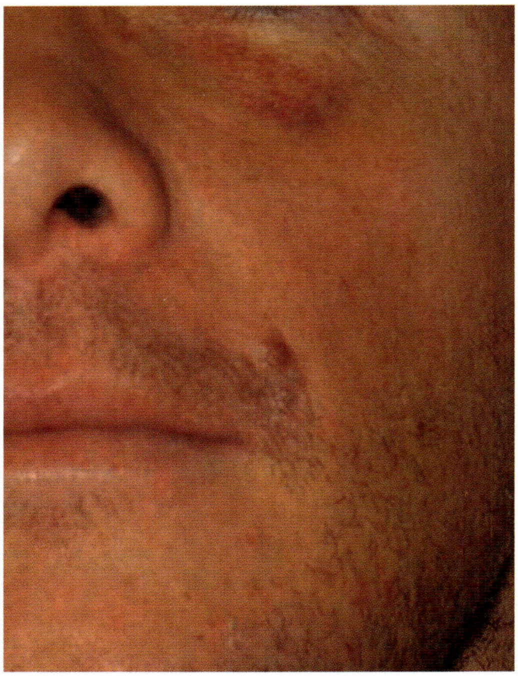

Fig 17.2 Infraorbital bruising 1 week following single implant placement with guided bone regeneration in the anterior maxilla.

common side effects may include skin or mucosal bruising due to haematoma and also the possibility of postoperative bleeding (Figure 17.2). Patients should be advised both verbally and in writing of what to expect and how to manage common side effects at home using simple remedies, such as cold compresses and over-the-counter analgesics.

There may be instances in which implant surgery carries a risk of more significant side effects, such as intraoperative bleeding or damage to a neurovascular bundle resulting in long-term pain and/or sensory deficit. Processes and procedures for minimizing the likelihood and managing these less common consequences must be in place.

◈ *Will treatment involve the use of animal-derived products?*

In order to try to optimize bone and soft tissue support for implant restorations, it is frequently necessary to carry out tissue augmentation using grafting materials. Patients need to be made aware of the origins of these materials because they may have objections to the use of animal- (xenogenic) and other human-derived (allogenic) products, and these objections need to be respected by the treating dentist.

◈ *What is the likelihood of being able to satisfy the aesthetic desires of the patient?*

This assessment requires a precise understanding of the desires and expectations of treatment outcome coupled with being able to predict situations in which suboptimal aesthetic outcome is possible or even likely.

To some degree, the difficulty in delivering satisfactory aesthetics is determined by how much of the teeth and surrounding gingiva (whether natural or prosthetic) the patient displays in day-to-day function. Those with lip morphology and function that hides the papillae and gingival margins may be more willing to accept aesthetic compromise at the white–pink junction than patients who display this area readily.

Patients who have thin periodontal biotype with long papillae and high gingival zeniths may be prone to gingival recession occurring both early on as a result of surgery and over time. Abutments and implants can sometimes be visible through thin tissues. These effects can significantly impair the aesthetic outcome.

Photographs and carefully produced diagnostic setups can be useful in order to demonstrate possible outcomes. If a compromise in aesthetics is predicted, it is very important that this information is communicated to the patient. In the latter circumstances, it is necessary to be satisfied that the patient's expectations have been moderated before proceeding with treatment.

Is it possible to communicate effectively to obtain a reliable history?

Does the patient have communication problems?

Effective clinical assessment, proposal of treatment plans, and receipt of valid informed consent rely to a large extent on effective interpersonal communication. Language barriers, visual and hearing impairment, as well as the ability of patient and dentist to be understood (intelligibility) affect the two-way process. Additional resources may be required, such as having an interpreter available.

Some psychiatric conditions impair a patient's ability to communicate, make judgements, or cooperate with treatment. Likewise, patients with learning impairment may not be able to comprehend treatment plans and risks.

Are there any pre-existing general factors that might compromise the establishment of bone and soft tissue integration?

The key feature of osseointegration is sustainable direct contact between living bone and the surface of an implant. A number of pre-existing general factors can interfere with the establishment of this phenomenon, and these need to be identified during the assessment. Some are very rare, and only the main factors are considered here. Local factors such as retained roots that might interfere with osseointegration are addressed elsewhere.

Does the patient smoke?

It is generally agreed that there is a relationship between patients who smoke and failure to achieve (primary implant failure) and maintain osseointegration (secondary implant failure). Smoking probably accounts for an approximate doubling of the failure rate up to 5 years after loading (5.5% for smokers compared to 2.9% in nonsmokers in one large retrospective study of more than 1500 patients) (Cavalcanti *et al.*, 2011). The risk is not clear-cut and is affected by factors such as the extent and duration of smoking, the type of bone being implanted, the type of implant, and whether any bone grafting has been carried out. Smoking is a risk factor for developing plaque-induced peri-implantitis, which can lead to secondary implant failure. These factors need to be carefully considered and discussed with the patient. It is an opportune time to counsel about the benefits of smoking cessation.

Has the patient had radiotherapy to the jaws?

Ionizing radiation is one of the primary modes of treatment for head and neck cancer. Bone exposed to therapeutic doses of radiation may undergo endarteritis obliterans, which results in bone marrow and mucosa having poor vascularity and impaired ability to repair. Not only is there a risk of failure to establish osseointegration but also the surgery to provide implant restorations could induce a process called osteoradionecrosis with potentially serious consequences. The crux of the dilemma lies in the fact that patients who have had radiotherapy sometimes have particular difficulties managing mucosa-borne removable dentures and stand to gain much from implant restorations. Each case must be considered individually to judge whether, with appropriate treatment protocols, risks can be kept acceptably low.

Have bisphosphonates ever been prescribed?

The bisphosphonates are a group of drugs used to reduce the risk of bone fracture in people with osteoporosis or to ameliorate some of the problems of malignant disease involving bone. Given the high prevalence of osteoporosis, particularly in postmenopausal women, it is likely that many patients of middle age or older will be taking bisphosphonates such as alendronate or zoledronate. Their prime mode of action is to slow bone turnover by inhibiting osteoclastic activity. In recent years, an association has been identified between bisphosphonates and a process known as osteonecrosis of the jaws. There are similarities to osteoradionecrosis with areas of bone becoming exposed and infected. Tooth extraction and jaw surgery, including implant surgery, are associated with an increased risk of osteonecrosis of the jaws that may not heal. The risk is much greater in patients who have an intravenous bisphosphonate administered to manage the side effects of malignant disease; implant surgery is contraindicated for these patients. Patients receiving bisphosphonates for osteoporosis carry a much lower risk of osteonecrosis of the jaws, with the risk being related to duration of use of the drug, extent of surgery, and the presence of additional risk factors such as smoking.

Does the patient suffer from diabetes?

Because diabetes can interfere with wound healing and resistance to infection, there is a low risk of failure of implant osseointegration in patients with diabetes. The risk is related to the level of diabetic (glycaemic) control.

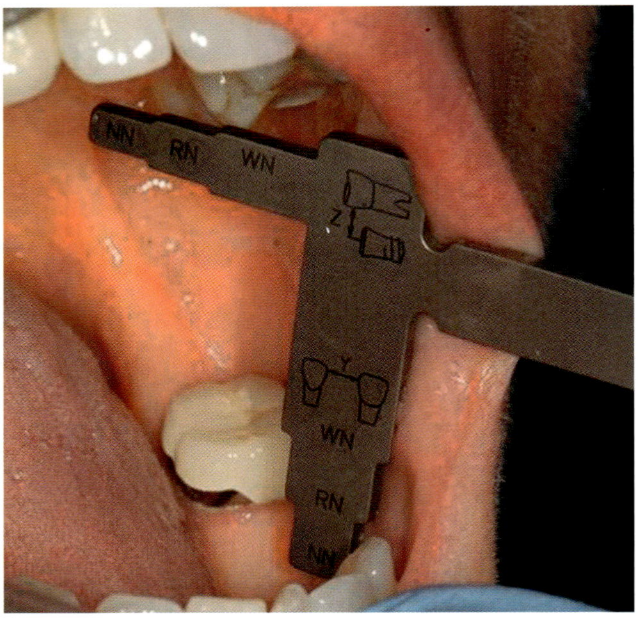

Fig 17.3 Assessing access for instrumentation to provide implant restoration in the posterior mandible.

Will it be possible to access the oral cavity to perform the required diagnostic, surgical, and prosthodontic procedures with acceptable risk?

Does the patient have a reduced oral aperture or mandibular opening range?

Implant dentistry involves the manipulation of small hand-held and machine-mounted instruments and implant components. Conditions such as scleroderma, arthritis, previous radiotherapy, and temporomandibular dysfunction may limit access. Assessment of access for instrumentation must be carried out at an early stage to gauge the feasibility of treatment (Figure 17.3).

Is the patient able to recline in the dental chair to allow the operator to work in a safe and acceptable position?

Patients who are unable to recline sufficiently make it very difficult to carry out operative dentistry, particularly in certain parts of the mouth. Patients with gastrointestinal reflux diseases, those with congestive cardiac failure, and women in the third trimester of pregnancy may fall into this category.

The first line of treatment for syncope is to lay the patient flat, and barriers to this manoeuvre, particularly in potentially anxiety-inducing situations such as implant surgery, carry risks of inadequate management of syncope and other medical emergencies.

Does the patient have a compromised airway protective reflex?

Implant dentistry requires a great deal of fine dexterity, and there is a real risk of dropping implant components and instruments in the mouth. Patients with certain neurological conditions or anatomical defects resulting from cancer surgery, for example, may not be able to mount an effective oropharyngeal reflex to prevent aspiration if an accident occurs.

Is the patient able to cooperate during assessment and treatment?

The degree to which the patient can remain relatively still during key moments of assessment and treatment will determine the extent of treatment that is possible. Some psychiatric and behavioural problems, epilepsy, and movement disorders such as Parkinson's disease may limit treatment options.

A common scenario is the patient who attributes his or her denture intolerance to a hypersensitive gag reflex and seeks treatment with fixed implant supported restorations. The difficulty for the implant dentist is to assess (1) whether the patient would tolerate the stages of assessment and treatment and (2) whether even fixed restorations would be tolerated once fitted.

Is the patient likely to tolerate surgery, anaesthetic, and anxiety management techniques with acceptable risk?

A regularly updated medical, drug, and allergy history is the key to identifying health factors that might compromise the ability of the patient to tolerate the surgery and anaesthetic techniques involved in placing dental implants. Communication with other health professionals may be necessary to clarify details and to request opinions about the fitness of the patient. Surgery for dental implants varies in extent from implant placement without the raising of a mucoperiosteal flap (transmucosal placement) to preparation of the alveolus with block bone grafts and multiple implant placements. It may be necessary to modify the treatment objectives in light of health risks.

How will the patient be anaesthetized?

For many patients undergoing single jaw implant placement, local anaesthetic alone is sufficient for intraoperative pain control. Intravenous sedation is a very useful anxiety management adjunct to local anaesthesia for implant surgery, and safe practice requires vital sign monitoring equipment as well as additional training and compliance with published protocols. General anaesthesia may be required for more extensive surgery, particularly for multiple implant placements in both jaws. The American Society of Anesthesiologists classification and body mass index are two ratings used to grade anaesthetic risk in preparation for intravenous sedation and general anaesthesia.

Is there a risk from ionizing radiation in pregnancy?

Radiography is an essential investigation during assessment, at certain stages of treatment, and for follow-up after completion of implant treatment. During the first trimester of pregnancy, the fetus is most at risk of damage caused by ionizing radiation. Most authorities agree that there is no risk to the fetus from dental diagnostic radiation. However, it is recommended that implant treatment be avoided during pregnancy to allay any concerns the patient may have about the effects of ionizing radiation. Delaying also avoids possible effects to the fetus from medications used around the time of implant surgery.

Is there any risk of compromised wound healing due to underlying medical conditions or the effect of current or past therapies?

General health factors may influence the ability to mount an effective soft and hard tissue healing response, thereby putting the patient at risk of postoperative infection or failure of osseointegration. For example, past radiotherapy, steroid, bisphosphonate, and immunosuppressant medications, as well as diabetes and disorders of haemostasis, all have the potential to interfere with wound healing. Once identified at the planning stage, decisions need to be made about whether risks are acceptable and whether specific precautions are required. Smokers are also at risk of compromised wound healing.

Is the oral environment stable and disease-free?

Is there any evidence of pulpal/periapical disease, active caries, heavily restored teeth at risk of mechanical failure, or tooth wear?

Dental implants are regarded as a long-term treatment modality and therefore require that the oral environment is disease-free and stable or that there is a plan to account for failure or removal of selected teeth or failing implants. A detailed oral assessment, which includes appropriate radiographs, is required. Deconstruction of questionable restorations may be required to establish individual tooth status and prognosis. Interventions may be necessary to attempt to establish an acceptable standard of oral health. In light of the oral assessment and initial therapies, it may transpire that the patient's best interests are to be managed with non-implant tooth replacement methods.

What is the risk of future peri-implantitis?

Does the patient have good oral hygiene?

Peri-implant and periodontal infection is related to the level of plaque control the patient is able to achieve. This is in turn related to the patient's dexterity and motivation. The patient should be able to demonstrate a good standard of oral hygiene before commencement of implant treatment, and this should be recorded using a plaque and bleeding index.

Is there a history of previous periodontitis or peri-implantitis?

The microflora associated with both periodontitis and peri-implantitis is similar. It has been established that both current and previously treated periodontitis are risk factors for future peri-implantitis. Smokers are at increased risk for future peri-implantitis. It is therefore important to ensure that existing periodontal disease is treated and disease control is documented prior to beginning implant treatment to reduce the risk of peri-implantitis.

Does the patient have a dry mouth?

Hyposalivation is a risk factor for caries and periodontal/peri-implant disease. The underlying cause should be identified and, if it is not possible to correct the cause, hyposalivation should be managed by saliva stimulation or replacement therapies before any implant treatment.

Has there been a course of orthodontic treatment?

Are tooth positions stable?

After completion of orthodontic treatment, there is a tendency for teeth to migrate back to where they were moved from (relapse tendency). The extent to which this unwanted movement may occur is related to the type of orthodontic movements that have taken place, the stabilizing effect of the final interocclusal contacts, the design of any restorations to replace missing teeth, and patient compliance with using a removable retainer to help stabilize tooth positions. Implant restorations that are not connected to natural teeth may not produce inherent tooth positional stability. This must be taken into account when planning the design and maintenance of implant restorations following orthodontic treatment (Figure 17.4).

Is gingival architecture mature?

Orthodontic treatment can also result in gingival architecture that is immature (incomplete passive eruption). Precise implant positioning for the best long-term result depends on stable adjacent landmarks at the time of implant placement. Preparatory mucogingival surgery may be needed to achieve mature gingival architecture at the outset.

Is the patient's age relevant?

Has craniofacial growth ceased?

Being effectively ankylosed to alveolar bone, dental implants will not change position in the way natural teeth do as the alveolus develops during growth or during postmaturational dentoalveolar compensation. In other words, the position of a dental implant relative to adjacent teeth will alter if local alveolar growth is incomplete at the time of osseointegration. Craniofacial growth completion varies according to jaw region and is substantially complete by early adulthood. An implant may become relatively malpositioned if placed too early, typically appearing infraoccluded with a gingival margin more apically positioned

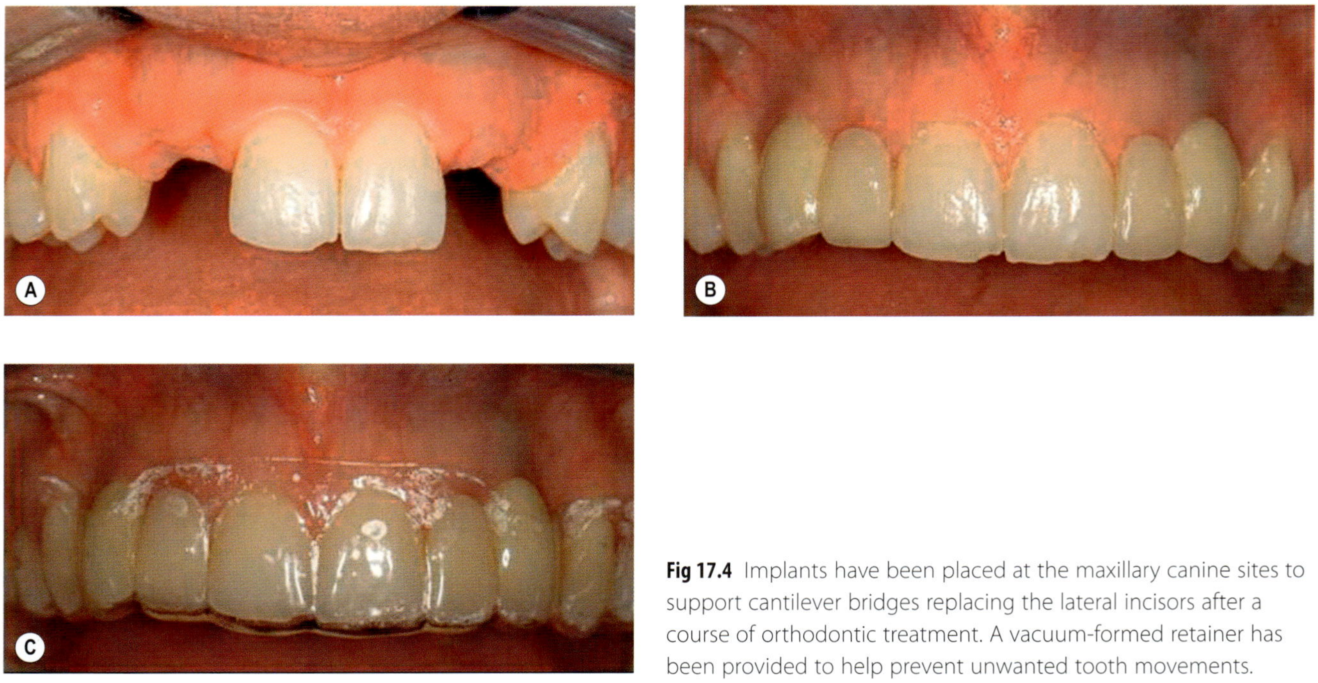

Fig 17.4 Implants have been placed at the maxillary canine sites to support cantilever bridges replacing the lateral incisors after a course of orthodontic treatment. A vacuum-formed retainer has been provided to help prevent unwanted tooth movements.

than adjacent natural teeth, resulting in possible aesthetic compromise and change in occlusal scheme.

Are there age-related co-morbidities?

Older age itself is not a risk factor for failure of osseointegration. However, age is important inasmuch as ill health, which may interfere with tolerance to implant procedures and compliance with maintenance regimes, is correlated with increasing age.

Are there any lifestyles or habits that might influence treatment options or that might pose a risk to implant restoration longevity?

Abnormally high occlusal loads acting over prolonged periods of time can have damaging consequences for the mechanical integrity of dental restorations and attachment mechanisms linked to implants. High loads may also jeopardize the bone–implant interface. Parafunctions such as daytime clenching and night bruxing are associated with abnormal load magnitude and loading direction and may be evident during assessment as attritive-type tooth wear.

Sudden loads—sustained, for example, through contact sports—may also put implant restorations at risk. If identified at the planning stage, alternatives to implants, design modifications, and protective appliances aimed at ameliorating the potential damage may be feasible.

The decision to proceed with treatment must consider the overall risks weighed against the likely benefits of implant restoration or alternative treatment options.

Chapter 18

Treatment planning

What is the overall treatment objective?

The key to developing any treatment plan is to have a clear objective. The terms *tooth-driven implant placement* and *prosthodontically driven implant placement* have been coined to emphasize this fundamental principle. Simply placing implants in any available bone without considering the restorative requirements risks restorations that have aesthetic and functional compromise, are difficult or impossible to keep clean, are prone to failure, or, at worst, are unrestorable and need to be removed.

This chapter discusses the key questions that need to be addressed during the planning process (Table 18.1). What follows is a series of theoretical planning steps. It is not intended that these steps are considered one after another in clinical practice. Rather, assessment of a case would involve a synthesis of these steps.

Is the final restoration to be fixed or removable by the patient?

Most patients have a desire for fixed restorations, and when small numbers of teeth are missing, this is usually feasible. However, for edentulous patients or when there is a large alveolar deficiency, detailed assessment may show that implant overdentures are the restoration of choice or may be the only realistic option.

What are the diagnoses and constraints for treatment and maintenance?

Chapter 16 considered the reasons why a patient may seek implant treatment and the oral diagnoses that need to be taken into consideration when planning and undertaking implant treatment. The holistic assessment described in Chapter 17 puts the patient's expectations and tolerance to treatment in perspective.

What are the aesthetic goals?

Which teeth are to be replaced in part-dentate patients?

If teeth have migrated or erupted into abnormal positions, or where there is marked dentoalveolar disproportion, the number and form of missing teeth to be replaced are not always clear-cut. This is quite often the case when teeth are missing for developmental reasons. Extractions or orthodontic tooth movements may be required to allow appropriate numbers and sizes of tooth replacements (Figure 18.1).

What is the ideal form and position of the individual teeth to be replaced?

The precise external form of a proposed tooth replacement has a major influence not only on the appearance of the final restoration but also on numbers of implants and their positioning. The space occupied by the proposed replacement, whether teeth or alveolus, is referred to as the *prosthetic envelope*. Several methods can be used to help establish this aspect of the proposed restoration from both the aesthetic and the occlusal standpoint (Figures 18.2 and 18.3). Stone casts and photographs of a previously satisfactory tooth arrangement as well as the form of failing restorations or teeth can give clues about the desired end result. In addition to assisting the dentist, diagnostic aids such as these assist dentist–patient communication and help the patient envisage what is proposed.

What is the ideal soft tissue frame of the teeth to be replaced?

The frame of gingiva around teeth is as important as the teeth in producing satisfactory aesthetics. Trial dentures and wax-based trial prostheses can help both dentist and patient visualize possibilities and limitations for the soft tissue frame around possible implant restorations (Figure 18.4).

Table 18.1 Questions that need to be addressed for planning dental implants

- What is the overall treatment objective?
- What are the diagnoses and constraints for treatment and maintenance?
- What are the aesthetic goals?
- What are the occlusal objectives?
- What are the requirements to facilitate access for oral hygiene?
- What are the ideal implant positions to satisfy the aesthetic, occlusal, and hygiene goals?
- What moderating factors point to a departure from "one implant per missing tooth" for fixed restorations?
- How many implants for overdentures?
- What are the ideal implant product features to satisfy the aesthetic, occlusal, and hygiene goals?
- Is satisfactory volume and quality of bone available to house the chosen implant products in the selected positions?
- Will the peri-implant soft tissue be appropriate?
- If bone and/or soft tissue is lacking, can it be created?
- If bone or soft tissue is lacking, is it possible to proceed accepting the risk of compromise?
- How will the patient make the transition to implant restoration?
- What is the stage-by-stage plan of treatment?

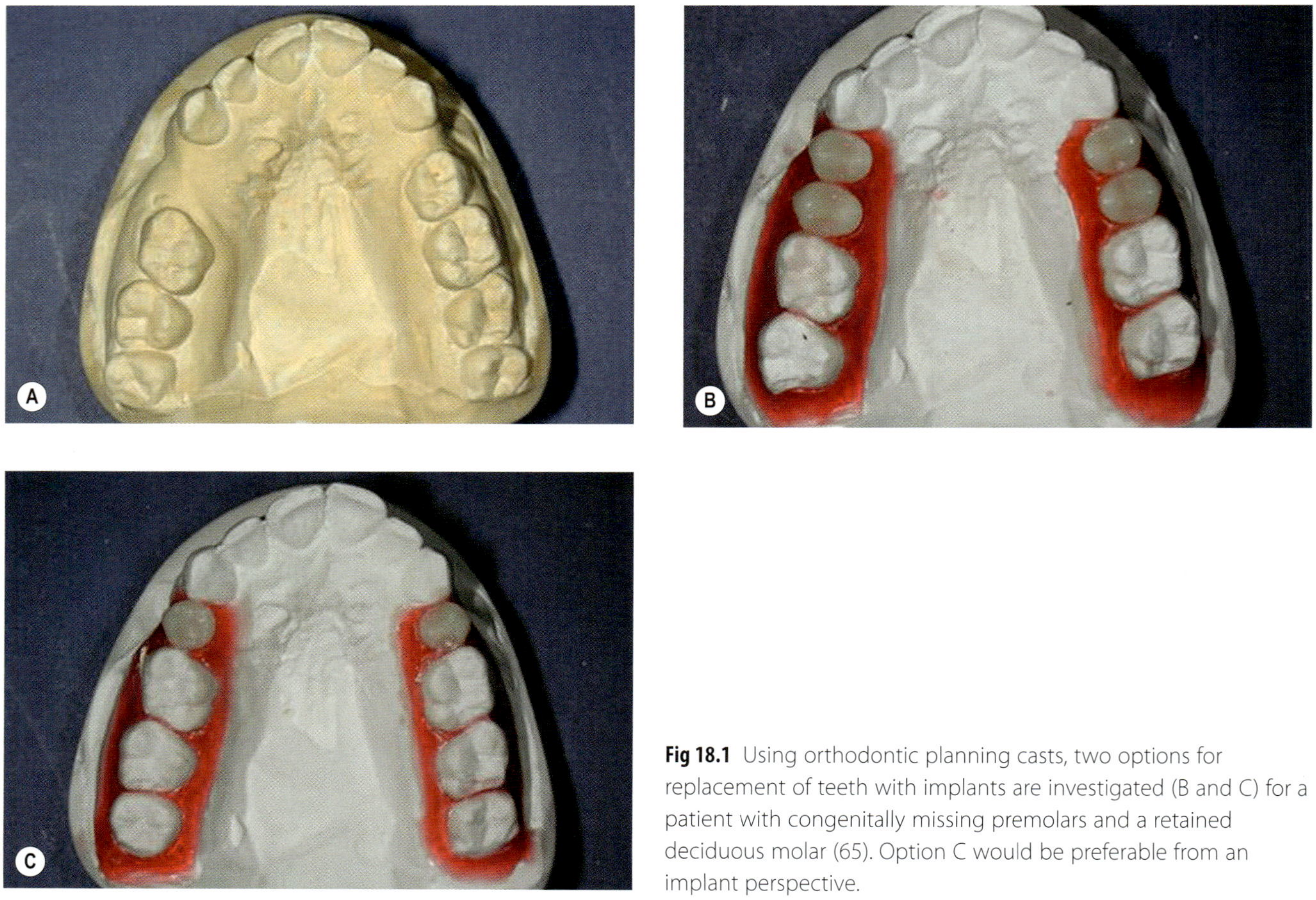

Fig 18.1 Using orthodontic planning casts, two options for replacement of teeth with implants are investigated (B and C) for a patient with congenitally missing premolars and a retained deciduous molar (65). Option C would be preferable from an implant perspective.

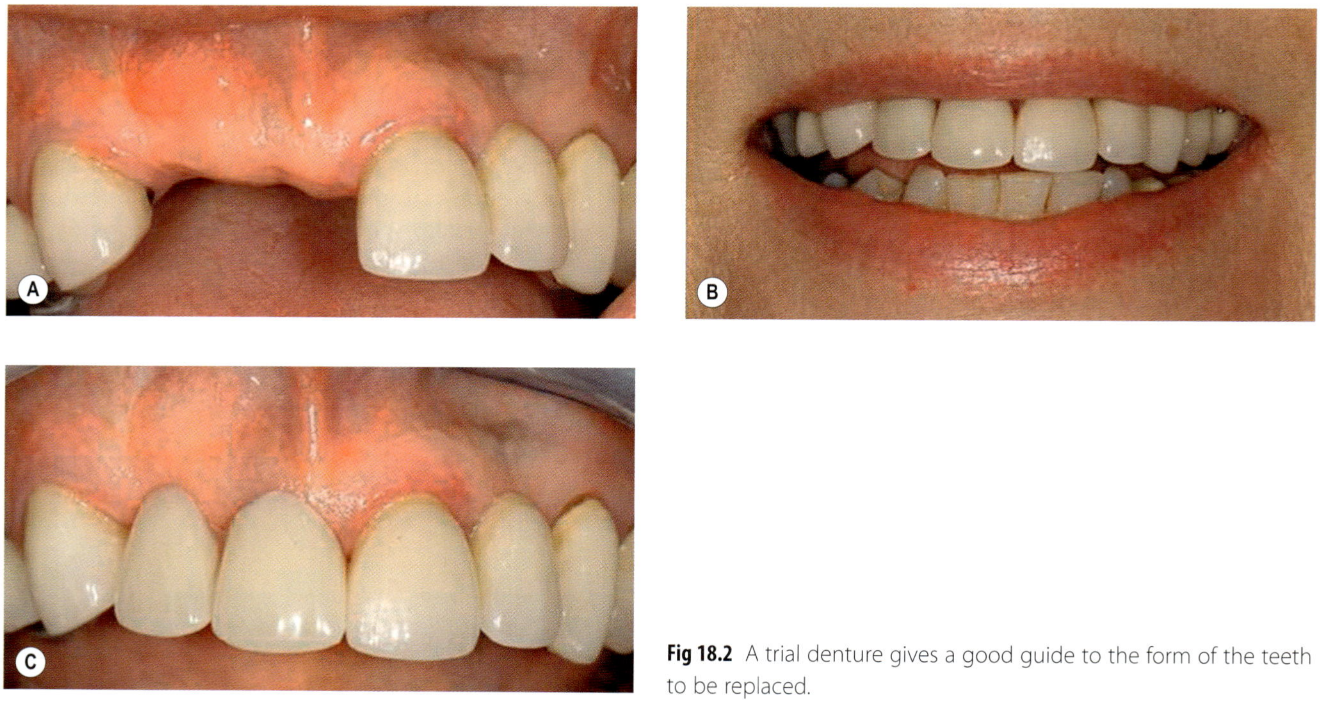

Fig 18.2 A trial denture gives a good guide to the form of the teeth to be replaced.

Does acceptable lip and facial support rely largely on the presence of a removable prosthesis?

Following tooth loss, it is usual for resorption in the maxilla to result in loss of buccal and vertical alveolar volume. Appropriately positioned maxillary artificial teeth come to lie in a buccal location relative to the resorbed alveolus (Figure 18.5). An idealized denture or wax trail denture provides a great deal of information about the missing dentoalveolar structures and the roles they play in providing facial support. Simple observations such as this help determine whether an implant overdenture is more realistic than attempting to provide fixed implant restorations that would require bone grafts to augment the alveolus.

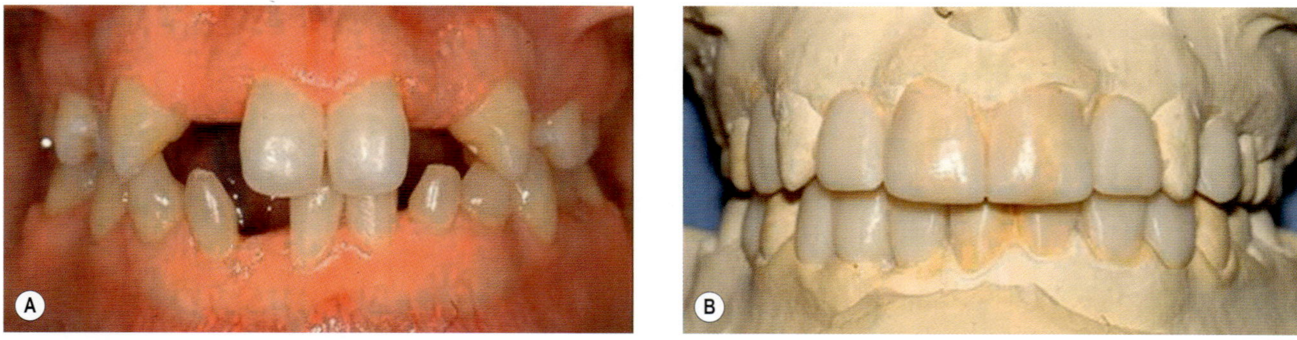

Fig 18.3 A wax-up of the proposed restorations has been made for a patient who has completed orthodontic treatment to realign teeth in preparation for dental implants. The wax-up helps to analyse the prosthetic envelope of the proposed restorations, which in turn directs the three-dimensional positions of dental implants.

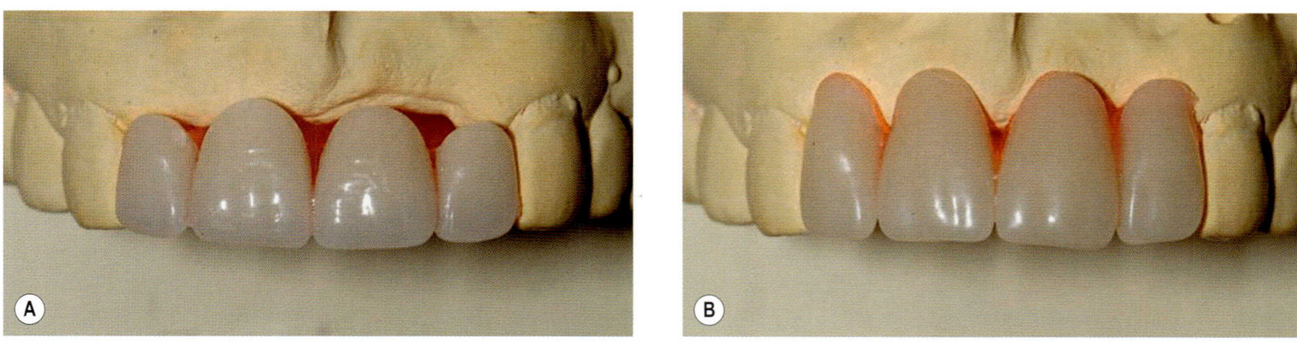

Fig 18.4 The trial tooth set up with well-proportioned teeth (A) shows that there is a significant alveolar deficit. If the deficit were to be replaced with teeth alone, they would have the appearance of gingival recession (B). If the compromise is unacceptable, this investigation reveals the need for exploring possibilities for replacement of alveolar tissue in the form of tissue grafts or by prosthetic means.

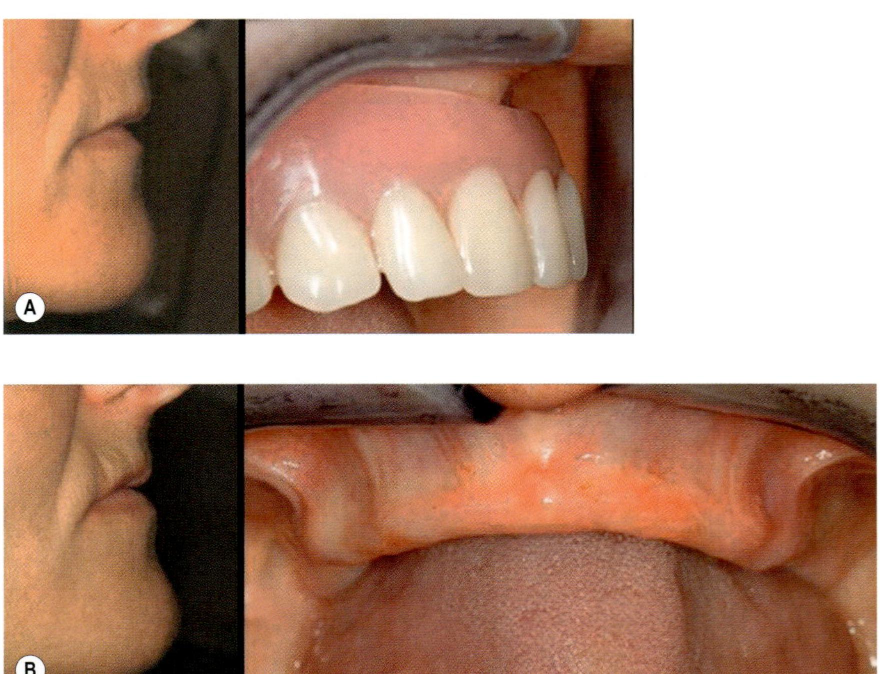

Fig 18.5 (A) Following loss of maxillary anterior teeth, tooth and flange elements of the denture are required to provide facial support. (B) There is a noticeable lack of upper lip support when the denture is removed.

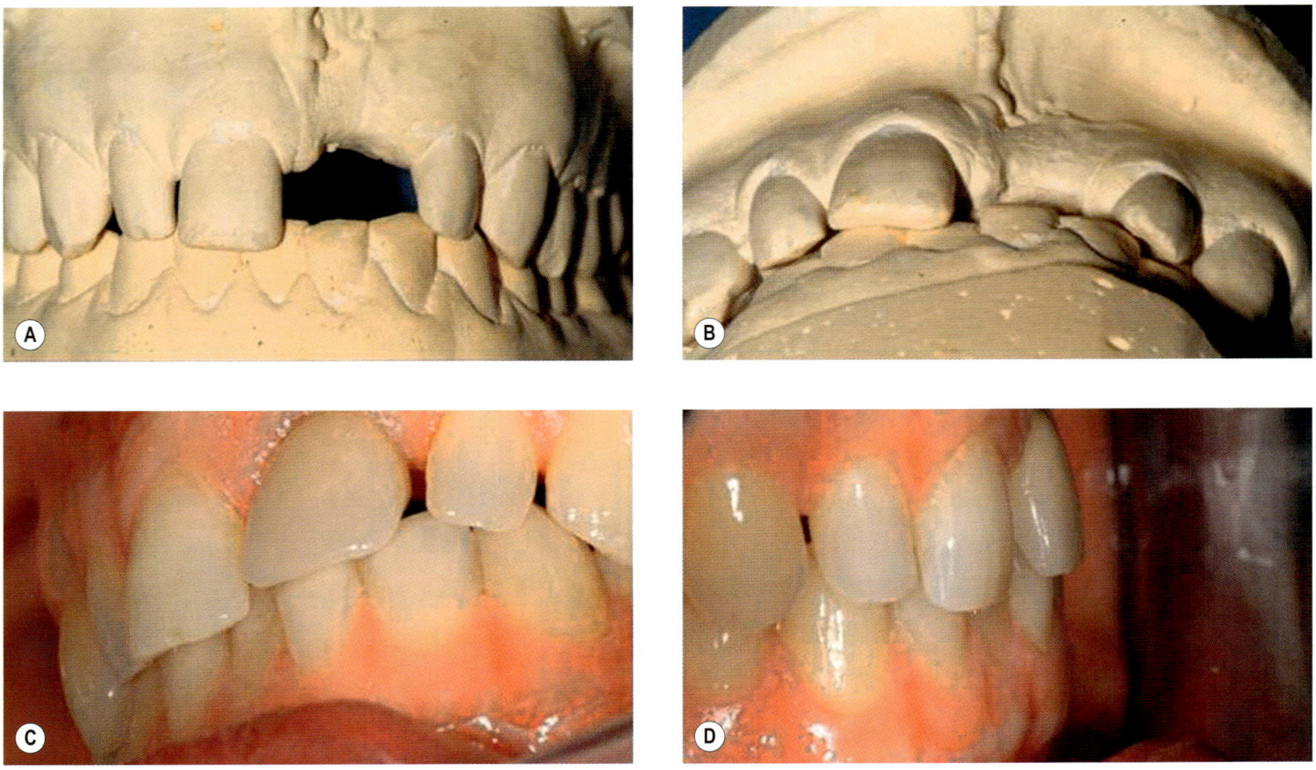

Fig 18.6 Failure to appreciate the prosthetic requirements for an implant restoration at the maxillary left central incisor. Although from the anterior view (A) there appears to be sufficient space, the occlusal view (B) shows that the mandibular incisors encroach on the required prosthetic envelope. It was not possible to simply adjust the mandibular incisors enough to create space, and the final restoration is significantly compromised (C and D). The patient declined orthodontic treatment to realign the mandibular teeth.

What are the occlusal objectives?

Is there space within an existing tooth-borne occlusal scheme to accommodate the proposed arrangement of teeth to be replaced?

Even a small amount of mandibular incisor anterior migration after maxillary tooth loss can create difficulties (Figure 18.6).

In addition to considering space for the external contours of the tooth replacement, it is necessary to decide whether there is sufficient internal volume to accommodate whatever method is chosen to attach the restoration to the implant (Figure 18.7). This is usually an easy clinical assessment to make in posterior regions but can be difficult anteriorly, where there is usually an overjet and overbite to be considered.

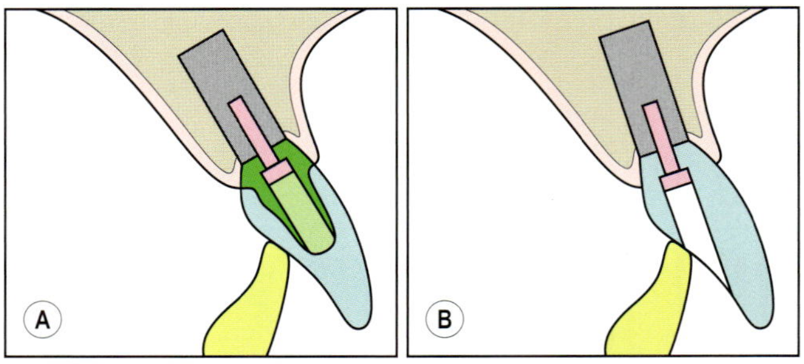

Fig 18.7 Examples of space requirements for implant-restoration attachment mechanisms for a maxillary incisor. (A) A cemented restoration requires sufficient volume to accommodate an abutment with adequate resistance and retention to be screwed into the implant. (B) A crown screwed directly into the implant without an intervening abutment may require less interocclusal volume than the cemented alternative. The position of the implant in panel A would make it difficult to provide the style of restoration shown in panel B because masking a visible screw access hole would be problematic.

Is the proposed restoration protected in excursions?

In addition to being accommodated in the static occlusion, the proposed restoration must integrate into the dynamic occlusion. Implant restorations can be designed to carry excursive contacts, share excursive contacts with natural teeth, or, if possible, to be clear of excursive contacts altogether. Philosophies for implant occlusion are drawn from conventional dental occlusal paradigms with the added precautionary principles, where possible, of axial loading of implants; excursions on teeth rather than implants; and sharing occlusal loads between implants, particularly in posterior areas of the mouth, where loads are higher.

In addition to clinical observation, trial dentures and wax-ups enable occlusal features to be identified and modifications in occlusion to be investigated.

It may be judged necessary to change occlusal relationships to achieve the occlusal goals, for example, by

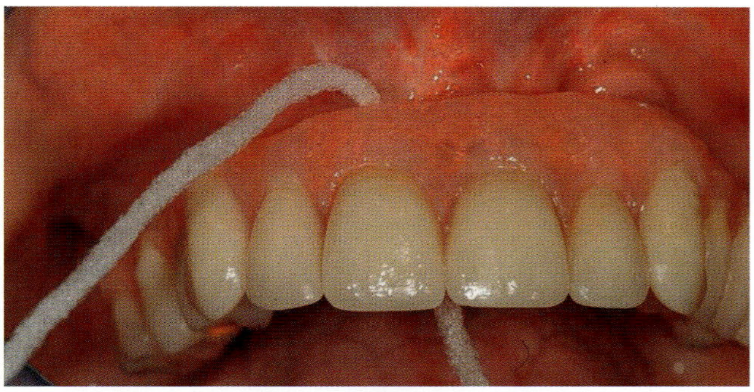

Fig 18.8 It is difficult for this patient to clean effectively around the implants that support a fixed restoration with a modest flange that provides lip support and gingival replacement.

recontouring of teeth, orthodontic movement, or reorganization of an existing occlusal scheme.

Is there space within the prosthetic envelope of a denture to accommodate overdenture attachments?

The size, shape, and position of the denture will be dictated largely by the anatomy of the patient. Clearly, the denture needs to be large enough in cross section to accommodate overdenture attachments.

What are the requirements to facilitate access for oral hygiene?

In order to reduce the risk of peri-implant inflammation, restorations must be designed to allow easy access for cleaning by the patient. Fixed restorations for the edentate maxilla in particular may not easily meet these objectives (Figure 18.8).

What are the ideal implant positions to satisfy the aesthetic, occlusal, and hygiene goals?

Having established the ideal features of the proposed fixed or removable restoration, it is necessary to envisage ideal positions for implants that might support the restoration. An understanding of the consequences of implant malposition is fundamental to the rationale for ideal implant positions.

How deeply placed should implants be?

A useful maxim is that an implant head needs to be as deep as necessary but as shallow as possible in relation to the restoration it supports.

If an implant is placed too deeply, there is a risk of developing a deep peri-implant sulcus or pocket that may be susceptible to infection or precipitate peri-implant recession. There is also a risk of magnifying the stress concentration at the implant–abutment interface due to a longer than necessary lever arm effect. Overly deep implants may also cause practical difficulties during the restoration phase of treatment. An unnecessarily deep implant implies an unnecessarily deep osteotomy, with potential for damage to adjacent structures, or the need for bone augmentation that might otherwise be avoided.

If an implant head is placed in too superficial a position, there may be difficulties making an abrupt transition in dimension from the implant head to the tooth cervix (which is usually larger). This is especially the case for "platform switched" implant–abutment interfaces where the diameter of the emerging abutment is smaller than the diameter of the implant head. If interocclusal space is limited, a superficially placed implant could leave insufficient space for an abutment or other tooth–implant attachment mechanism (see Figure 18.7). Even a small degree of gingival margin recession at a superficially placed implant over time could expose the implant body, with detriment to the aesthetic result and possible precipitation of peri-implant inflammation associated with plaque retention on the threads of a microrough implant surface.

Two-part implant systems that recommend placement of the implant head at bone level suggest that approximately 3 mm clearance should be provided between implant head and proposed gingival margin of the restoration. This satisfies the requirements of implant depth to be as deep as necessary but as shallow as possible.

Alveolar resorption usually results in there being adequate space within a proposed denture for overdenture attachments. However, if the prosthetic envelope is limited, it may be necessary to envisage implants placed more deeply than would be immediately apparent. The implication is that some ridge reduction may be necessary in order to position the implant heads at the correct depth.

What should the mesiodistal position of implants be?

In order to maintain or form papillae between implants and teeth, or between adjacent implants, it is important that implants emerge correctly. Encroaching on the space required for papillae and their supporting bone runs the risk of serious aesthetic compromise.

The establishment of the peri-implant biologic attachment zone at the neck of an implant can manifest as a narrow zone of bone loss, particularly for products with a flat implant–abutment interface. If this physiologic bone resorption is accompanied by retraction of overlying soft tissue, the result can be a lack of papilla filling the gingival embrasure space. Minimum dimensions of 1.5 mm between tooth and implant and 3 or 4 mm between implants have been suggested in order to accommodate the biologic attachment zone(s) and maintain papillae.

When the plan is to replace soft tissue by prosthetic means, mesiodistal implant positioning can be determined more by the biomechanical requirements of optimizing load dissipation and avoidance of cantilevers.

If implants are to support/retain an overdenture, a fundamental requirement is that they are far enough apart to accommodate attachments that are housed within the prosthesis (Figure 18.9).

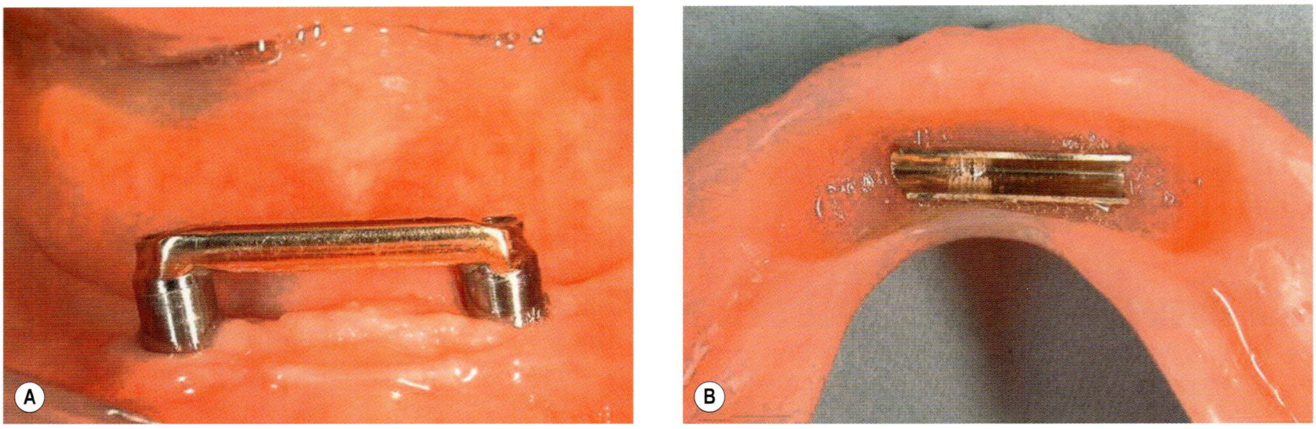

Fig 18.9 (A) A bar attached to two implants in the anterior mandible. (B) The implants need to be sufficiently far apart to allow an adequately long clip to be processed into the overdenture.

What should the buccolingual position of implants be?

If an implant is placed too far to buccal, there is a risk that the crestal bone and soft tissue remodelling that commonly occurs at the neck of an implant may manifest as buccal vertical alveolar loss. This can cause the gingival margin at an implant crown to develop the appearance of recession compared to adjacent teeth. Too lingual an emergence makes it necessary to cantilever the restoration toward the buccal with potentially difficult access for adequate hygiene, aesthetic compromise, and unfavourable load dissipation. As a general rule, the ideal position is for the long axis of the implant to be just lingual to the long axis of the tooth to be replaced by a fixed restoration.

Implants intended for use as overdenture abutments must emerge through the mucosa, allowing for attachments to be contained within the prosthetic envelope of the proposed denture.

What should the trajectory of the implants be?

The trajectory of implants has a major bearing on the design choices of the final restoration.

If the long axis of an implant closely approximates the long axis of the tooth being replaced, not only might restoration of the implant be simplified but also off-axis occlusal loads will be minimized, thereby reducing the risk of mechanical damage to components such as abutment attachment screws.

The ability to screw-retain a restoration rather than cement it over an abutment has advantages, including making the restoration more easily retrievable and avoiding the risk of peri-implant cement entrapment, which is a cause of peri-implantitis. Screw retention is most easily accomplished when the trajectory of the implant leaves a screw access hole hidden from view on an anterior tooth or on the occlusal surface of a posterior tooth (see Figure 18.7).

Multiple implants for overdentures used to carry individual (nonlinked) attachments such as the ball-and-socket type need to be mutually aligned with reasonable harmony to allow the attachments to function as intended.

What moderating factors indicate a departure from "one implant per missing tooth" for fixed restorations?

If planning proceeds with the intention to place one implant per missing tooth in the ideal positions discussed previously, the final number of implants will be influenced by moderating factors. This stage in planning is carried out before considering bone volume and adjacent anatomical structures. It may reveal that implant placement is not possible.

Narrow teeth

Planning one implant per tooth when replacing small-diameter units such as maxillary lateral incisors and mandibular incisors may reveal that implants would be positioned very close together or very close to adjacent teeth. In addition to making implant placement particularly challenging, this can result in aesthetic compromise because of a lack of papillae, as discussed previously.

Realization of this phenomenon can mean that pontics are more appropriate than overly close implants (Figure 18.10). A strategy to avoid overly close implants is to plan fewer but wider teeth (Figure 18.11).

Edentate fixed restoration

It would be unusual to place one implant per tooth to be replaced for an edentate fixed restoration. It appears that as few as four strategically positioned anterior/premolar region implants can be sufficient to provide a fixed restoration that supports cantilevered posterior teeth. A detailed discussion of implant positioning for edentate fixed restorations is beyond the scope of this chapter.

How many implants for overdentures?

What support is intended for the overdenture?

If an overdenture is to rely entirely on implants for support, four or more well-spaced implants are required (Figure

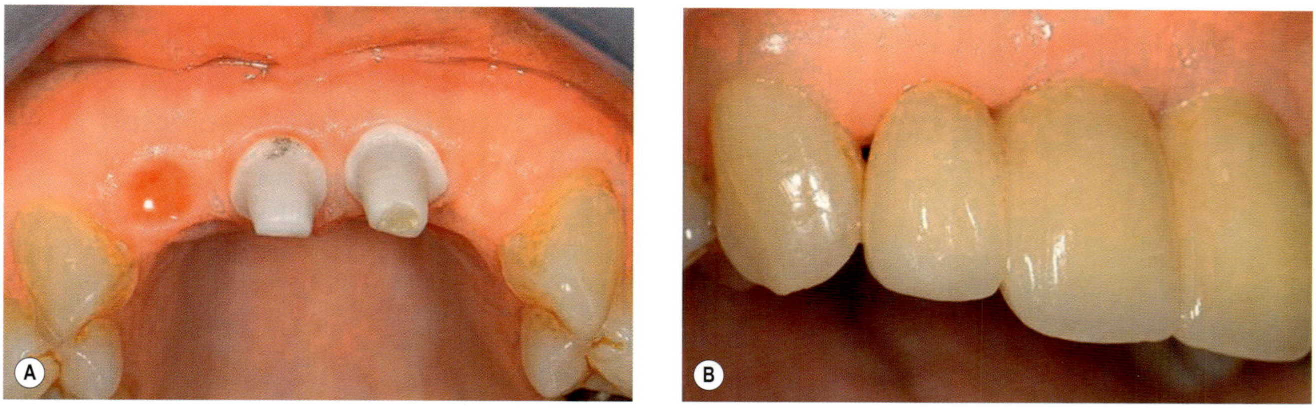

Fig 18.10 (A) Two implants used to replace four missing teeth by means of cantilevered pontics. Four implants would not have allowed for adequate interimplant and tooth–implant space. (B) The contact points have been taken further toward the gingiva to reduce the space that papillae should fill.

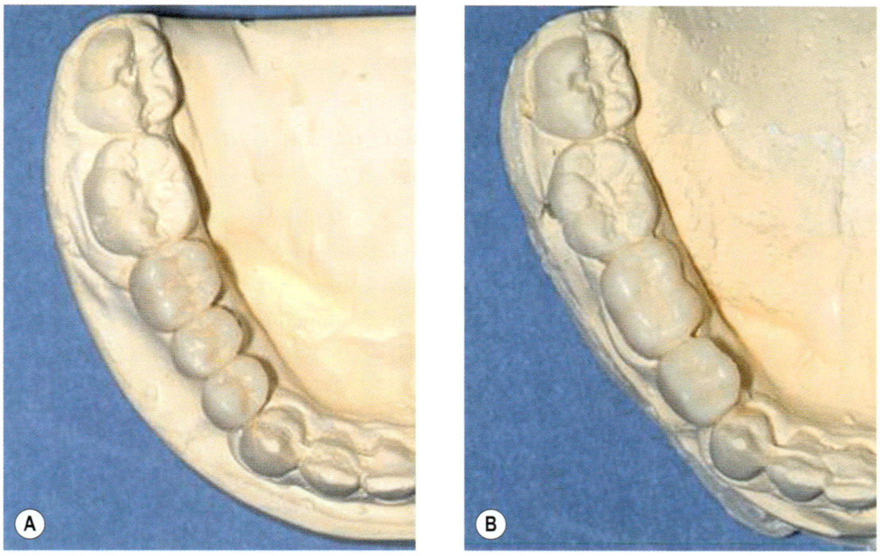

Fig 18.11 Diagnostic wax-ups used to investigate alternative numbers of replacement teeth. It may be more difficult to achieve adequate implant spacing with the three-teeth option (A) than with the two-teeth option (B).

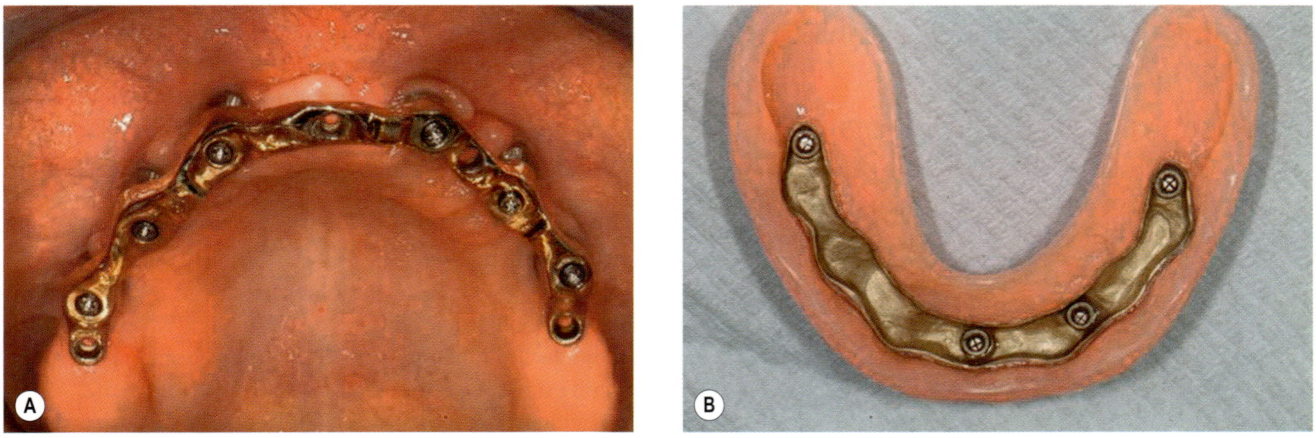

Fig 18.12 Six implants used to support a metallic framework that houses attachments (A) for both support and retention of an overdenture (B).

18.12). If support is to be provided primarily by mucosa such that the function of the implants is mainly to retain the denture, then fewer implants are required. Two implants placed anteriorly in the edentate mandible to retain an overdenture is an effective design (Figure 18.13). Two implants satisfy the requirement to resist horizontal rotational displacement that could occur around a single implant. A single axis of vertical rotation between two implants allows for the inevitable displacement that occurs due to posterior mucosal compression when the denture is in function.

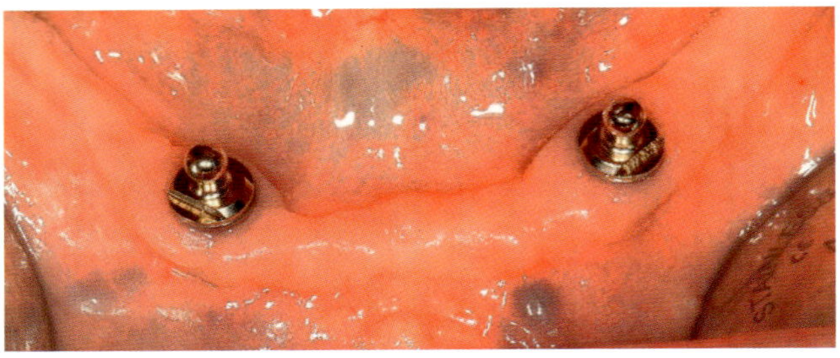

Fig 18.13 An implant overdenture that houses attachments will clip onto the ball abutments that have been screwed on to the underlying implants.

What are the ideal implant product features to satisfy the aesthetic, occlusal, and hygiene goals?

Much of what guides the following discussion is drawn from basic biomechanics and a precautionary approach. Evidence of high occlusal forces suggests it would be prudent to incorporate as much mechanical protection as possible, such as fewer cantilevered pontics and wider implants and abutment retaining screws.

How wide should implants be?

The wider the implant, the greater the surface area available for tissue integration. The converse is true for narrower implants. Wider implants may also be stronger and have more robust abutment attachment screws than narrower implants. Bearing this in mind, the size of the teeth being replaced tends to govern the width of implants chosen: an implant of 3-mm diameter may well be appropriate for maxillary lateral incisors and mandibular incisors, whereas one of 5-mm diameter or more is appropriate for a molar. Even if it were robust enough, making the transition from a 3-mm-diameter implant to a 10-mm-wide molar could result in plaque retentive problems unless the implant is deeply placed.

How long should the implants be?

It is important to achieve an adequate degree of stability in bone at the time of implant placement (primary stability). Many factors influence this goal, and implant length is a major factor. For example, placement into a fresh extraction socket, where immediate restoration of the implant is planned, will require a longer implant to engage the residual socket walls and bone beyond the socket than if an implant is placed in mature bone and left to heal submerged below the sutured gingiva.

What about other implant product features?

For each diameter and length, implants are available in a large variety of body shapes, neck configurations, abutment connection mechanisms, surface configurations, and microtopography and biochemical properties. Each design has purported advantages in different situations.

Is satisfactory volume and quality of bone available to house the chosen implant products in the selected positions?

Thorough clinical and radiographic evaluation is necessary to assess bone volume in relation to the ideal implant positions and chosen product features.

Where teeth are already missing, clinical examination may show that adequate mesiodistal and buccolingual bone is likely to be present. A denture, failing bridge, or wax-up can assist in relating the residual alveolus to the proposed implant and restoration. Careful measurements are needed, particularly where mesiodistal space appears to be limited. Even when teeth are still present, assessment of alveolar contours may reveal concavities that could encroach on proposed implant positions. Mapping the residual ridge with calipers, for example, can give useful information about bone volume.

How much bone will remain after a tooth is extracted?

If teeth are still present but destined for replacement with implants, an assessment of tissue thickness referred to as periodontal biotype can give an indication of how much the alveolus is likely to be damaged at the time of extraction and how much is likely to be lost in association with socket healing. People with a thin periodontal biotype tend to have thin or even absent cortical bone buccal to tooth roots in the anterior maxilla. A history of periradicular infection or root surgery could also mean that there is a bone deficit in the vicinity of a remaining root that may persist after extraction—the very bone that may be required to enable adequate primary stability of the implant.

What can radiography show?

Radiographs are required to evaluate anatomy not visible to the naked eye. Two-dimensional images, such as panoramic and periapical radiographs, help to show vertical and mesiodistal anatomical limitations: adjacent tooth roots, neurovascular bundles, and sinus and nasal floors, for example. Pathology may also be evident on radiographs. Transparent overlays can be used with two-dimensional radiographs to assess bone availability in relation to specific implant products (Figure 18.14).

Lateral and occlusal radiographs can give limited information about buccolingual bone shape. Two-dimensional image techniques are prone to magnification and/or orientation effects, which need to be taken into account.

Tomographic radiographic techniques such as cone beam computed tomography (CBCT) enable three-dimensional visualization of the anatomy, including evaluation of the alveolar cross section (buccolingual volume). Implant planning information from CBCT images can be greatly enhanced by having the patient wear a radio-opaque simulation of the proposed restoration. Implant planning software then allows virtual implants that match the chosen products to be positioned on-screen (Figure 18.15). This provides the final link in the planning sequence: being able to evaluate

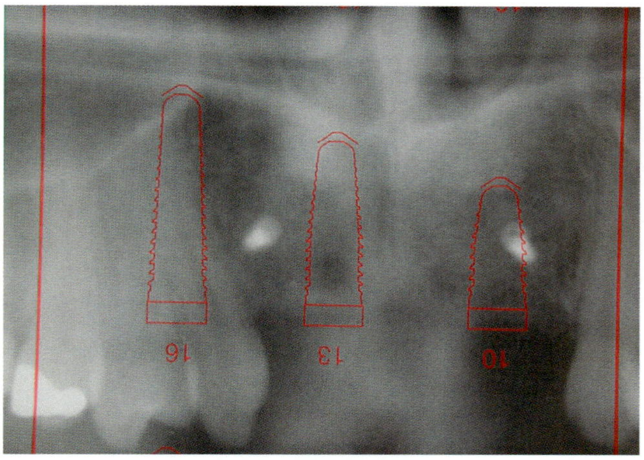

Fig 18.14 Transparent overlays matched to the magnification of a panoramic radiograph used to help select implant sizes.

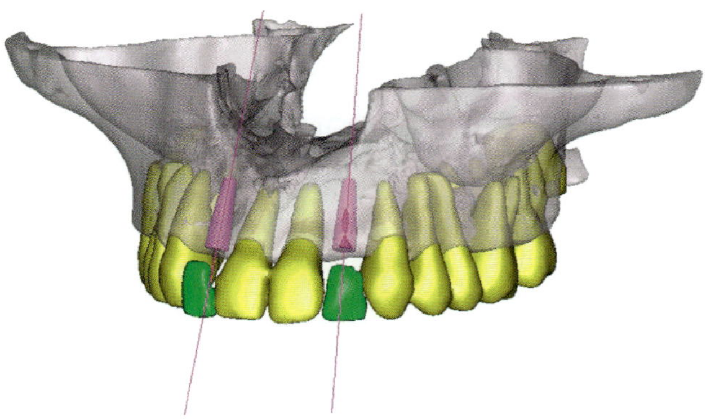

Fig 18.15 Virtual implant placement performed on an image obtained by CBCT.

the proposed restoration in relation to the available bone and chosen implant products.

Bone density is related to achievement of primary stability at the time of implant placement. Assessment using two-dimensional radiography is imprecise. Computed tomography and virtual implant planning software allow for quantification of bone density at the proposed implant site (the Hounsfield number). Implant type and placement technique may be modified according to bone density.

Will the peri-implant soft tissue be appropriate?

Having decided whether sufficient bone volume exists to house the proposed implants in the ideal positions, the features of the soft tissue through which the implants will emerge need to be considered.

Is the peri-implant tissue attached mucosa or mobile alveolar mucosa?

It is possible to maintain peri-implant soft tissue health when implants emerge through alveolar mucosa. However, attached mucosa as peri-implant mucosa is likely to make it easier for the patient to perform the required oral hygiene, less likely to allow foreign body entrapment in the peri-implant sulcus, and be better able to withstand physical pressure that can be associated with insertion and withdrawal of overdentures (Figure 18.16).

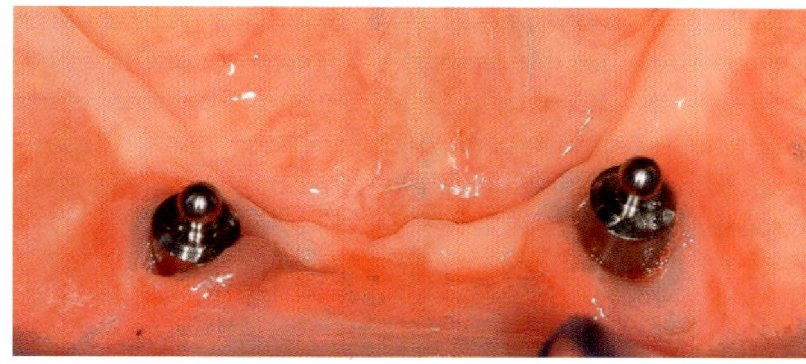

Fig 18.16 Where the buccal aspects of these overdenture abutments emerge through mobile alveolar mucosa there is peri-implant inflammation.

If bone and/or soft tissue is lacking, can it be created?

The assessment carried out so far may reveal that bone and/or soft tissue of adequate volume or quality is lacking. If this is the case, consideration should be given to augmenting the tissues in order for the implant objectives to be achieved.

It is anticipated that the implant will gain adequate primary stability from existing bone

If it is decided that there is enough bone present of adequate density to enable the implant to be inserted with good primary stability but not enough to house the implant sufficiently for soft tissue coverage, then it may be possible to augment the missing bone by carrying out a bone graft at the same time as the implant placement. A popular technique in this circumstance is to utilize the guided bone regeneration (GBR) method that allows new bone to grow into a space created by a barrier that occludes faster-growing soft tissue from the area. Filler material is often used in the space beneath the membrane, both to prevent the barrier (which is often a membrane) from collapsing and to encourage osteogenesis by virtue of osteoconductive or osteoinductive properties. GBR is most effective for augmenting small buccal alveolar deficits.

Bone can also be manipulated using various dilatation and ridge-splitting techniques to increase its volume simultaneous with implant placement.

It is anticipated that initial implant stability in existing bone cannot be achieved

Bone augmentation prior to implant placement may be the only way to position implants in ideal locations for the restorations they will support. GBR for pre-implant augmentation may be feasible, and it has the advantage that it may be possible to avoid a second surgical site (intra- or extraoral), which is often required if a larger volume of bone is harvested for use as a graft. In this so-called staged approach, the graft is left for a period of months for it to be remodelled before implants are placed.

Distraction osteogenesis is a technique that uses a mechanical device to transport a segment of bone to a new position without separating it from its nutrient periosteum. Segmental osteotomy, orthognathic surgery, and orthodontic tooth movement are additional methods of generating increased bone volume.

It is anticipated that peri-implant soft tissue will be lacking

It is possible to augment attached tissue by embellishments to flap design, pedicle grafts, free partial-thickness epithelial or connective tissue grafts, or by using non-autogenous graft materials.

If bone or soft tissue is lacking, is it possible to proceed, accepting the risk of compromise?

There are risks related to accepting suboptimal implant positions or product dimensions at the planning stage. Considerations at this stage are similar to those when implants have already been placed in less than ideal positions and design modifications and changes to patient expectations are required.

What are the aesthetic risks?

The influence of lip morphology and periodontal biotype on aesthetic risk was discussed in Chapter 17. Surgery to place implants and to connect abutments can result in recession of gingiva at adjacent teeth. This outcome can be a particular problem if dark root dentine is exposed apical to a crown margin necessitating replacement restoration. Formation of papillae is more difficult to achieve between adjacent implants than between implants and teeth (Figure 18.17).

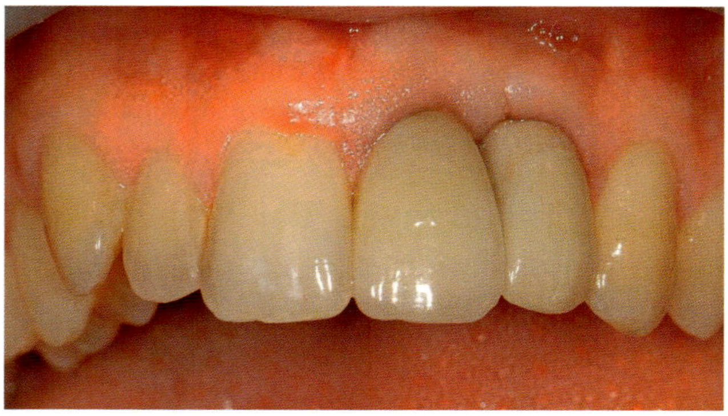

Fig 18.17 Implant crowns at left central and lateral incisor sites. The contrast in the gingival architecture compared with the right-hand side is quite evident. Implants that are positioned without accommodating long-term tissue requirements make achieving satisfactory results in these already challenging situations even more difficult.

What are other possible compromise outcomes?

Accepting suboptimal implant positions, product dimensions, or tissue coverage may also result in restorations with increased risk of mechanical failure, phonetic interference, and the consequences of oral hygiene difficulty. It is particularly important to be able to identify when it would no longer be possible to provide a fixed restoration and have to resort to a removable overdenture for an edentulous arch.

How will the patient make the transition to implant restoration?

The treatment plan must consider what kind of provisional restoration is to be used and whether it is possible to utilize implants as soon as they are inserted.

Provisional fixed restoration borne by teeth

This design of provisional restoration avoids loading a surgical site; loading can cause wound breakdown, particularly in the early stages of healing.

A minimal preparation adhesive restoration or a denture tooth simply bonded to an adjacent tooth may be possible, although there are drawbacks of having to spend time removing the restoration on one or more occasions and of possible unexpected debonding. The pontic should be made from a material such as acrylic or composite resin that allows easy adjustment to accommodate for swelling and for any healing abutments.

A provisional bridge may also be an option when there is a plan to place crowns at the abutment teeth or to extract them at a later stage.

Provisional removable restoration

This straightforward option allows easy adjustment. A vacuum-made design that fits over the teeth prevents mucosal loading and can accommodate deep complete overbites when there is not enough interocclusal space for a denture connector.

Provisional fixed restoration borne by implants

With good implant primary stability and careful attention to avoiding unfavourable occlusal loading, a provisional implant-borne restoration is possible.

Immediate final restoration using implants

It may be possible to provide the final restoration at or within a short time after implant insertion. Developments in computer-aided design/computer-aided machining technologies have helped make this possible.

No provisional restoration

Short periods without replacement are often accepted in nonaesthetic locations. For other locations, even a short period without tooth replacement is unacceptable for some patients, who may even decline implant treatment if this is unavoidable.

What is the stage-by-stage plan of treatment?

Once design, implant product choices, surgical procedures, method of provisionalization, and risks have been decided, then a detailed treatment sequence can be drawn up and presented to the patient.

Chapter 19

Basic surgery for implant placement

This chapter discusses the surgical techniques for implant placement. Three different cases demonstrate individual techniques that can be considered when replacing teeth in different areas of the mouth.

Surgical placement of an implant to replace an upper first molar

Summary

A 55-year-old female presents with pain from UR6, which had been endodontically treated and crowned more than 10 years ago.

History

◇ ***Complaint***

The patient is complaining of pain from UR6, particularly when biting.

◇ ***History of complaint***

The tooth was endodontically treated and a porcelain-fused-to-metal crown provided, which had remained functional for approximately 10 years. The patient first started to experience pain when biting on this tooth approximately 1 week ago; since then, the pain has become progressively worse.

◇ ***Dental history***

The patient has been a regular dental attendee and has had several restorations and extractions throughout the years. The patient is now concerned about the long-term prognosis for her dentition. She is keen to avoid a removable prosthesis.

Examination

◇ ***Intraoral examination***

The dentition is heavily restored. Most of the posterior teeth are crowned or have intracoronal restorations (Figure 19.1). The upper central incisors are crowned, and the lateral incisors are restored with labial porcelain veneers. The restorations are functional, albeit with minor defects.

UR6 has a porcelain-fused-to-metal crown. The tooth is tender to percussion.

◇ ***Radiographic examination***

UR6: Single-cone root fillings are noted in the two buccal canals, and obturation voids are noted in the palatal canal. A slight widening of the lamina dura is noted in the mesiobuccal canal (Figure 19.2).

UR7: Single-cone root fillings are present in the buccal canals. The tooth has been restored with cast post and core crown.

UR5: Has a distal–occlusal restoration, with no periapical pathology.

What is the diagnosis and what factors will determine the prognosis of this tooth?

Diagnosis: Chronic periapical periodontitis in UR6.

The prognosis depends on two main factors:

1. Endodontic retreatment
2. Restorability of the tooth

Endodontic retreatment is possible and has a predictable outcome. The removal of existing obturation seems straightforward. However, one should be suspicious of a possible fourth canal (second mesiobuccal). A conscious effort to identify it and, if present, instrument appropriately is imperative in achieving success.

Moreover, the restorability of the tooth has to be determined. Although the tooth may be successfully treated after endodontic retreatment, the long-term prognosis will also depend on the underlying restorability of the tooth. It is advisable to dismantle the extracoronal restoration to investigate the amount of remaining tooth structure.

Once the crown was removed, underneath was primarily a core of composite resin. The mesial margin was subgingival (Figure 19.3), and it would not have been possible to achieve a crown margin on sound tooth structure without carrying out a surgical crown-lengthening procedure.

After discussing the risks and benefits, it was decided to extract the tooth.

What replacement restorations would you consider and why?

1. Conventional three-unit bridge (UR5 to UR7)

   Overall, a conventional bridge has a 10-year survival rate of 89.2% and would be cost-effective. However, UR7 is already restored with a post–core crown and would therefore be prone to a higher failure rate. In addition, UR5 has a small intracoronal restoration, and preparing it for a bridge would result in significant loss of healthy tooth tissue.

2. Single-tooth implant crown

   A single-tooth implant restoration is independent and does not require support from adjacent teeth. It would provide a long-term successful restoration, with a reported survival rate of 89.4% after 10 years. However, an implant requires a surgical procedure with its related postoperative complications, protracted treatment time,

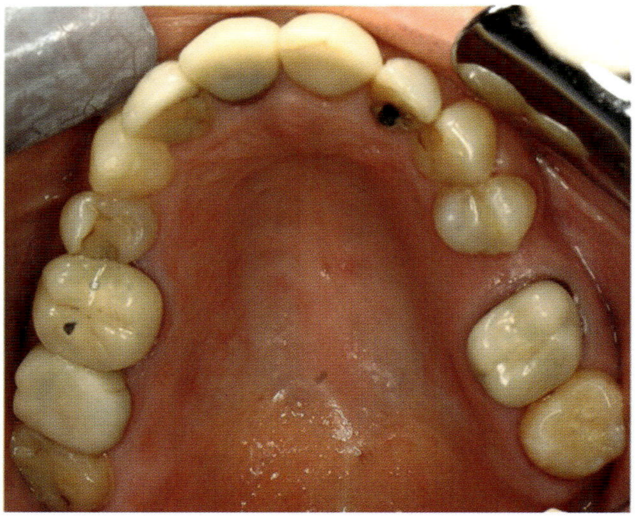

Fig 19.1 Occlusal view of maxillary dentition.

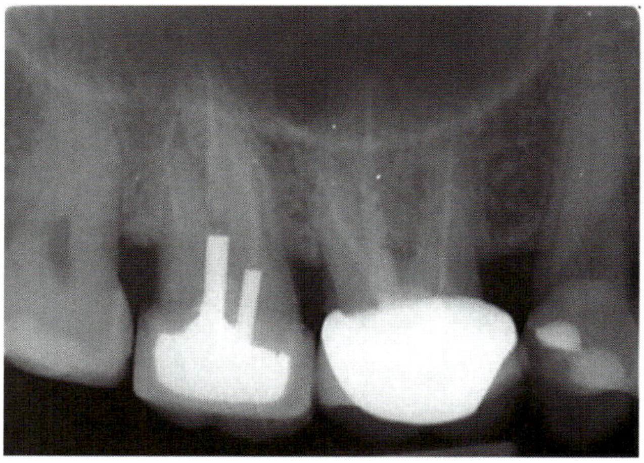

Fig 19.2 Radiograph of UR6 showing undercondensed root fillings with radiolucency in the furcation area.

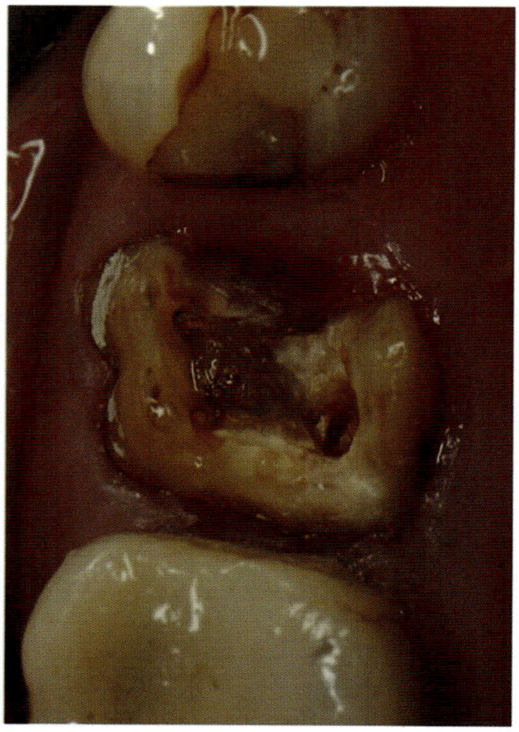

Fig 19.3 Removal of the existing restoration and underlying core, demonstrating lack of adequate coronal dentine.

and it is expensive in comparison to conventional options.

After a detailed discussion about the options, the patient chose to have the tooth replaced by an implant-retained crown.

Preimplant assessment

◈ ***What factors would you consider when planning an implant to replace a maxillary and a mandibular molar?***

See Table 19.1.

◈ ***Describe the surgical technique pertinent to molar region***

As outlined in Table 19.1, the maxillary sinus and the mandibular canal are two important limiting anatomical landmarks when surgically placing implants in maxilla and mandible, respectively. It is necessary to drill short of these structures, and in order to prevent damage to the inferior dental nerve, drilling is carried out at least 2 mm short of the canal.

The patient should sign an informed consent prior to surgery. The surgery can usually be performed under local anaesthesia. A crestal incision is extended to include a tooth on either side. A vertical releasing incision can also be made

Table 19.1 Factors to assess when considering implant replacement of molar teeth

Factor	Comments
Anatomical structures	Maxillary molar: maxillary sinus (Figure 19.4) Mandibular molar: inferior dental canal and mandibular foramen (Figure 19.5)
Bone height	Adequate bone height for the selected implant length using plain radiograph paralleling technique or a cone beam CT scan. In the mandible, watch for lingual concavity
Bone width	Clinical assessment and cone beam CT scan
Functional and aesthetic outcome	Although it is a molar, the final restoration should blend with the adjacent teeth
Implant selection	Implant with a wider body diameter is selected. It is desirable to choose an implant with a wider restorative head (platform), which will facilitate a good crown emergence for a molar tooth (Figure 19.6)

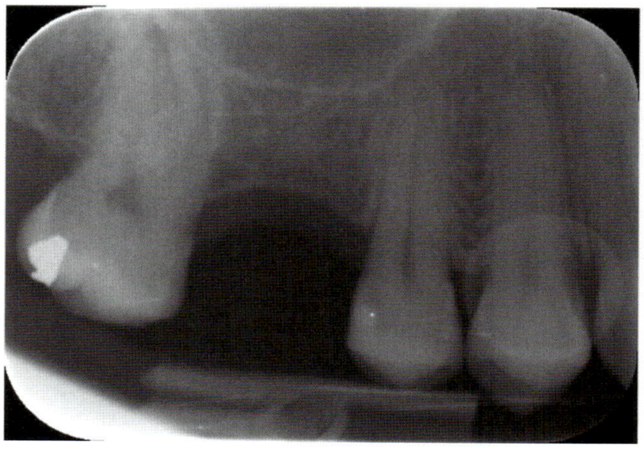

Fig 19.4 Radiograph showing limited alveolar ridge height due to position of the maxillary sinus floor.

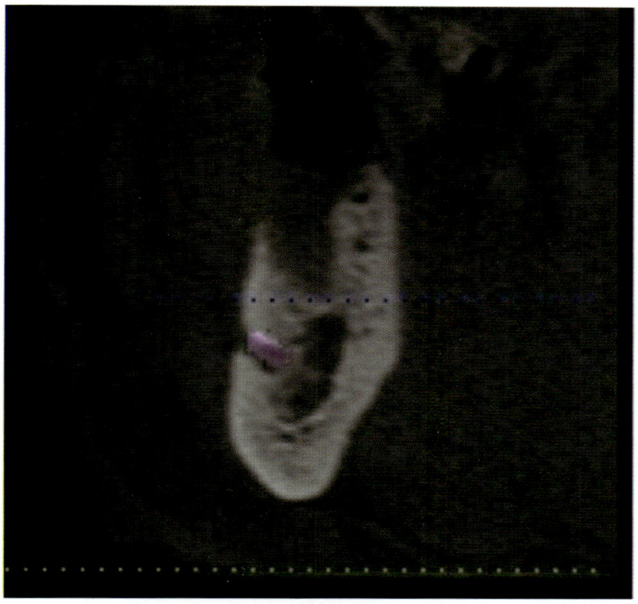

Fig 19.5 A cross-sectional view of mental foramen and mandibular canal.

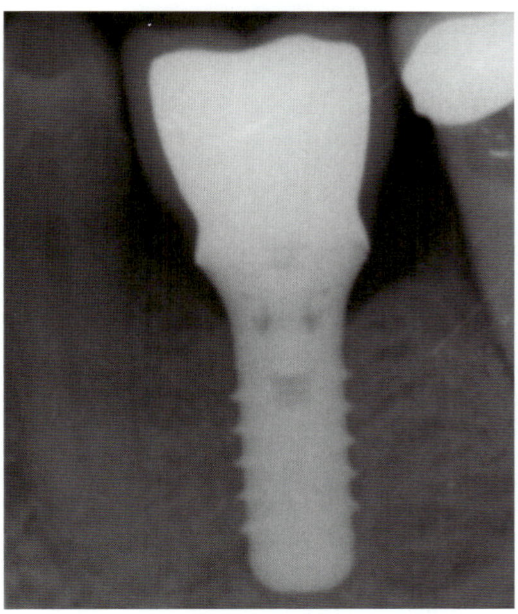

Fig 19.6 An appropriate-diameter implant to replace a molar tooth. The shape of the implant allows an ideal emergence for a molar tooth to be developed.

to gain better access. A surgical template is advisable and fabricated using an appropriate technique. A series of drills of widening diameters (Figure 19.7), as supplied by each implant manufacturer, are used to prepare the implant site (Figure 19.8) to the desired length and diameter under copious irrigation, at a low rpm of approximately 700–900. Finally, the implant is inserted using a gentle insertion torque.

A healing cap is attached to the implant. Depending on the type of implant used, it can either be buried or left transmucosal (exposed) for the period of healing during which osseointegration takes place (Figure 19.9).

After a period of healing, if the implant is buried, a second surgical procedure is necessary to expose the top of the implant and a taller healing cap is placed.

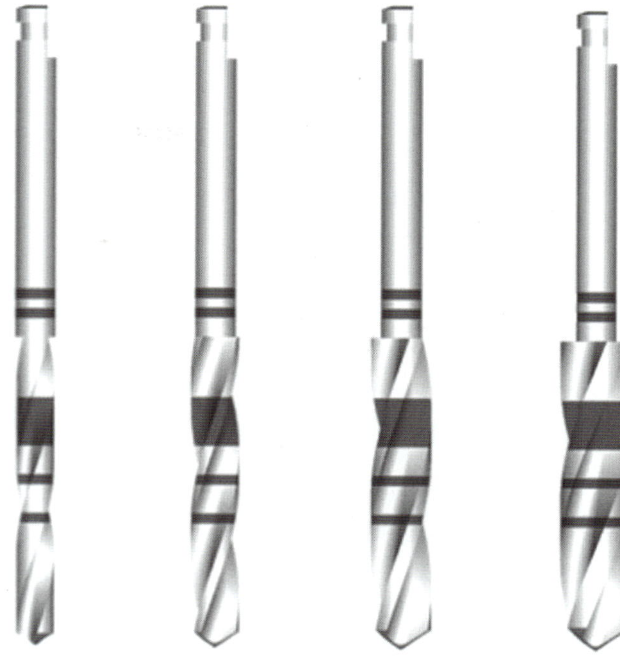

Fig 19.7 System-specific drills for preparing the implant osteotomy sites. Each manufacturer offers drills specifically for its implant system.

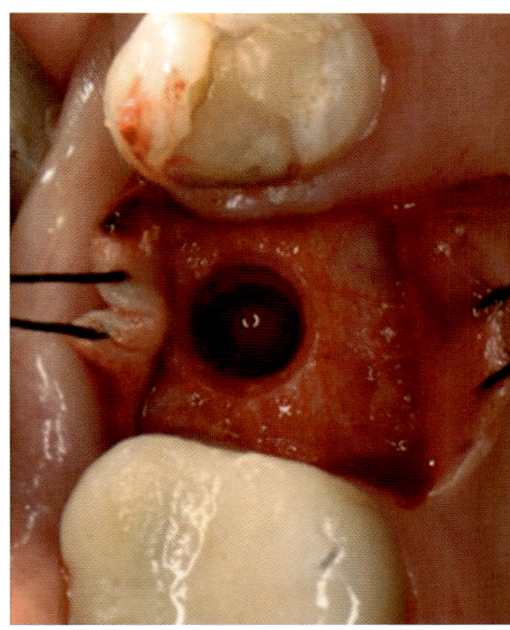

Fig 19.8 A typical implant site prepared in a correct three-dimensional position.

The implant is now ready for restorative treatment (Figures 19.10 and 19.11), which is described in detail in Chapter 21.

Immediate implant placement to replace two upper premolars

Summary

A 58-year-old male presents with fractured UL4 and UL5 seeking restoration of these teeth.

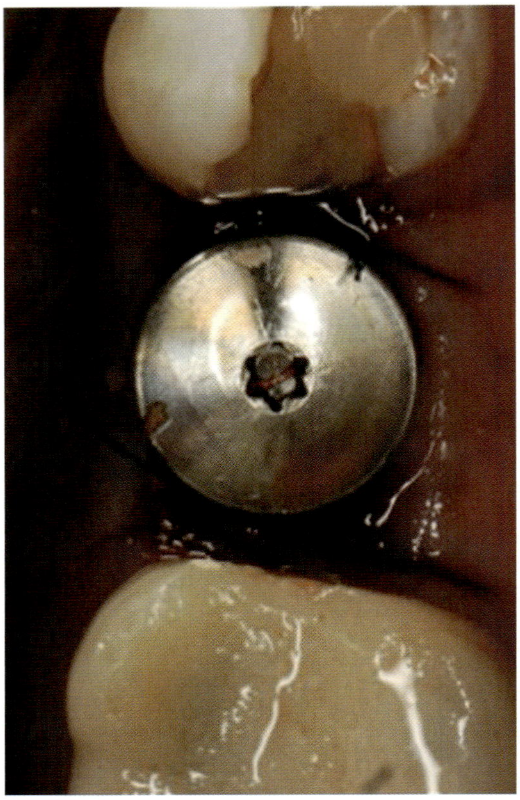

Fig 19.9 A transmucosal implant immediately after placement.

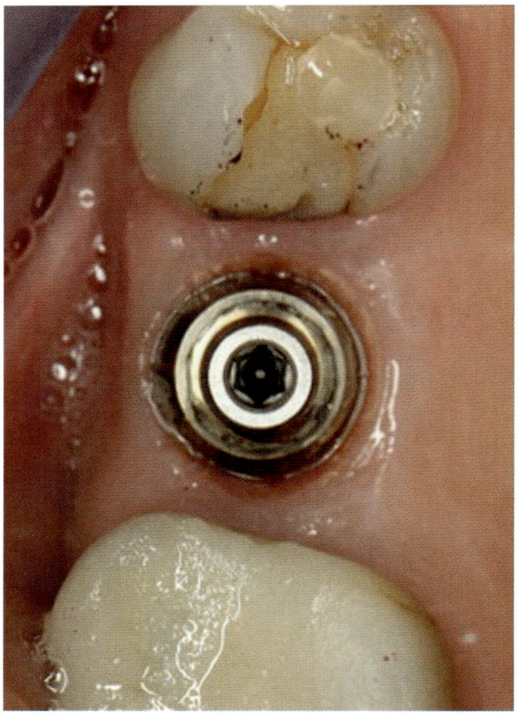

Fig 19.10 Implant abutment screwed in place and ready for restoration.

History

Complaint

The patient complains of fractured UL4 and UL5. The teeth are not associated with any pain, but he is concerned about function and aesthetics. He is inquiring about the possibility of restoring the fractured teeth with crowns.

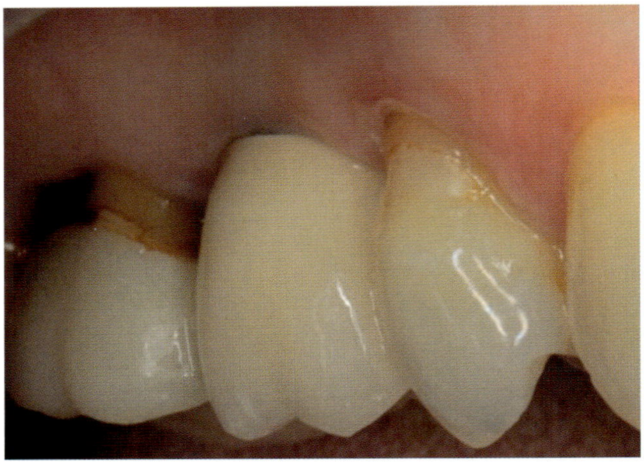

Fig 19.11 Definitive restoration showing a good aesthetic outcome.

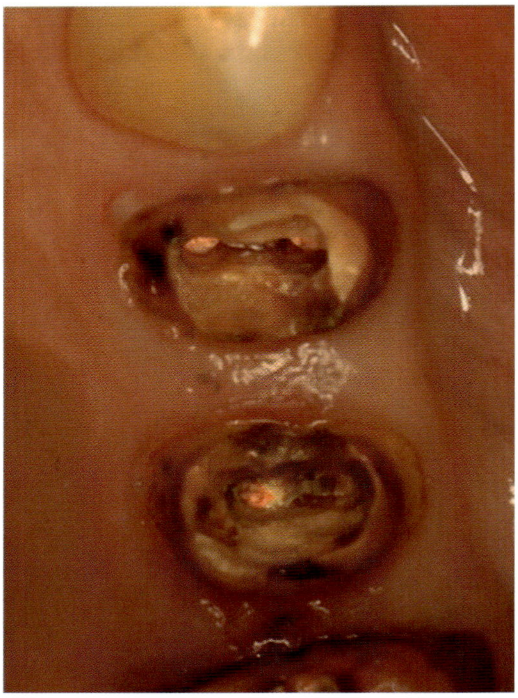

Fig 19.12 Occlusal view of UL4 and UL5 showing gingival-level fracture in both teeth.

History of complaint

The UL4 and UL5 fractured while the patient was eating approximately 2 months ago. The teeth had large restorations and had been endodontically treated approximately 4 years ago.

Dental history

The patient has been a regular dental attendee and has had several restorations and endodontic treatments throughout the years.

Examination

Intraoral examination

The dentition is heavily restored with several intra- and extracoronal restorations, which remain functional.

UL4 and UL5 have both fractured at the cervical margin. The root canal fillings are exposed with no coronal seal (Figure 19.12).

◈ ***Radiographic examination***

Both UL4 and UL5 have been endodontically treated and a peri-apical pathology is noted in UL6 (Figure 19.13).

What is the prognosis for these teeth?

Endodontic retreatment is possible with a predictable outcome. Because the coronal seal has been missing for at least 2 months, endodontic retreatment would be advisable if the teeth were to be restored. However, restorability of these teeth is the major hurdle with a poor long-term prognosis. Surgical crown lengthening would be necessary to increase the available sound tooth tissue for provision of predictable crowns.

After discussing the various risks and benefits, it was decided to extract the UL4 and UL5 roots.

What replacement restorations would you consider and why?

1. Conventional four-unit fixed–fixed bridge (UL6 to UL3)

   Such a long-span bridge would not be advisable due to a limited long-term success being anticipated. UL6 will require a root canal filling and UL3 is unrestored and would result in loss of substantial healthy tooth tissue.
2. Conventional cantilever bridge (UL5 off UL6)

   A cantilever bridge has 80% chance of survival after 10 years and would be cost-effective. However, UL6 will be a root filled abutment and would negatively influence the long-term success, especially as a cantilever design. The cantilever designs are advantageous because a bridge debond is immediately evident and replacement restorations of smaller units are cost-effective.
3. Resin-bonded cantilever bridge (UL4 off UL3)

   A distal cantilever resin-bonded bridge in the posterior area would be unpredictable and more likely to debond and fail. The advantages are no or minimal preparation in UL3 and it is a cost-effective restoration.
4. Implants to replace both UL4 and UL5

   Single-tooth implant restorations of UL4 and UL5 would be independent and do not require involvement of adjacent teeth. These would provide predictable long-term successful restorations. The two implants can be linked together, but this is not always necessary. Separate units would minimize future maintenance costs if and when replacement of restoration(s) is necessary. However, implant requires a surgical procedure with its postoperative complications, protracted treatment time, and it is expensive in comparison to conventional treatment option.

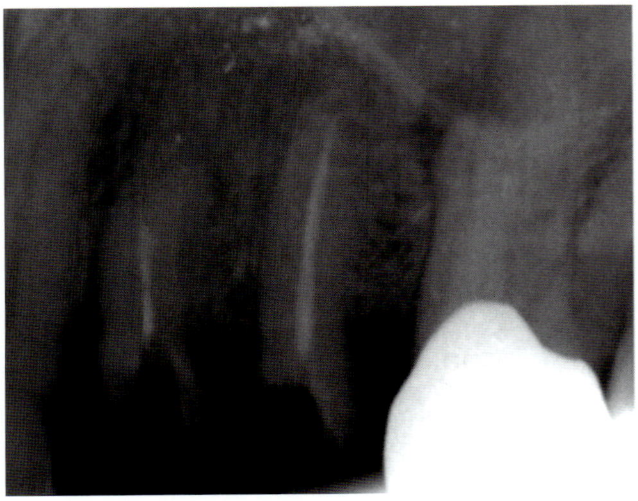

Fig 19.13 Failed endodontic treatment in both UL4 and UL5 with periapical pathologies.

After a detailed discussion about the options, the patient opted to have the teeth replaced by two implant-retained crowns.

What surgical protocols would you consider for implant placement? Discuss the risks and benefits

See Table 19.2.

Preimplant assessment

As outlined in preceding chapters, preimplant assessment requires a thorough clinical and radiographic analysis. Bone height and width availability, proximity of maxillary sinus, and any existing periapical infections have to be considered in planning.

◈ ***Describe the surgical technique, with particular consideration for immediate implant placement***

A detailed written consent form is signed by the patient. Adequate local anaesthesia is achieved, and surgical isolation procedures are followed.

The teeth need to be extracted using an atraumatic technique. It is imperative to avoid damaging the alveolar socket during extraction. This requires special skills, instruments, and technique. Periotomes, which are very fine elevators, are used to sever the periodontal ligament fibres. This loosens the root within the socket for an easy extraction without fracturing the labial bone. The socket is thoroughly debrided off any periodontal ligament fibres and granulation tissue. The intact socket walls are inspected.

In the premolar and molar region, the implant has to be positioned in the centre of the extraction site. A well-controlled implant bed preparation is necessary to achieve accurate implant positioning (Figure 19.14). If bone height is available, the implant length should exceed the apical tip of the extracted root because most of the primary stability is achieved from this apical part of the implant. Furthermore, a tapered (conical) shaped implant with a more aggressive

Table 19.2 Comparison of immediate and delayed implant placement protocols

Immediate placement protocol	Delayed placement protocol
Technically demanding surgery	Technically an easier procedure
Reduced primary stability	Improved primary stability
Reduced treatment time	Protracted treatment time
Slightly reduced success and survival rate	Highest reported success and survival rates
More risk of complications and recession around crowns	Better control on final restorative outcome
Possible need for bone grafting at surgery	If ridge width and height maintained, uncomplicated surgical procedure

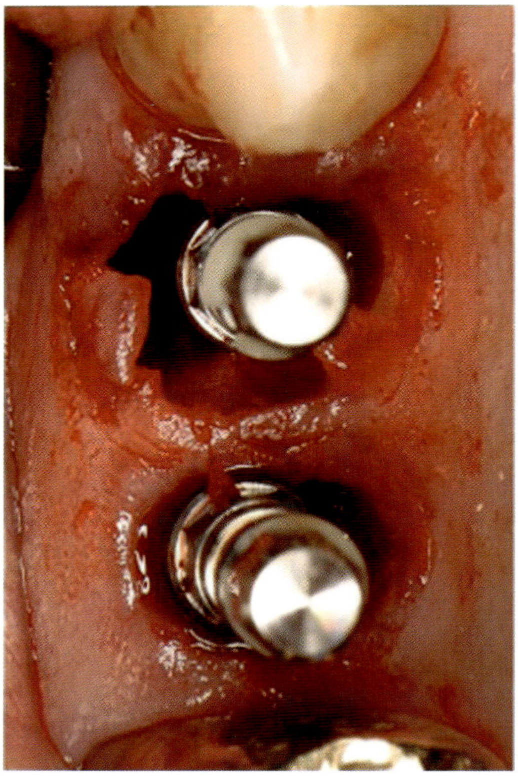

Fig 19.14 Two implants in correct position to facilitate future restorations.

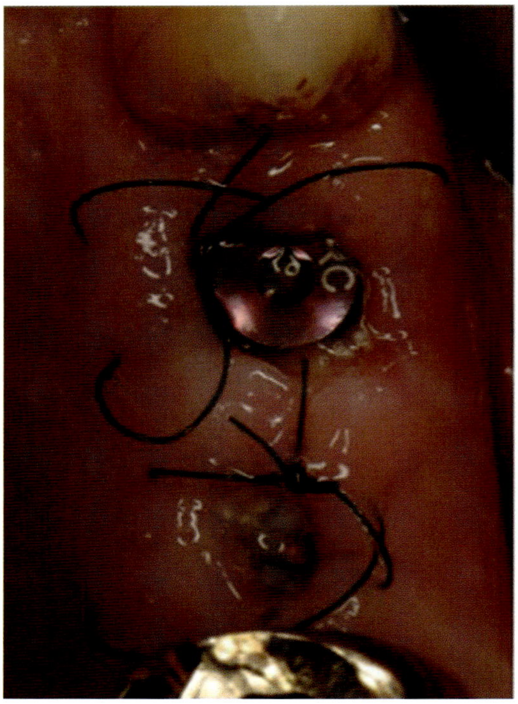

Fig 19.15 Implants are transmucosal to allow single-stage surgical procedure.

thread pitch is desirable in an extraction socket to improve primary stability. This procedure can be performed without raising the flap; thus, it is described as a "flapless" procedure.

Once the correct depth and diameter are prepared with the implant drills, the implant is inserted. This requires precise control because the coronal part of the extraction socket will be larger in diameter than the chosen implant and the implant might end up in an undesirable position. A correctly positioned implant will generally have a gap at the coronal aspect between the socket walls and the implant (see Figure 19.14). If this gap is less than 2 mm, the defect will regenerate with new bone by simply allowing the clot to fill the defect. However, if the gap exceeds 2 mm, some form of bone graft should be used to occlude the defect and prevent soft tissue ingress, which can compromise osseointegration.

A healing cap is attached to the implant. Depending on the type of implant used, it can either be buried or left transmucosal (exposed) for the period of healing during which osseointegration takes place (Figure 19.15).

After a period of healing, if the implant was buried, a second surgical procedure is necessary to expose the top of the implant, and a taller healing cap is placed.

The implant is now ready for restorative treatment (Figure 19.16), which is described in Chapter 21.

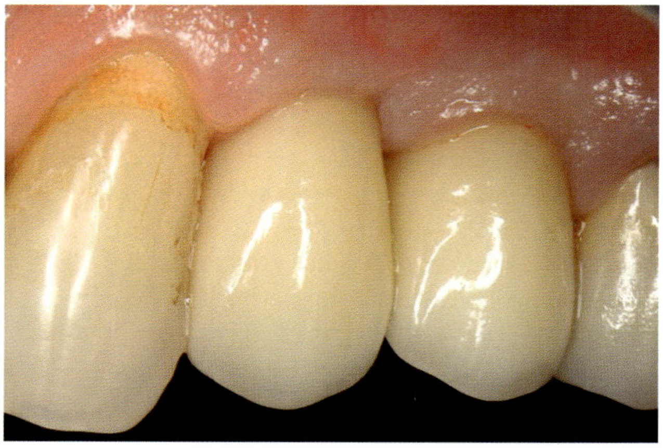

Fig 19.16 Definitive screw-retained crowns on UL4 and UL5. Note the excellent peri-implant soft tissue health and aesthetic outcome.

Replacement of an upper central incisor with a dental implant

Summary

A 45-year-old female presents with missing UR1 and would prefer a fixed option to replace the tooth.

History

◈ *Complaint*

The patient complains of missing UR1. The tooth was extracted 6 months ago, and she had been provided with a removable acrylic partial denture.

◈ *History of complaint*

The patient reported a history of trauma 15 years ago, which resulted in coronal fracture in UR1. At the time, endodontic treatment was carried out and a crown was fabricated. Six months ago, the crown fractured, and the root was extracted due to an untreatable root canal infection. She was provided with a removable acrylic mucosa supported partial denture. The denture is loose, and she is unable to function satisfactorily with the denture.

◈ ***Dental history***

The patient has been a regular dental attendee.

Examination

◈ ***Intraoral examination***

The dentition is moderately restored but well maintained.

UR1 is missing (Figure 19.17), and the adjacent UR2 and UL1 are unrestored. A class I incisal relationship is noted. She has a high smile line and a medium gingival biotype.

◈ ***Radiographic examination***

No abnormality is noted.

What replacement restorations would you consider and why?

1. Resin-bonded cantilever bridge (UR1 off UL1)

   A cantilever resin-bonded bridge in the anterior area in a class I incisor relationship would be a predictable option with a 65% survival after 10 years. The abutment tooth requires minimal or no preparation and would maintain the long-term health even if the bridge debonds. This option would be cost-effective, quick, and painless. However, there is a likelihood of failure by debond.
2. Single-tooth implant to replace UR1

   A single-tooth implant restoration replacing UR1 would be independent and does not require involvement of adjacent teeth. It would provide the most predictable long-term restoration (89.4% survival after 10 years). However, an implant requires a surgical procedure with postoperative discomfort, protracted treatment time, and it is expensive in comparison to the resin-bonded bridge option.

After a detailed discussion about the options, the patient decided to have a single-tooth implant crown.

Preimplant assessment

◈ ***What important factors would you assess when replacing implants in the aesthetic zone?***

See Table 19.3.

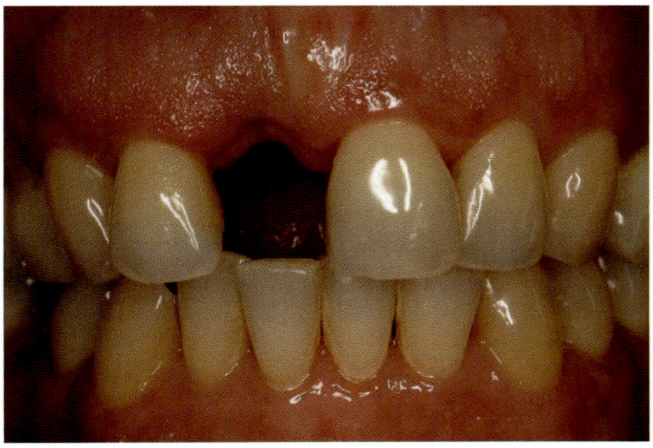

Fig 19.17 Pre-op frontal view. UR1 is missing, and there is a minor vertical soft tissue deficiency.

As outlined in the preceding chapters, preimplant assessment requires adequate clinical and radiographic analysis. Thorough planning includes a diagnostic wax-up, which will form the basis of a surgical guide. The surgical guide is used at the time of surgery to place the implant in an ideal restoratively determined position.

◈ ***Describe the surgical technique most appropriate for the highly demanding aesthetic zone***

A detailed written consent form is signed. Adequate local anaesthesia is achieved, and surgical isolation procedures are followed.

The presurgical assessment has revealed an adequate bone height (Figure 19.18) and soft tissue volume (Figure 19.19). Nonetheless, in the aesthetic zone, especially in a patient with a high smile line, a cautious surgical approach is recommended for optimal aesthetic outcome. A crestal incision and vertical relieving incisions are made to raise a full mucoperiosteal flap.

Table 19.3 Factors to assess when considering implants in the aesthetic zone

Factor	Findings in this case
Smile line	High
Space for restoration	Adequate (>7 mm)
Gingival biotype	Medium
Condition of adjacent teeth	Unrestored
Infection at implant site	None
Bone width	Adequate
Bone height	Adequate
Bone level at adjacent teeth	No bone loss
Soft tissue defect	None
Patient expectation	High

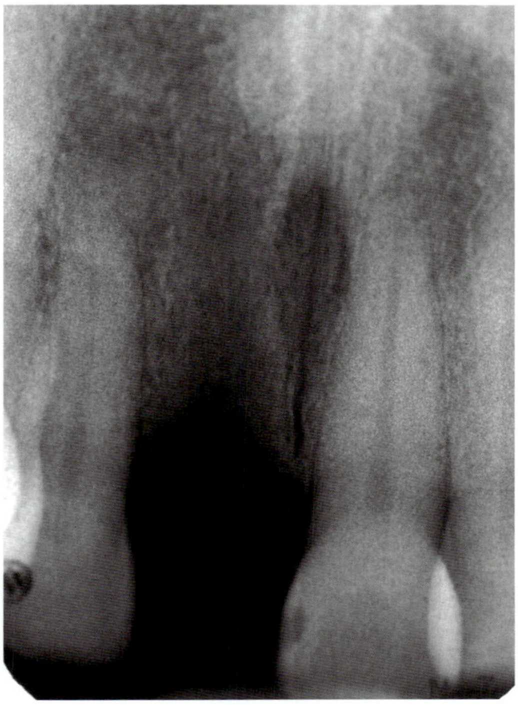

Fig 19.18 Pre-op radiograph of the implant site.

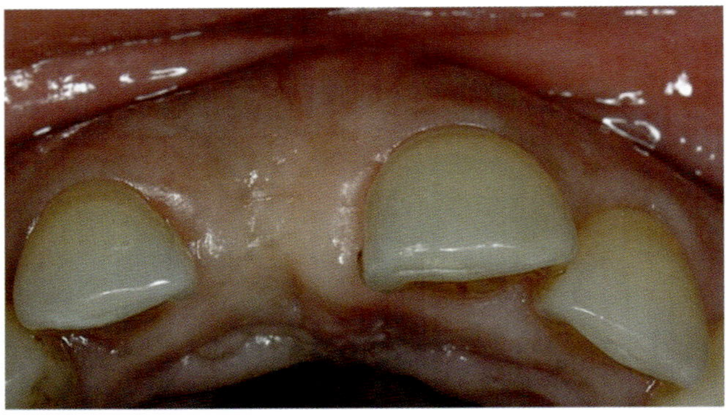

Fig 19.19 Pre-op photo showing adequate tissue volume.

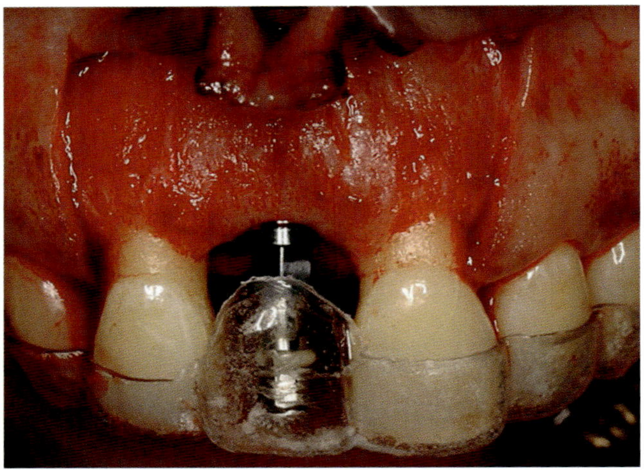

Fig 19.20 Implant depth being confirmed with a surgical guide.

The surgical guide is positioned, and implant bed preparation is carried out using the implant drills. A correct position of the implant is verified with the surgical guide (Figures 19.20 and 19.21). An appropriate-size closure screw is placed, and a tension-free primary closure is achieved. In the aesthetic zone, it is desirable to bury the implant for ideal healing conditions. After 2 or 3 months of healing, a second surgical procedure is necessary to expose the top of the implant.

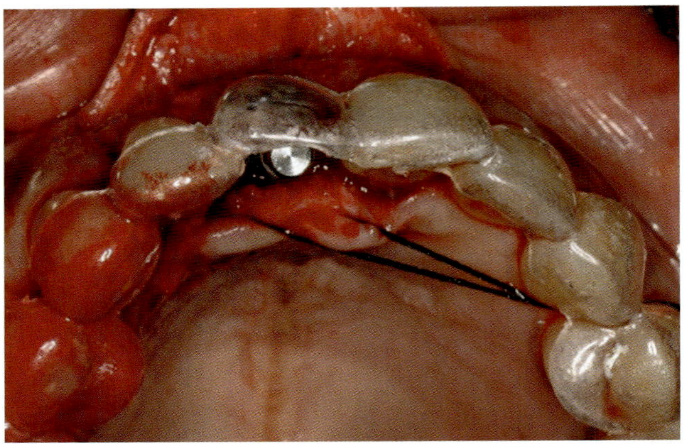

Fig 19.21 Ideal three-dimensional labiopalatal position being verified by the surgical guide.

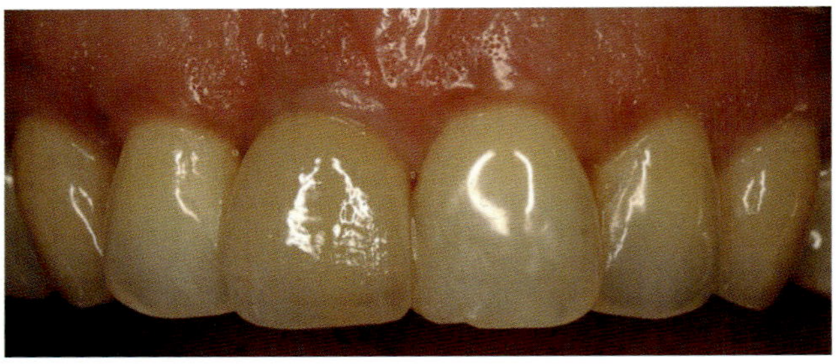

Fig 19.22 Post-op view of single-tooth implant restoration in UR1.

A well-planned and executed implant placement and subsequent restorative treatment will predictably result in a successful outcome (Figure 19.22).

Summary

This chapter focused on various surgical prerequisites that should be considered when planning for and placing dental implants. In particular, the reader should remember and reinforce the principle that "implant placement should be restoratively driven." An implant placed within the described three dimensions will normally result in a successful functional and aesthetic outcome.

Chapter 20

Managing bone deficiencies for implant surgery

Chapter 19 illustrated three cases in which implants were placed in sites with adequate bone volume (i.e., height and width). This chapter discusses the surgical technique most widely recommended for sites where resorption of alveolar ridge after tooth extraction has been significant, leaving insufficient bone width for placement of a dental implant in an ideal prosthetically driven position. Often, there is simply insufficient bone width to even place an implant within the bony housing.

Rebuilding alveolar bone width is more predictable than vertical bone grafting. The focus of this chapter is limited to bone grafting in cases with inadequate bone width.

Generally, two different surgical approaches are indicated in cases with inadequate bone width: simultaneous or staged bone grafting (Table 20.1). As the name implies, simultaneous bone grafting is carried out at the same time the implant is placed, whereas in the staged approach, the ridge is grafted first in a separate surgical procedure. After a healing period of 4–6 months, the implant is placed in a second surgical procedure.

The former technique, also called simultaneous guided bone regeneration (GBR), is carried out using particulate bone, which is protected under a barrier membrane during healing. This is based on similar principles as guided tissue regeneration in periodontal defects, which was discussed in Chapter 12. The most predictable technique in implants involves use of autogenous bone chips collected during the surgical procedure combined with deproteinized bovine bone granules, which are then covered with a resorbable porcine-derived collagen membrane.

On the contrary, if the ridge defect is significant, a staged approach is necessary. This involves grafting with a block of bone of appropriate dimension to rebuild the surgical site. Autogenous bone is still considered to be a gold standard, and this can be harvested from either the mandibular ramus or the symphysial area. The former allows a limited size of bone block, whereas the latter can offer a larger size extending from lower right to left canine.

This chapter discusses two cases illustrating the previously mentioned techniques.

Surgical placement of an implant with simultaneous guided bone regeneration

Summary

A 20-year-old female presents with a failing resin-bonded bridge (RBB) replacing the UR1.

History

Complaint

The patient is complaining of repeatedly debonding RBB.

History of complaint

The tooth had a previous history of trauma and reimplantation following avulsion, subsequently developed root resorption, and was extracted when the patient was 16 years old.

Dental history

The patient has been a regular dental attendee and had had several years of endodontic treatment in UR1 before its extraction. The patient is now concerned about the long-term prognosis of UR1 and wishes to have a more predictable solution for the missing tooth. She has lost confidence due to repeated failure of the RBB.

Examination

Intraoral examination

The dentition is minimally restored, with a good level of oral hygiene.

UR1 is missing (Figure 20.1), and the adjacent UR2 and UL1 are unrestored. A class I incisal relationship is noted. She has a high smile line and a thin gingival biotype.

A detailed examination and assessment as discussed in Chapter 17 was carried out. Assessment of alveolar ridge confirmed lack of adequate ridge width (Figure 20.2); however, it was considered feasible to manage implant placement with simultaneous GBR. The patient consented to have this tooth replaced with a dental implant.

Radiographic examination

No abnormality is noted (Figure 20.3).

What important factors would you consider when placing implants with simultaneous GBR?

In order to achieve a successful functional and aesthetic result, several surgical factors must be considered:

1. Implant position

   It is imperative that the position of the implant is not compromised due to lack of optimal bone volume. For a successful outcome, prosthetically driven ideal three-dimensional position should be the goal.
2. Primary stability

Table 20.1 Advantages and disadvantages of staged and simultaneous bone augmentation

	Staged (block graft)	Simultaneous (particulate bone)
No. of surgeries	Two-stage procedure involving separate grafting and implant placement surgery	Single procedure in which implant is placed and bone grafted
Morbidity	Higher because two separate surgical sites, including risk to lower anterior teeth	Reduced
Predictability	Predictable	Predictable
Scope of grafting	Potentially greater than simultaneously using particulate bone	Predictable in horizontal but unpredictable in vertical augmentation
Treatment time	Significantly increases treatment time	Much shorter treatment time
Cost	Higher	More cost-effective for the patient

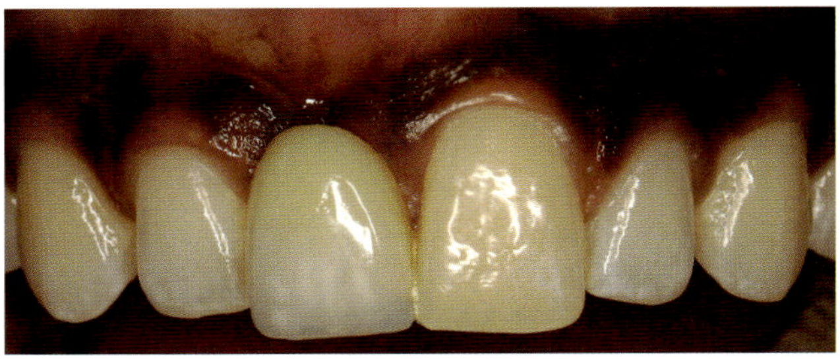

Fig 20.1 A missing UR1 that has been replaced with a resin-bonded cantilever bridge from UL1.

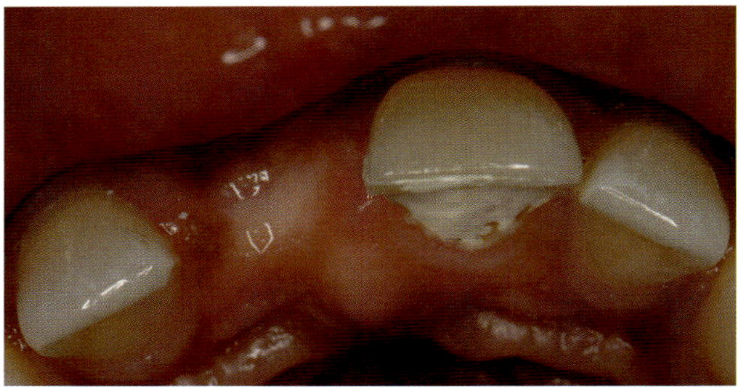

Fig 20.2 Alveolar ridge assessment shows lateral ridge resorption.

A good primary stability is necessary for this surgical approach.

3. Principles of GBR
   Angiogenesis and space maintenance are two important prerequisites for successful GBR. Angiogenesis is promoted by carrying out corticotomy holes. These are holes drilled with a small bur perforating the cortical plate to encourage bleeding from the bone trabeculae. When using particulate bone under a resorbable and malleable membrane, overcontouring with bone graft is recommended to maintain adequate long-term bone volume.
4. Tension-free primary closure
   A tension-free primary closure is of significance to ensure the flap remains completely closed during submerged healing. Dehiscence is the most common postoperative complication, which is primarily attributed to forced flap closure as opposed to tension-free primary flap closure.

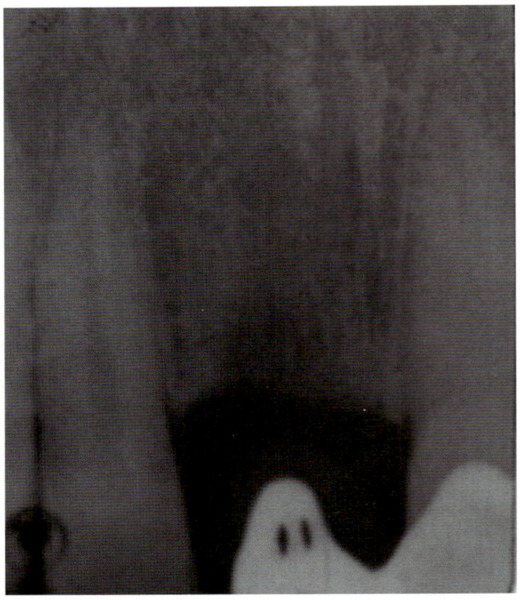

Fig 20.3 A periapical radiograph confirming satisfactory vertical bone level.

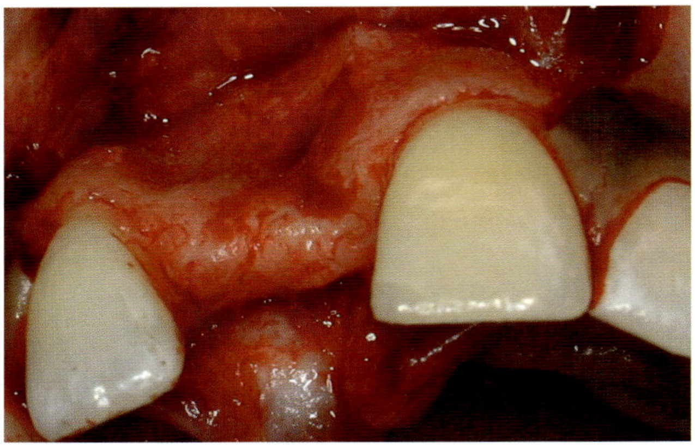

Fig 20.4 A narrow ridge is confirmed at the time of surgery.

5. Healing time
   A healing period of 2 or 3 months is adequate if the surgery for exposure of the implant is minimal. Provided the flap is not raised beyond the shoulder of the implant, early exposure can be performed. However, when an extensive flap has to be raised—for example, if soft tissue grafting is indicated—then a longer healing period of 6–9 months is recommended to allow a better bone integration.

Describe the surgical technique of simultaneous GBR

A detailed written consent form is signed. Adequate local anaesthesia is achieved, and surgical isolation procedures are followed.

A crestal incision and vertical relieving incision(s) are made to raise a full mucoperiosteal flap. The presurgical assessment has revealed inadequate bone width, which is confirmed when the flap is raised (Figure 20.4).

The surgical guide is positioned, and implant bed preparation is carried out using the implant drills. A correct position of the implant is verified with the surgical depth and direction indicator (Figure 20.5). The lack of bone width becomes clearly evident; however, the ideal implant positioning is not compromised.

The implant is placed with a good primary stability. A large dehiscence-type defect is noted (Figure 20.6). The smallest closure screw is placed to facilitate primary closure. Corticotomy holes are drilled in the cortical plate. Bone chips are scraped from the adjacent area or collected in a bone trap, which is connected to a special surgical aspirator. The autogenous bone is laid as a first layer over the exposed implant surface (Figure 20.7), which is covered by a generous layer of deproteinized bovine bone particles (Figure 20.8). The granules of bone can be presoaked in the patient's blood collected locally from the surgical site, which helps to make the granules sticky and easy to manipulate.

A resorbable collagen membrane is then cut to size and laid over the bone graft. Ideally, the membrane should extend at least 2 or 3 mm beyond the bone graft to achieve good stability. It is claimed that a second layer of collagen membrane laid on top also helps to improve membrane stability and reduce the speed of resorption (Figure 20.9). Alternatively, the membrane can be tacked in place using special titanium or resorbable tacks.

A generous periosteal release is achieved by using a fresh scalpel blade to carry out periosteal incision running from the mesial vertical relieving incision to the distal. This will facilitate tension-free primary closure, which can be confirmed by lack of blanching in the flap (Figure 20.10). In the aesthetic zone, it is desirable to bury the implant for ideal healing conditions.

The patient is instructed on postoperative care, and appropriate antibiotics and analgesics are prescribed. For immediate postoperative use, 0.2% chlorhexidine is

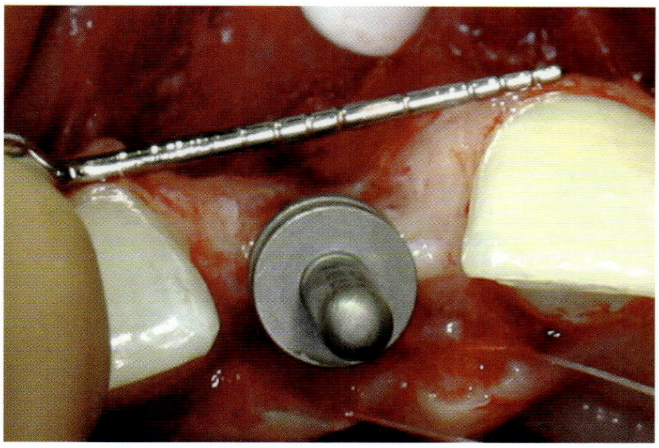

Fig 20.5 Direction indicator confirming the position of prepared implant site.

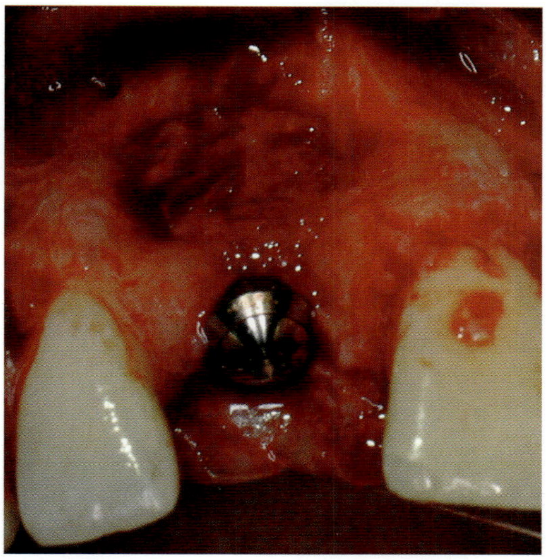

Fig 20.7 GBR procedure with initial layer of autogenous bone chips over the exposed implant surface.

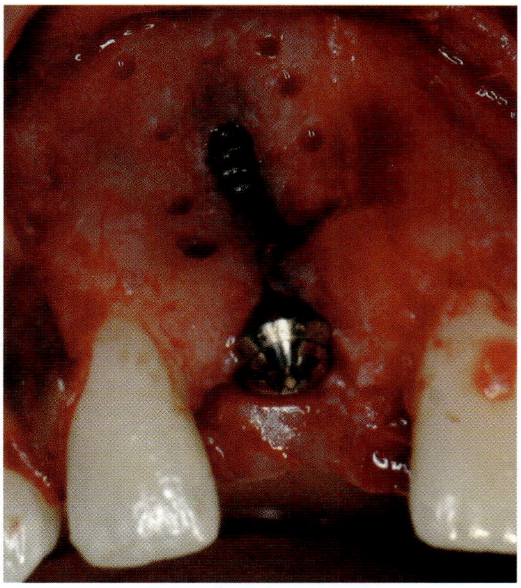

Fig 20.6 A large dehiscence-type defect on the labial aspect. Corticotomy holes prepared for GBR procedure.

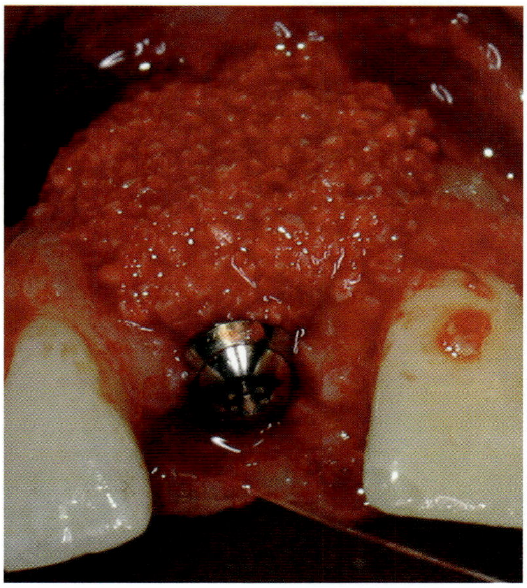

Fig 20.8 Alveolar ridge contour redeveloped using particulate bovine bone substitute.

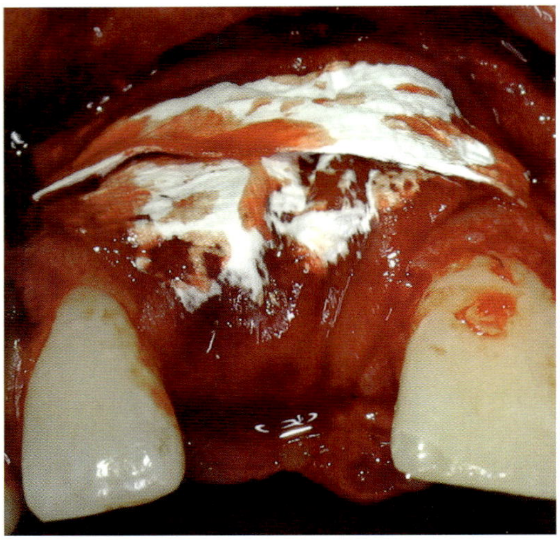

Fig 20.9 Bilayer porcine collagen membrane applied over the bone graft.

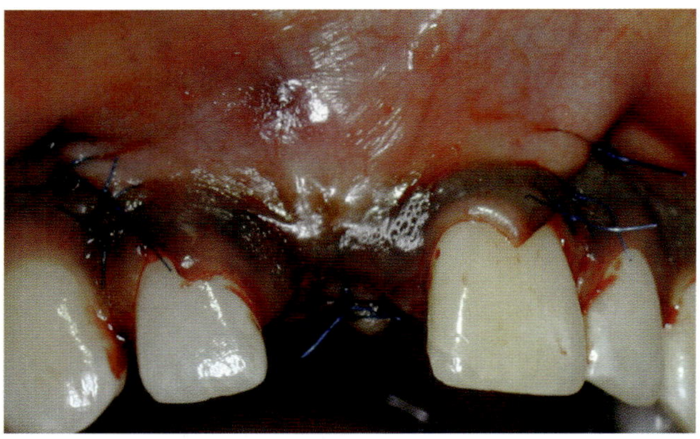

Fig 20.10 Tension-free primary closure is essential to ensure success of GBR procedure and prevent flap dehiscence.

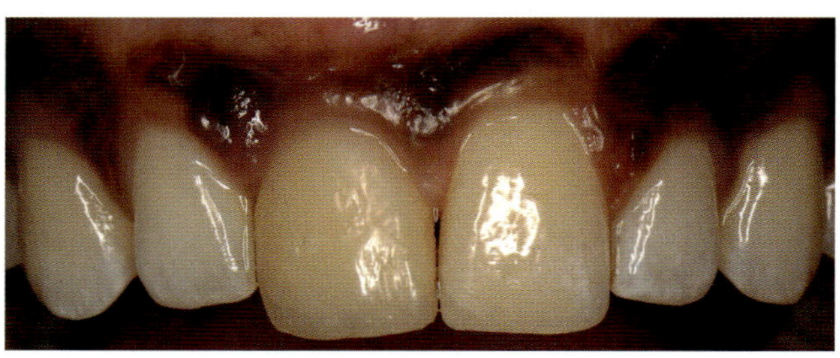

Fig 20.11 Provisional restoration allows soft tissue moulding to optimize pink aesthetics.

recommended. Care is taken to prevent any trauma to the surgical site from the provisional restoration. If a removable prosthesis is used, it should be avoided for at least 1 week postsurgery, and following the resolution of swelling, the denture will require trimming to prevent trauma. Because the site has been grafted, naturally, the denture will require much trimming to re-seat. The denture should be flangeless. If the patient has a fixed provisional restoration, the pontic will need adjustment. The sutures are usually removed after 7–10 days.

After 2 or 3 months of healing, a second surgical procedure is necessary to expose the top of the implant, and a taller healing abutment is attached. The restorative phase of treatment commences with provision of a temporary crown (Figure 20.11), which is used to mould the peri-implant soft tissues (Figure 20.12). Finally, a screw-retained definitive

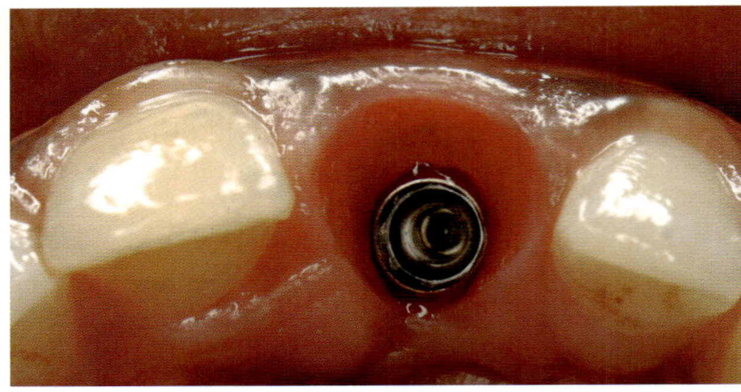

Fig 20.12 Ideal emergence created with the help of the provisional restoration.

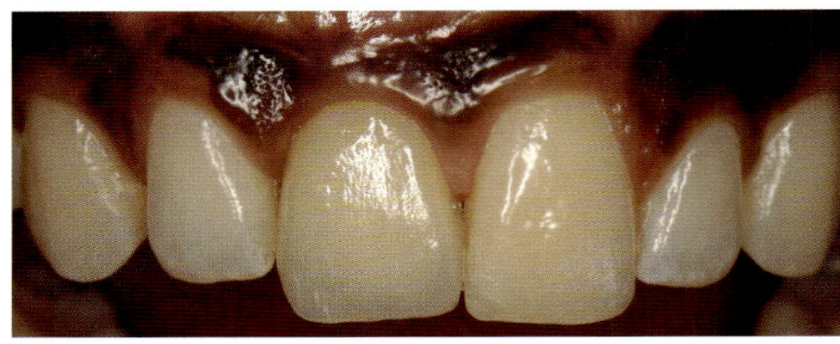

Fig 20.13 Definitive crown restoring both pink and white aesthetics.

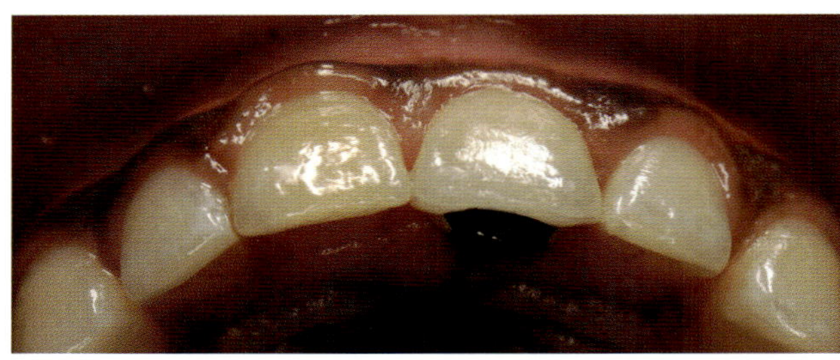

Fig 20.14 Note the alveolar contour that has been redeveloped with the GBR procedure.

restoration is provided, resulting in excellent aesthetic and functional outcome (Figure 20.13). The restorative stages of a single-tooth implant crown are discussed in detail in Chapter 21.

Figure 20.14 shows how GBR with particulate bone substitute has been successful in rebuilding the previously resorbed labial bone contour.

Surgical placement of an implant after staged augmentation with block bone graft

Summary

A 28-year-old female presents with missing UL1 requesting replacement with a dental implant.

History

Complaint

The patient is complaining of missing UL1.

History of complaint

UL1 had been extracted 2 years ago. Previous history of trauma in teenage years resulted in endodontic treatment and a restoration with a cast post-crown. A chronic draining sinus and an isolated periodontal pocket ensued due to root fracture. The tooth was extracted, and an immediate acrylic mucosa-borne partial denture with a labial flange was provided.

◈ *Dental history*

The patient is a regular dental attendee and has no other restorations.

Examination

◈ *Intraoral examination*

The dentition is unrestored, with a good level of oral hygiene.

UL1 is missing (Figure 20.15), and the adjacent teeth are unrestored. A class I incisal relationship is noted. She has a high smile line and a thin gingival biotype.

A detailed examination and assessment as discussed in Chapter 17 was carried out. Assessment of the alveolar ridge confirmed a significant narrowing of the ridge (Figure 20.16) and need for a block bone graft to reconstruct the ridge for future implant placement.

◈ *Radiographic examination*

No abnormality is noted. Cone beam computed tomography examination confirms lack of adequate bone width for implant placement (Figure 20.17).

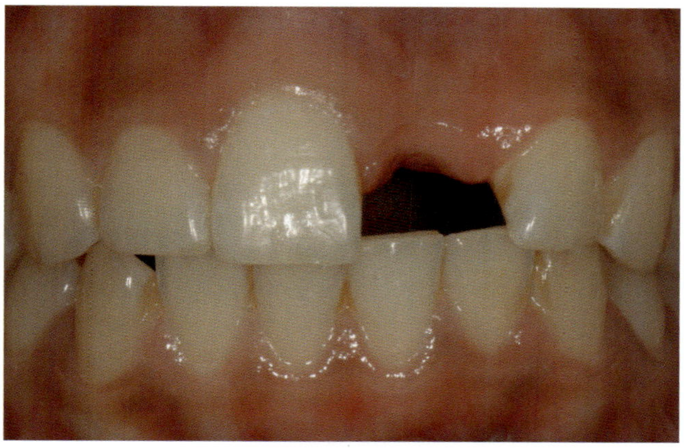

Fig 20.15 Pre-op view of missing UL1.

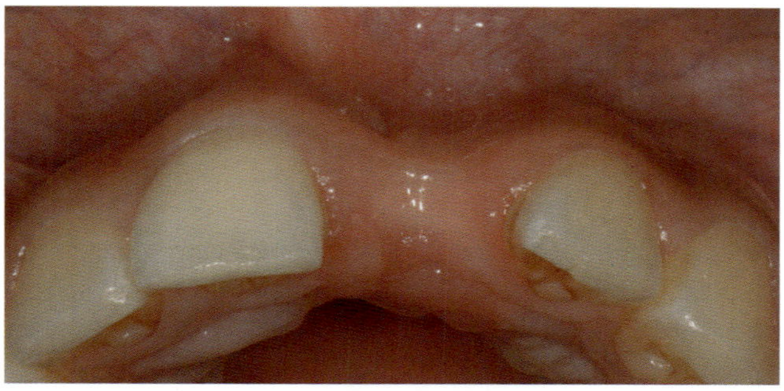

Fig 20.16 Occlusal view showing the extent of lateral ridge resorption.

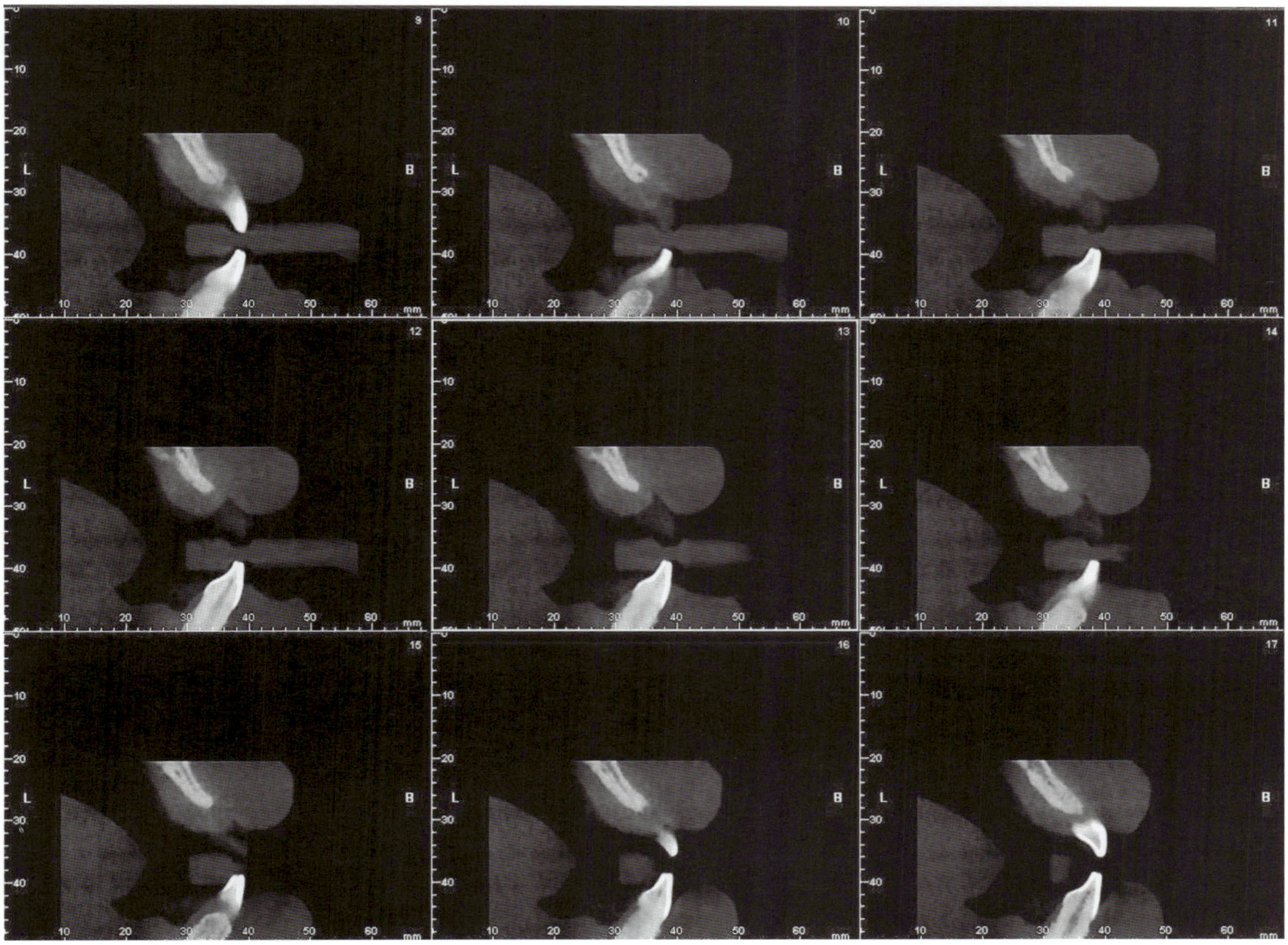

Fig 20.17 Cross-sectional views of UL1 confirming lack of alveolar ridge width.

Describe the surgical technique for block bone grafting

A detailed written consent form is signed. Adequate local anaesthesia is achieved, and surgical isolation procedures are followed. Two surgical sites, the recipient site and the donor site, need to be anaesthetized.

First, the recipient site is investigated. A crestal incision and vertical relieving incision(s) are made to raise a full mucoperiosteal flap. The presurgical assessment has revealed inadequate bone width, which is confirmed when the flap is raised (Figure 20.18). Although the ridge is narrow, there is no vertical bone loss (Figure 20.19). The size of the graft needed is measured using a template, which can be cut and shaped utilizing any sterile material.

Once the graft size and volume requirements are established, the donor site is prepared. In this case, the symphysis was chosen as the preferred site. A flap extending from the right to the left canine is usually desired in order to gain adequate access to the site. A full mucoperiosteal flap is raised, extending to the lower border of the mandible. The template is used to mark the outlined size of the graft. Cuts are made in the bone using either a fine fissure carbide bur or peizo-surgical instruments (Figure 20.20). The bone cuts should be deep enough to traverse the thickness of the cortical part of the labial bone. Finally, the block is released using a chisel to detach the block from its underlying cancellous bone bed.

The donor site can then be sutured and pressure applied to eliminate any blood clot between the flap and the bone. Meanwhile, the block of bone is kept wrapped in moist gauze.

Next, the recipient site is prepared by drilling corticotomy holes to encourage angiogenesis underneath the bone block (Figure 20.21). It is recommended to use the implant surgical guide to inform the correct position for the block (Figure 20.22) in order to facilitate the intended future implant surgery (Figure 20.23). The block is then stabilized using special bone screws (Figure 20.24). Occasionally, two screws are necessary to ensure stability of the graft. There should be no movement in the graft during healing, which may otherwise lead to graft failure. Sharp edges are smoothened,

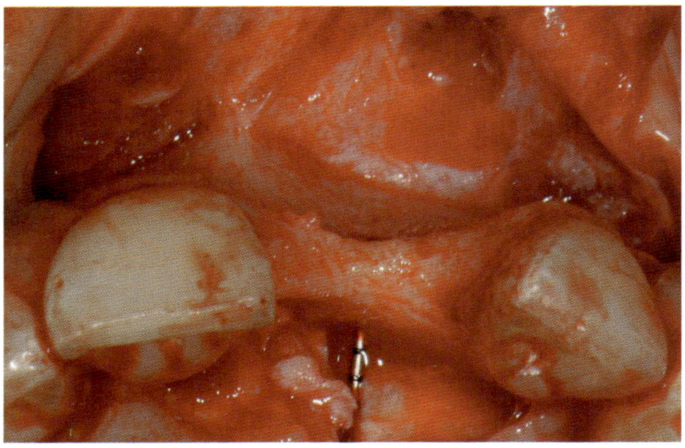

Fig 20.18 A narrow ridge in UL1.

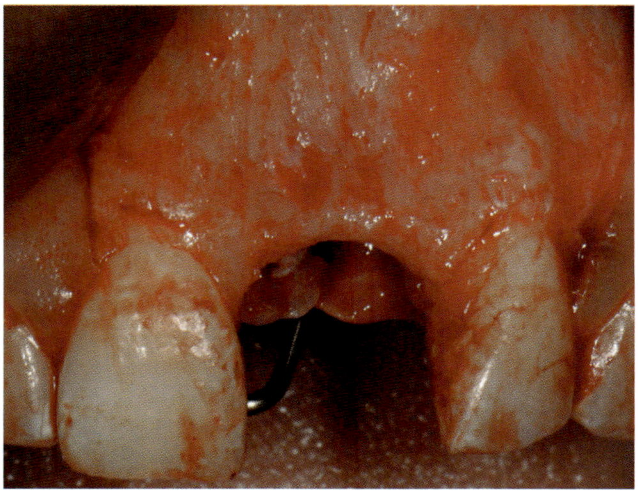

Fig 20.19 Despite lateral resorption, vertical bone height is maintained.

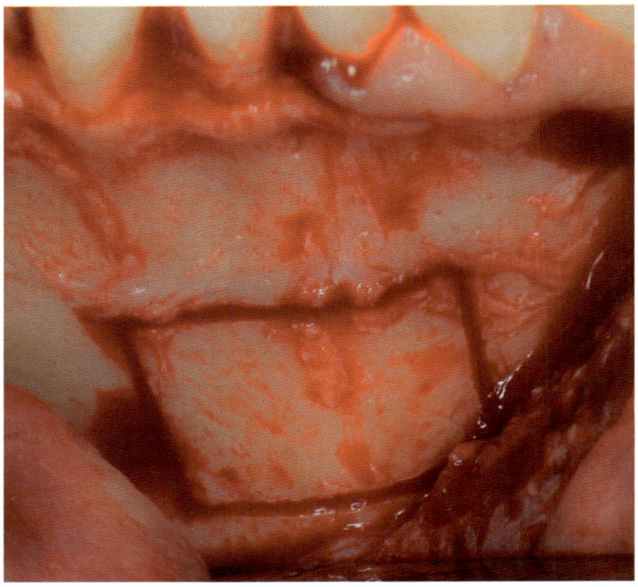

Fig 20.20 Corticocancellous bone block is harvested from anterior symphyseal region.

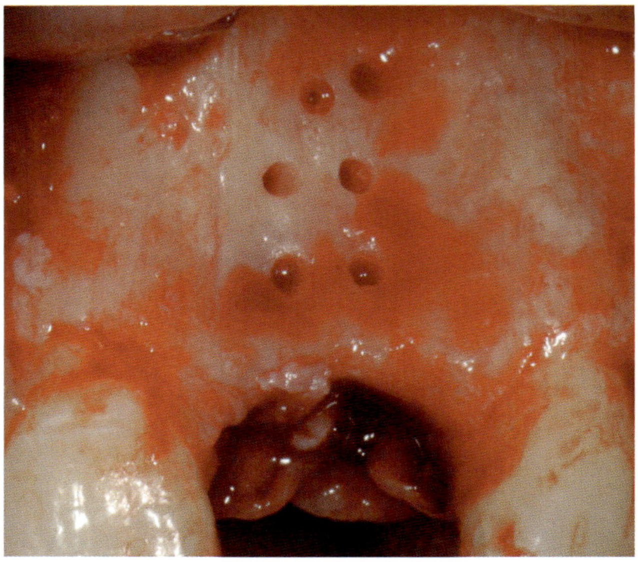

Fig 20.21 Corticotomy holes to promote angiogenesis in the recipient site.

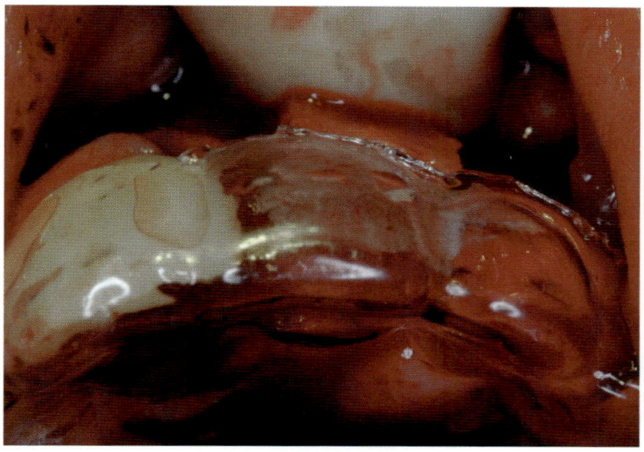

Fig 20.22 Surgical template used to confirm graft positioning.

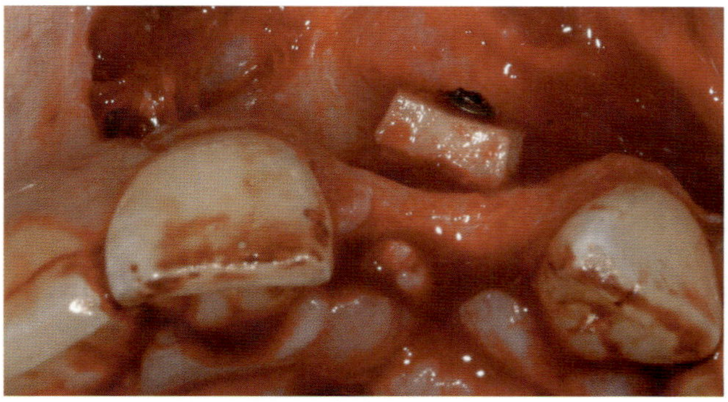

Fig 20.23 Occlusal view of the secured bone graft. It is desirable to overaugment the site to compensate for graft remodelling.

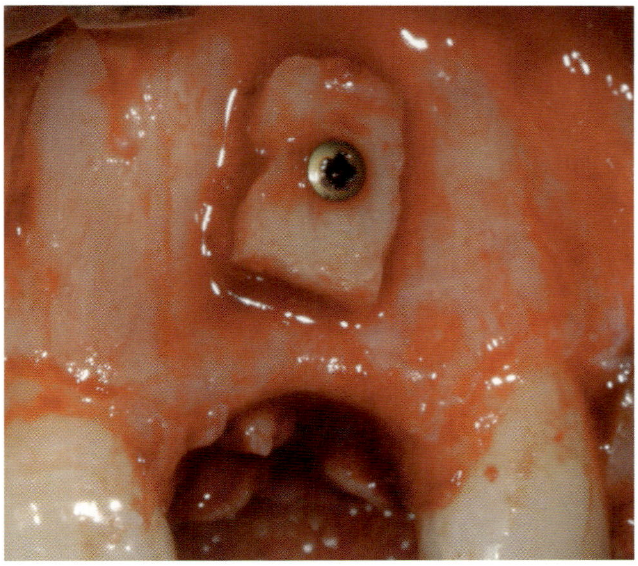

Fig 20.24 Facial view of the bone block that has been screwed in place for stability.

and the flap can be closed by using appropriate sutures and ensuring a tension-free primary closure.

The patient is instructed on postoperative care, and appropriate antibiotics and analgesics are prescribed. For immediate postoperative use, 0.2% chlorhexidine is recommended. Care is taken to prevent any trauma to the surgical site from the provisional restoration, as described in the previous clinical case. The sutures are usually removed after 7–10 days.

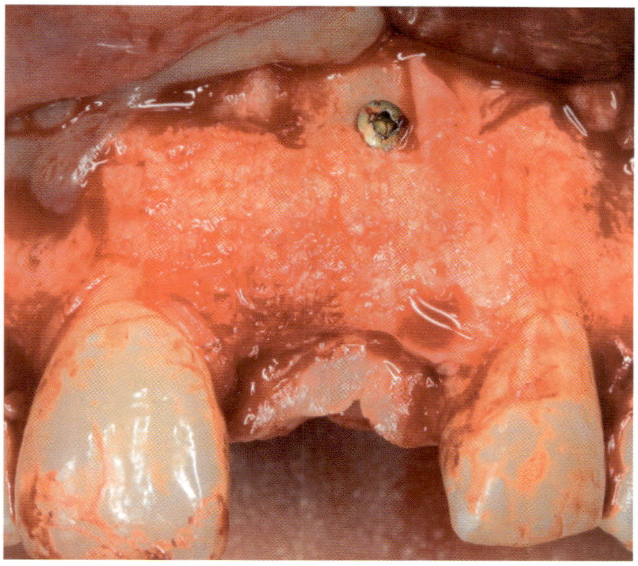

Fig 20.25 Successful graft integration at the time of implant placement surgery after 5 months.

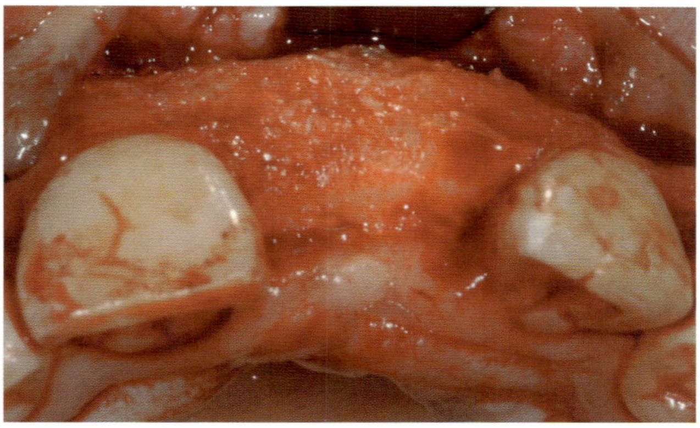

Fig 20.26 Occlusal view showing excellent ridge width reconstruction.

When using autogenous bone block, a healing period of 4–6 months is recommended as ideal. After 6 months, the graft starts to resorb, and up to 60% of graft resorption has been reported within the first year. However, the bone block can be covered with particulate bovine bone substitute to protect the autogenous bone from resorption.

Following 5 months of healing, a full mucoperiosteal flap is raised, the bone screw is removed, and the stability and integration of the graft is assessed (Figures 20.25 and 20.26). The surgical guide is positioned, and implant bed preparation is carried out using the implant drills. A correct position of the implant is verified (Figure 20.27). In the aesthetic zone, it is desirable to bury the implant for ideal healing conditions.

After an additional 2 or 3 months of healing, a second surgical procedure is necessary to expose the shoulder of the implant, and a taller healing abutment is attached prior to commencement of prosthetic treatment.

Conclusion

This chapter describes the two techniques most commonly used to augment missing bone in an implant site. A

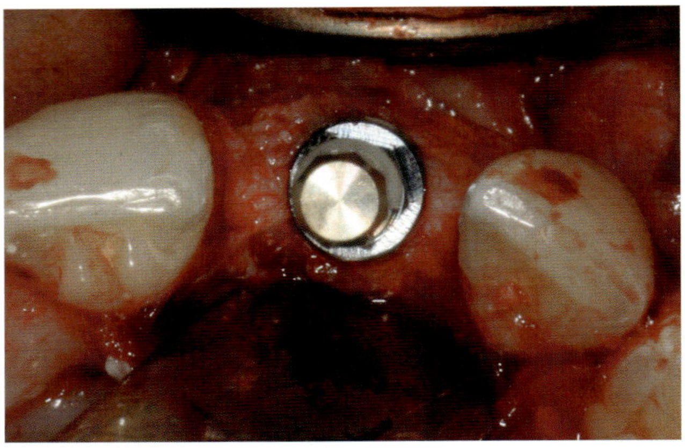

Fig 20.27 Adequate bone volume allows an ideal implant position.

two-stage procedure using a block of autogenous bone has been considered the gold standard for many years; however, with the established predictability of the guided bone regeneration procedure with particulate bone, clinicians can now successfully choose a simultaneous bone grafting procedure. The advantages of this approach are numerous; however, its limitations should be carefully considered when assessing potential patients.

Chapter 21

Restorative options in implant dentistry

After successful surgery and osseointegration, the restorative phase involving fabrication of the prosthesis commences. For this, the laboratory requires an impression that accurately captures the position of the implant in the mouth. The laboratory can then produce an ideal restoration that fits accurately on the implant.

This chapter discusses the various stages involved in the process of fabricating a screw- or a cement-retained prosthesis, single- or multiple-unit prosthesis, and prosthetic options for an edentulous patient. The following questions are addressed.

1. What are the techniques for transferring the implant position to a working cast?
2. What is an implant abutment and what are the various available types?
3. What are the methods of attaching a restoration to the dental implant?
4. What restorative options can be considered for an edentulous patient?

Several clinical case examples are presented to illustrate the various restorative options.

What are the techniques for transferring the implant position to a working cast?

In order to record an accurate impression of the position of an implant, specially designed components called impression copings or transfer aids are used. All implant manufacturers have their own corresponding impression copings, which are machined to fit accurately over an implant. These are either screwed or press-fit (snap-on impression copings) on the implant and are used for open-tray or closed-tray impression techniques, respectively.

Accurate seating of impression coping is important, and the coping has to engage the internal or external antirotational features of the implant. For example, in Figure 21.1, the Straumann implant has an octagonal antirotational configuration. Its corresponding impression coping has a similar octagonal configuration so that, when inserted accurately, these configurations should slot into each other. If the implant is subgingival and there is doubt about complete seating of the impression coping, a radiograph should be taken to check the seating prior to taking an impression (Figures 21.2 and 21.3, respectively, show incomplete seating of the impression coping and the same impression coping when correctly seated). When the implant is subgingival, snap-on impression copings should not be used.

Following confirmation of complete seating of the impression coping, an accurate impression is recorded using either a polyether or addition-cured silicone impression material. It is important to handle the impression tray with care to ensure an accurate impression. It is particularly relevant when using snap-on impression copings because they can be easily dislodged if the tray is forced into position.

Although it is advisable to have a special custom tray made for an implant impression, for a single-tooth and a short-span restoration, a correctly selected stock tray can be adequately used. The author prefers to use a lower impression tray without palatal coverage when recording an impression for a fixed restoration.

As the name implies, an open-tray impression tray has an opening to access the screw head in order to unscrew the impression coping after the material has set (Figure 21.4). After the tray is selected, a wax lid can be added using a warm sheet of modelling wax to prevent outflow of impression material through the window.

After the impression material is fully set, the tray is removed. The snap-on impression coping will snap off the implant and remain embedded within the impression material. In contrast, the screwed type will need to be unscrewed to detach the coping from the implant, and the tray is removed from the mouth (Figure 21.5). The impression is checked for its accuracy, and seating of the coping can be verified (Figure 21.6). If impression material is overflowing the fitting surface of the coping, then it is fair to assume that the impression coping was either not fully seated or dislodged during the procedure.

The next stage involves attaching an implant analogue (replica implant) to the impression coping within the impression (Figures 21.7 and 21.8). The analogues are also accurately machined to replicate a particular implant type.

In order to easily develop the subgingival emergence of the implant restoration, the peri-implant gingivae is mimicked using pink-coloured silicone material (Figure 21.9). This creates an accurate representation of the clinical situation after the model is poured in stone and allows easier subgingival manipulation than if only stone is used.

What is an implant abutment and what are the various available types?

The implant abutment has a very important role to play and constitutes a critical interface between the implant and the prosthesis. An abutment connects the implant to the restoration and also interfaces with the peri-implant soft tissue as it emerges through these tissues. Therefore, abutments should be biocompatible, stable in the oral environment, allow an intimate soft tissue attachment, and withstand occlusal forces.

Abutments can be classified according to their fabrication techniques:

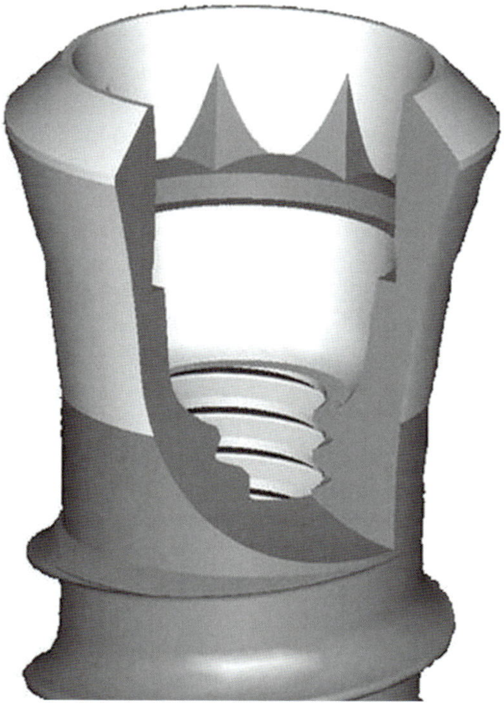

Fig 21.1 A cross section of an implant showing the internal antirotational feature.

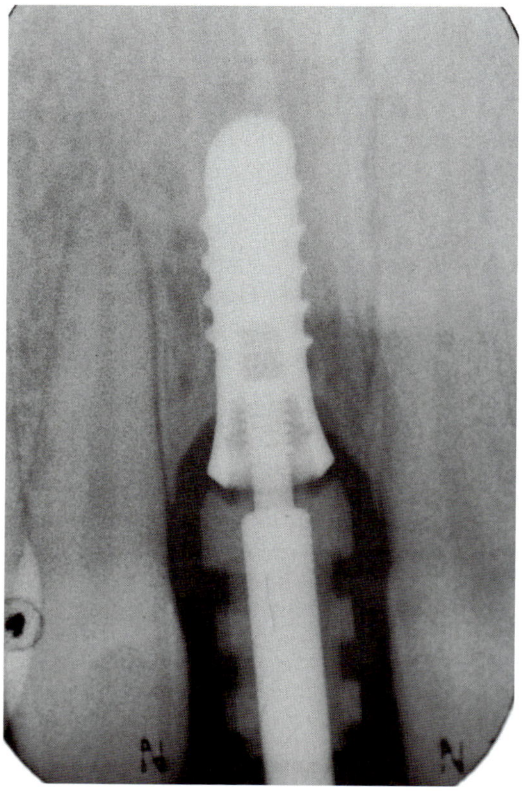

Fig 21.2 Screw-retained impression coping that is incompletely seated.

- Prefabricated abutments
- Cast to abutments
- Computer-aided design/computer-aided manufacturing (CAD/CAM) abutments

Implant manufacturers offer prefabricated abutments in various shapes, sizes, and angulations (Figure 21.10). These

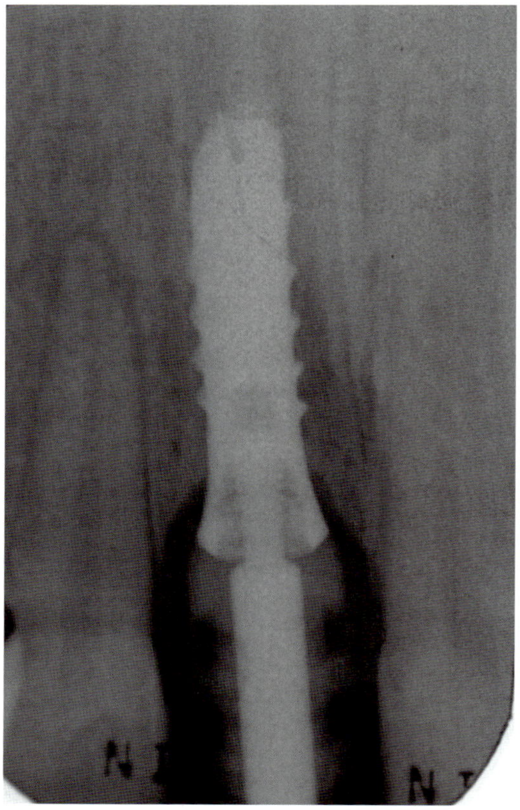

Fig 21.3 Screw-retained impression coping fully engaging the internal antirotational features and fully seated for accurate impression.

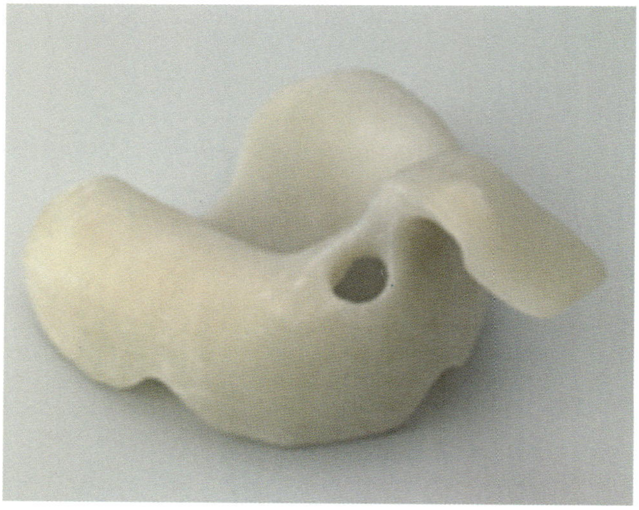

Fig 21.4 Custom tray with an opening allowing access to impression coping to facilitate removal after setting of the material.

are suitable for certain clinical situations and can be a cost-effective option.

Although most of the prefabricated types are noncustomizable, some can be customized, albeit after a time-consuming process. Blocks of titanium or zirconia are available that can be trimmed to shape and desired size (Figure 21.11). These have largely been superseded by CAD/CAM-based customized abutments.

The castable abutment (also widely known as the UCLA-type abutment) offers a reasonable alternative. These are manufactured with a precise machined connection to fit the implant and a plastic sleeve (Figure 21.12A), which the

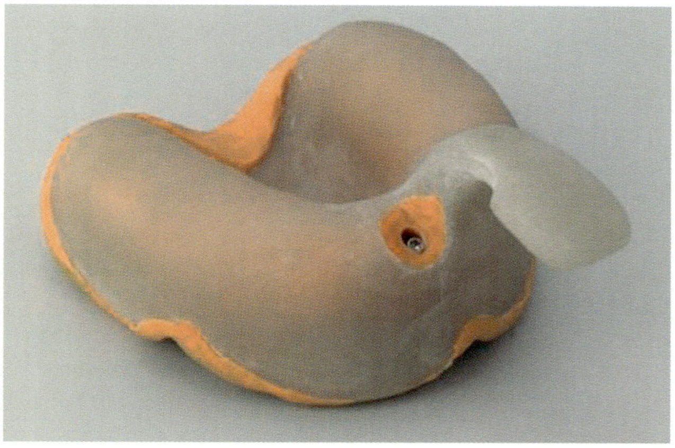

Fig 21.5 The impression coping retained within the set impression material.

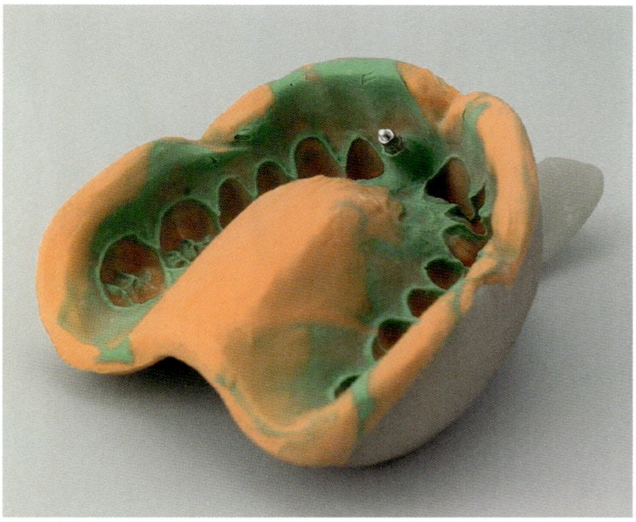

Fig 21.6 Inside view of the impression with an embedded impression coping.

laboratory technician can modify to an ideal geometry (Figure 21.12B,C). It is then cast in precious metal using the conventional lost wax technique.

In recent years, CAD/CAM technology has been at the forefront of development in the dental industry. The two main materials used in implant dentistry are zirconia and titanium. Special scanners are used to scan the working cast. Abutment designing is carried out on the computer, and the data generated are used to mill the abutment. The majority of the milling is carried out in dedicated manufacturer's milling centres. The zirconia coping for the overlying crown or a bridge framework is also designed and milled using a similar procedure (Figure 21.13).

What are the methods of attaching a restoration to the dental implant?

In order to address this question, we consider a few clinical situations that illustrate the various restorative options for a single-tooth and a short-span implant bridge.

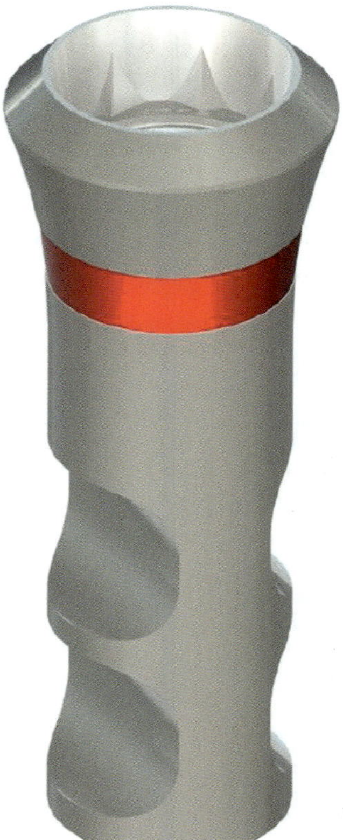

Fig 21.7 A typical implant analogue that mimics the shape of a particular implant system and type.

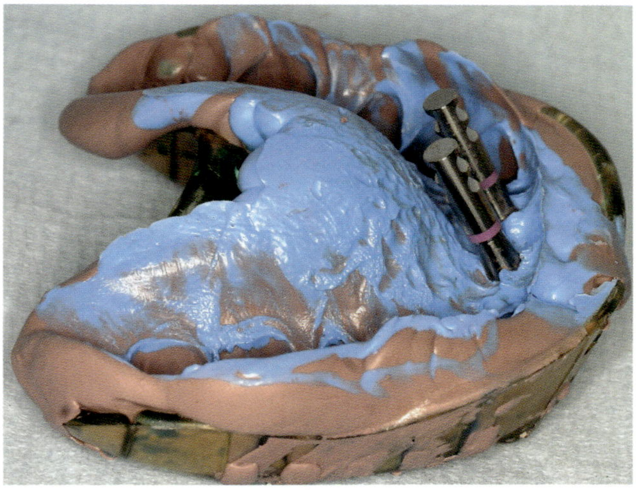

Fig 21.8 Two implant analogues are attached to the two impression copings in this particular case.

Single-tooth posterior replacement

Posterior cement-retained crown

A 55-year-old male patient had an implant placed in the LL6 region (Figure 21.14A). The implant was placed using a transmucosal approach, and after an adequate healing period it is now ready for restoration. The implant shoulder is at the gingival level, and excess cement removal is easily accessible. The angulation of the implant is favourable for both screw- and cement-retained crown. A closed-tray impression technique is used (Figure 21.14B).

A prefabricated cementable abutment was chosen (Figure 21.14C). The abutment height had to be adjusted in the laboratory, and a well-fitting metal ceramic crown is made. The abutment is screwed on the implant, and final tightening to recommended torque is carried out (Figure 21.14D). The screw access hole is sealed, and the crown is cemented using a soft (temporary) cement. The excess cement is removed, resulting in a very natural-looking restoration that does not have a screw access hole (Figure 21.14E).

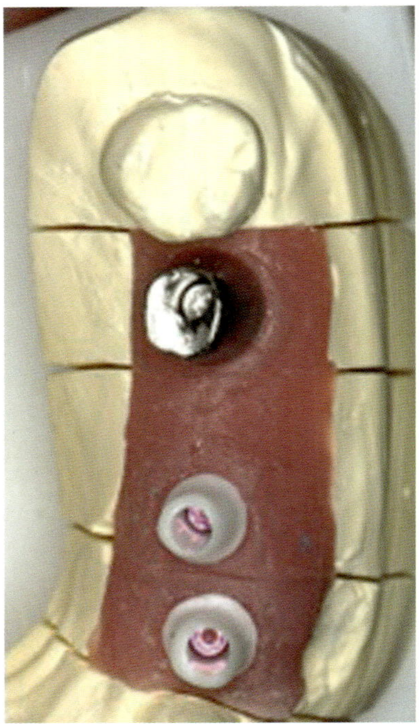

Fig 21.9 A working cast with pink-coloured silicone gingival mask and implant abutments.

Posterior screw-retained crown

A 43-year-old female patient had an implant placed in the LL5 region (Figure 21.15A). The implant placement was transmucosal; however, the implant shoulder is a few millimetres subgingival (Figure 21.15B). A cement-retained crown on prefabricated abutment would be inappropriate because adequate access to removal of excess cement would be highly unlikely. Leaving residues of cement subgingivally around the implant–abutment junction will cause peri-implantitis and complications. In order to provide a cement-retained restoration, the abutment in this case should be customized to create a restoration finish line at or just below the gingival level. Alternatively, if the angulation of the implant permits, a screw-retained crown would be desirable (Figure 21.15C). Such a crown can be a metal ceramic cast

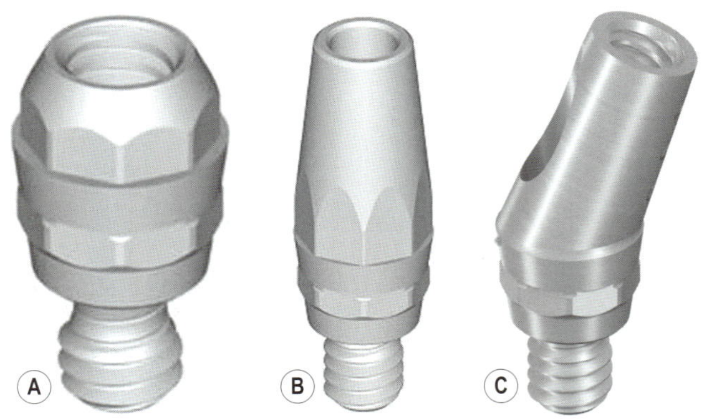

Fig 21.10 Prefabricated (A) screw-retained abutment, (B) straight-cemented abutment, and (C) angled abutment.

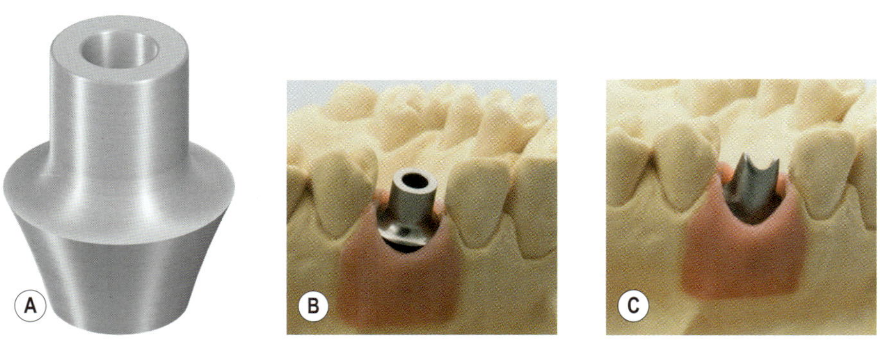

Fig 21.11 (A–C) Customizable titanium abutment can been trimmed to shape and margins are placed at or just below the gingival level. A cementable crown can be fabricated, allowing easy access to cement.

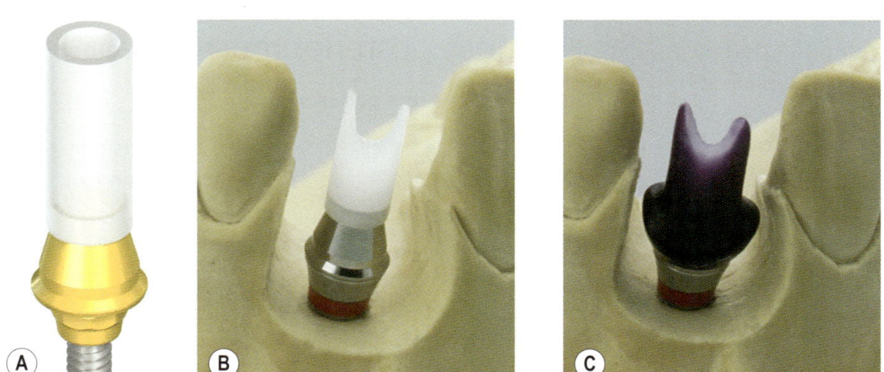

Fig 21.12 (A) An example of a castable abutment. (B and C) The burnout plastic sleeve is trimmed and an abutment is designed in wax prior to casting.

crown, or the abutment can be manufactured using CAD/CAM followed by direct lamination of ceramic to create a one-piece screw-retained crown (Figure 21.15D).

Anterior cement-retained crown

A 25-year-old female patient had an implant placed in the UR1 and UL1 region (Figure 21.16A) using an early-delayed approach as described in Chapter 19. Following a healing period of 10 weeks, the implants were exposed and healing abutments were attached. Note the flat gingival profile in comparison to the adjacent teeth. Implants in the aesthetic site add an additional aesthetic dimension and challenge clinicians to produce imperceptible restorations. In order to achieve this aim successfully, a very measured and a patient approach is recommended. Provisional crowns were provided to commence moulding of peri-implant soft tissues to optimize the pink aesthetics (Figure 21.16B). Several appointments may be necessary to achieve the end result. The subgingival transitional zone is the area of interest, and appropriate modification of this zone is carried out for desirable soft tissue moulding (Figure 21.16C).

After the pink aesthetics are optimized, a new impression of the implant is recorded. The open-tray impression coping is used as the implant in the aesthetic zone and is usually subgingival. The soft tissue emergence does not match the shape of the impression coping and therefore modification or customization of impression coping should be carried out (Figure 21.16D), or else the soft tissue will collapse readily, resulting in loss of detail of the previously moulded tissue emergence shape. This technique allows accurate recording of the emergence profile and the subsequent laboratory procedure is facilitated with great accuracy.

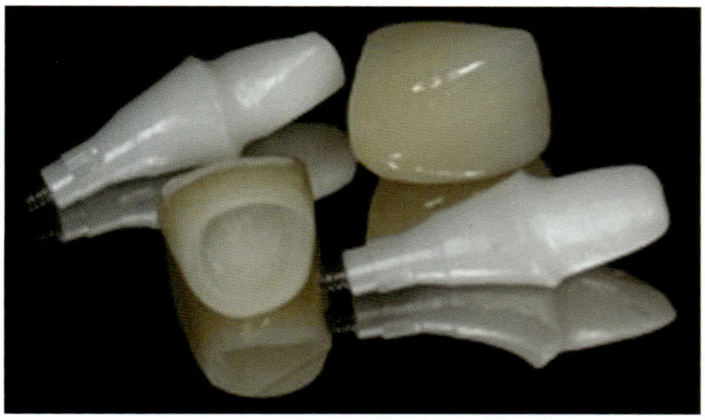

Fig 21.13 Zirconia abutments and two corresponding crowns with zirconia inner copings.

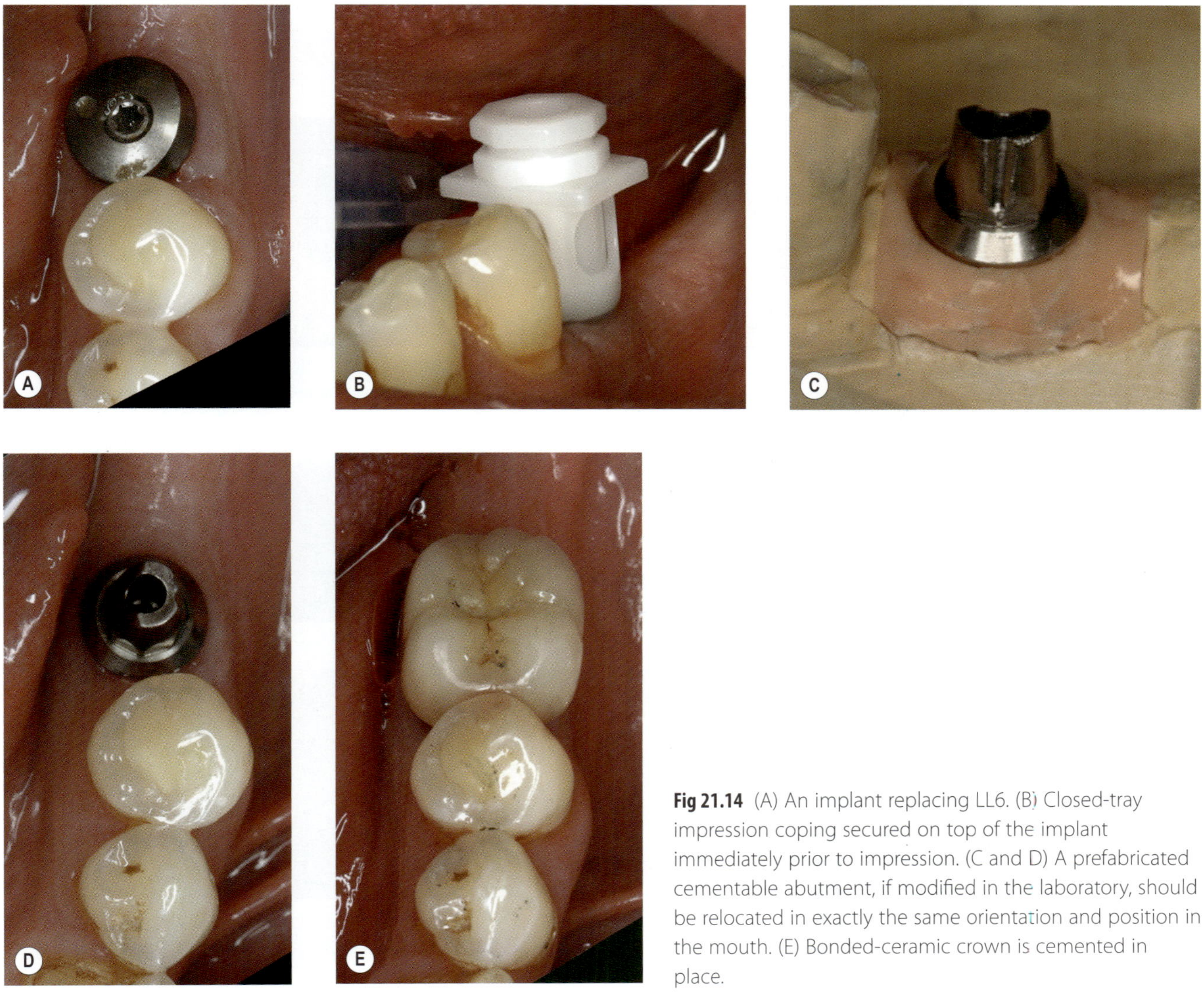

Fig 21.14 (A) An implant replacing LL6. (B) Closed-tray impression coping secured on top of the implant immediately prior to impression. (C and D) A prefabricated cementable abutment, if modified in the laboratory, should be relocated in exactly the same orientation and position in the mouth. (E) Bonded-ceramic crown is cemented in place.

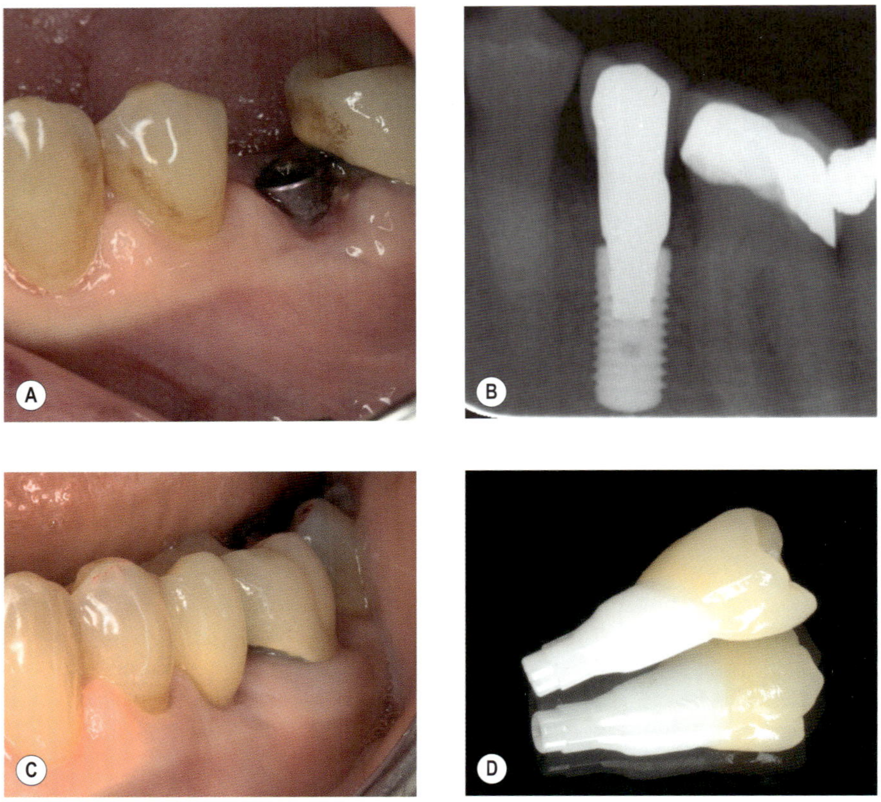

Fig 21.15 (A) Implant replacing LL5. (B) A periapical radiograph shows that the implant shoulder is subcrestal. (C and D) A screw-retained crown is fabricated in this case, and the ceramic is directly laminated on the zirconia abutment.

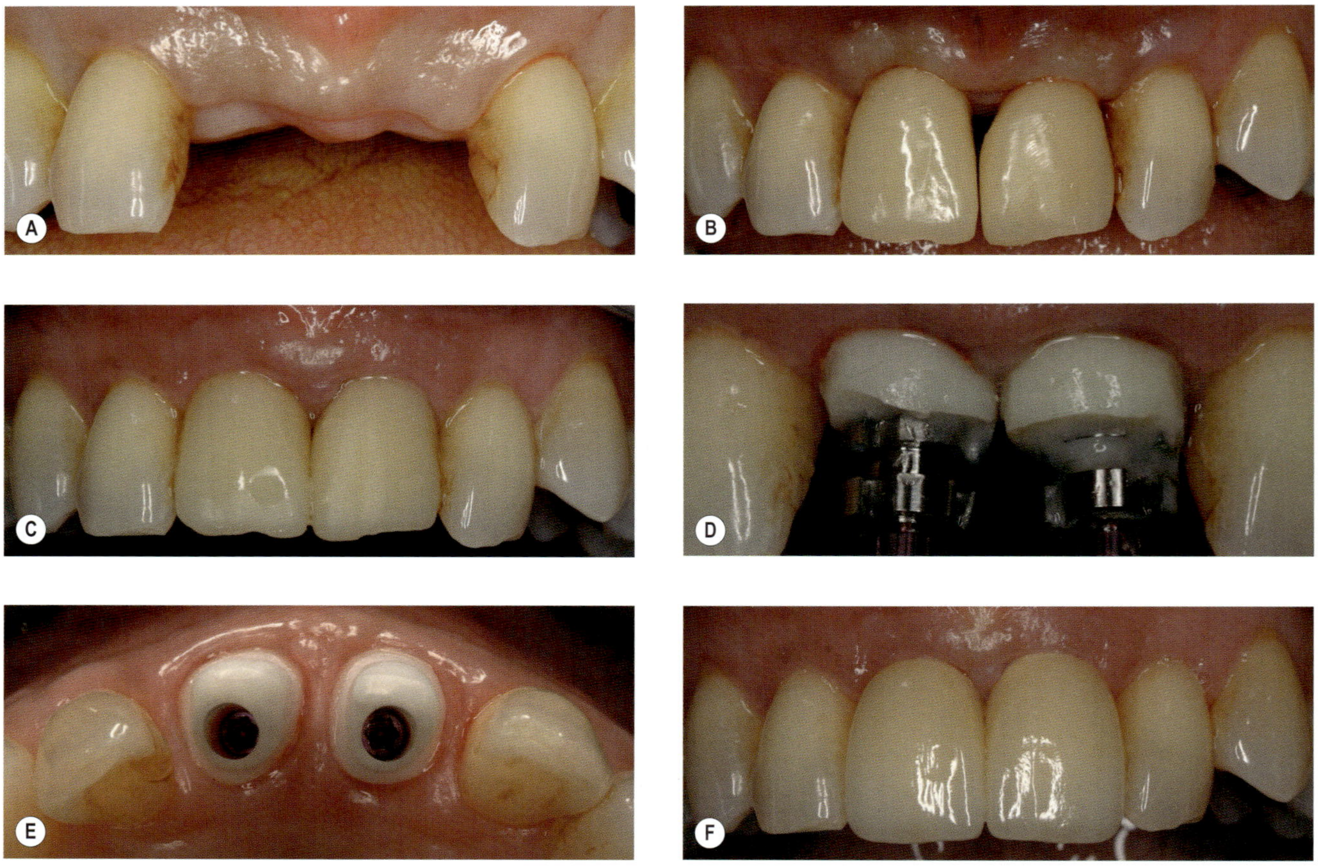

Fig 21.16 (A) Preoperative view of missing upper central incisors. (B and C) Provisional crowns used for peri-implant soft tissue moulding and optimization of pink aesthetics. (D) Impression copings are customized to copy the crown emergence. (E) Zirconia abutments are torqued to 35 N cm. (F) All-ceramic crowns replacing the two central incisors.

The angulation of the implant does not allow a screw-retained crown because the screw access hole is emerging close to the projected incisal edge. Therefore, a cement-retained crown is prescribed. A prefabricated abutment should not be selected because the cement margin will be subgingival. A customized abutment that will place the cement margin at or just below the gingival level should be designed. Furthermore, because the impression is customized, the size and shape of the transitional part of the abutment should closely conform to the size and space created in the emergence zone of the impression.

The abutment is inserted, and after confirming fit of the crown, it is tightened to the final recommended torque (Figure 21.16E). The screw access hole is sealed, and the crown is cemented in place (Figure 21.16F).

◇ *Anterior screw-retained crown*

A 30-year-old male patient had an implant placed to replace UR1 using an early delayed implant placement technique (Figure 21.17A). Following the implant exposure surgery, a provisional restoration was placed to mould the peri-implant soft tissues (Figure 21.17B). As described in the previous case, a customized impression technique was used to create an accurate impression of the clinical situation.

The screw access hole is ideally emerging through the cingulum, and the occlusion of the patient allows for a screw-retained crown. In this case, a UCLA-type castable abutment was used to provide a one-piece screw-retained crown (Figure 21.17C), resulting in a very natural-looking restoration (Figure 21.17D).

Alternatively, zirconia abutments can also be fabricated using CAD/CAM and ceramic laminated directly on the abutment (Figure 21.18).

What restorative options can be considered for an edentulous patient?

- Edentate
  - Removable
    - Locator and ball
    - Bar
    - Milled bar
  - Fixed
    - Screw retained
    - Cement retained

The assessment and a variety of treatment options were discussed in Chapter 17. Therefore, this section highlights a few clinical case examples only. In general, edentulous patients can be restored with either a removable or a fixed implant prosthesis. The most obvious determining factor is the number of available implants to support a prosthesis. Although two implants in the mandible and four in the maxilla are sufficient to support a removable overdenture, a greater number are required if a fixed prosthesis is desired.

Implant-retained removable overdenture options

◇ *Locator attachment*

A variety of attachment systems can be used to retain a removable implant overdenture. In recent years, the Locator attachment has become increasingly popular due to its ease of use and cost-effective long-term maintenance. The implants need to be reasonably parallel to each other to facilitate path of insertion. Locator attachments are available in different lengths, so an appropriate length is selected. The

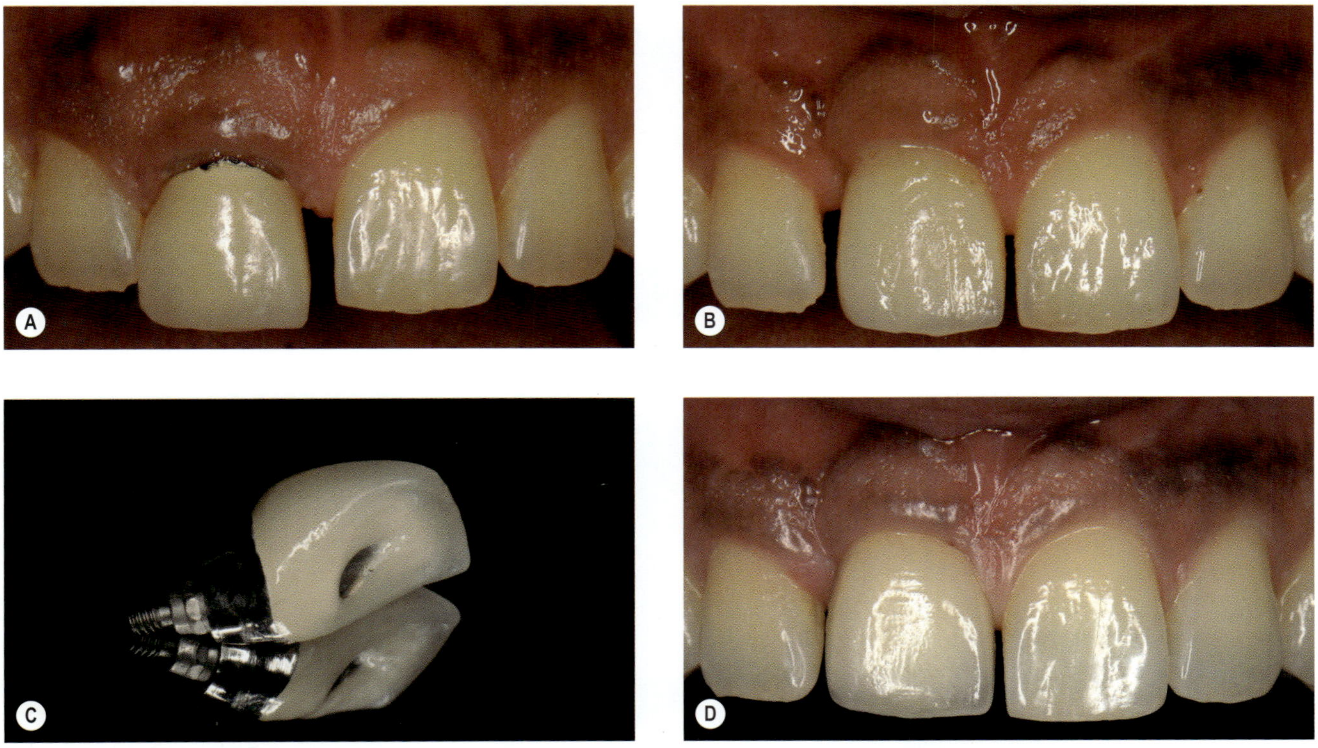

Fig 21.17 (A) A failing post–crown in UR1 is planned for replacement with dental implant. (B) Provisional crown allowed shaping optimal pink aesthetics. (C and D) One-piece screw-retained crown fabricated as definitive restoration.

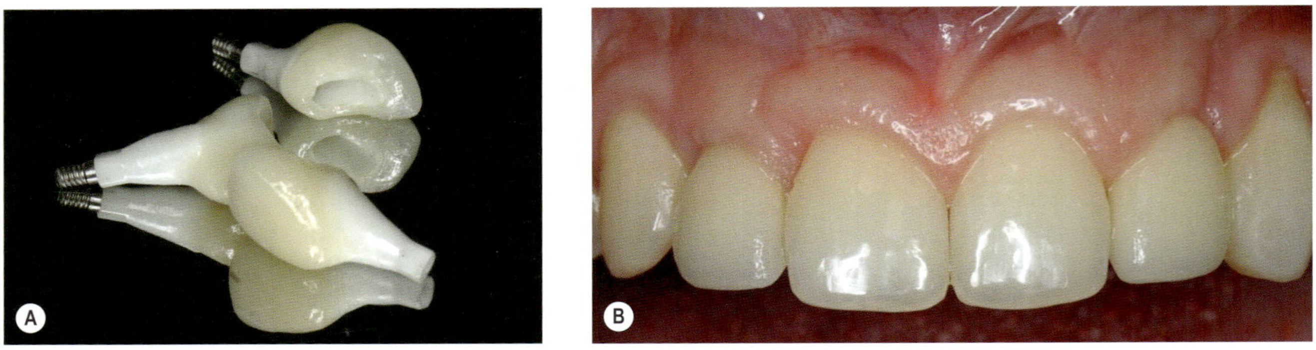

Fig 21.18 (A and B) Zirconia abutments have been laminated with ceramic to create screw-retained aesthetic restorations replacing the two lateral incisors.

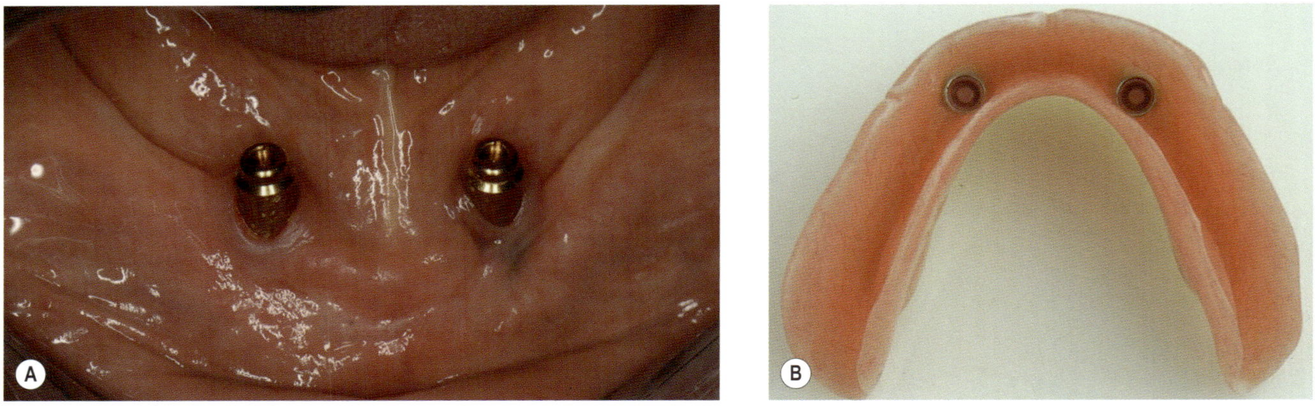

Fig 21.19 (A) Locator attachment on implants and (B) nylon male components within the denture.

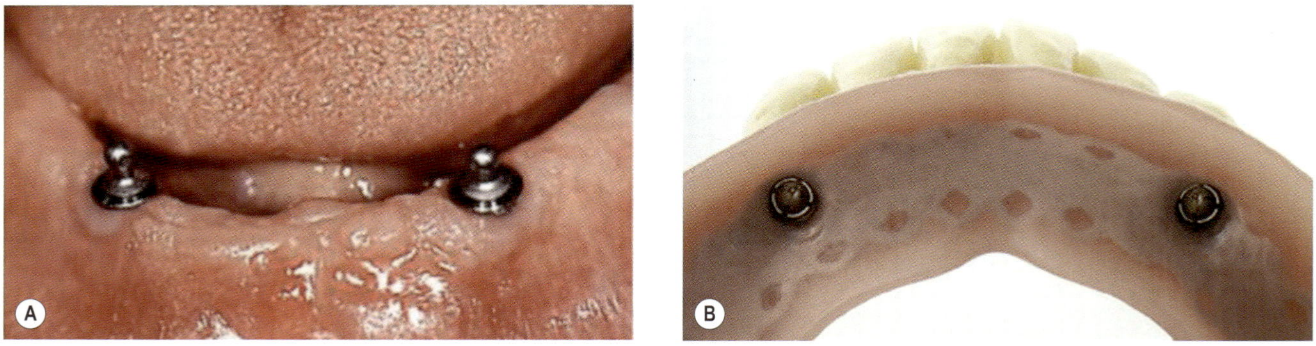

Fig 21.20 (A) Ball anchors or attachments secured on implants and (B) female matrices within the denture.

metal cap is incorporated within the denture into which a nylon male component is inserted (Figure 21.19A). The retention is derived from the nylon component, which engages the Locator on the implant (Figure 21.19B). In the future, when the nylon component wears, resulting in loss of retention, a new one can be easily inserted without having to replace the whole assembly, thereby resulting in cost-effective long-term maintenance.

Ball attachment

Among the nonsplinted group, a ball-type attachment is another popular attachment system. A ball anchor is attached to the implant (Figure 21.20A), and a female matrix is attached to the denture, providing retention (Figure 21.20B).

Bar attachment

The other alternative is to splint the two implants with a bar (Figure 21.21A) and have a matching female matrix within the denture to provide retention and stability to the overdenture (Figure 21.21B). This option can allow correction of nonparallel implants to some degree.

Milled bar

Occasionally, despite having adequate implants that could have supported a fixed prosthesis, it might become necessary to opt for a removable option. It may be necessary to provide adequate lip support with a denture flange, or the implant position and angulations may be inappropriate for a fixed prosthesis. In such cases, a milled bar can be fabricated to splint the implants together (Figure 21.22A), and the overdenture can gain significant support and retention from this milled bar. It may also be possible to minimize the palatal coverage of the denture (Figure 21.22B).

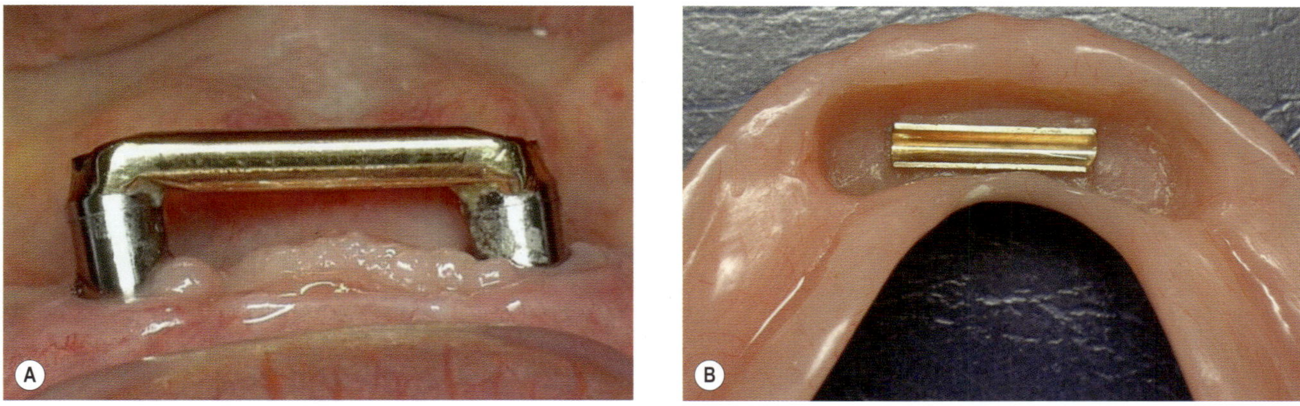

Fig 21.21 (A) A bar splinting the two implants and (B) a gold matrix within the denture that rides and clips around the bar to provide retention.

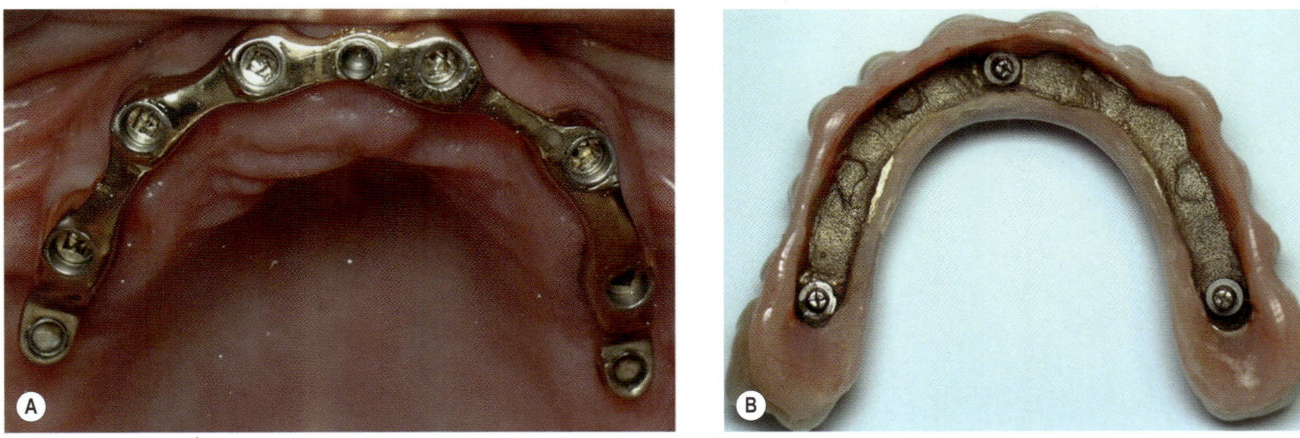

Fig 21.22 (A) A milled bar on six implants with (B) a minimal coverage maxillary prosthesis.

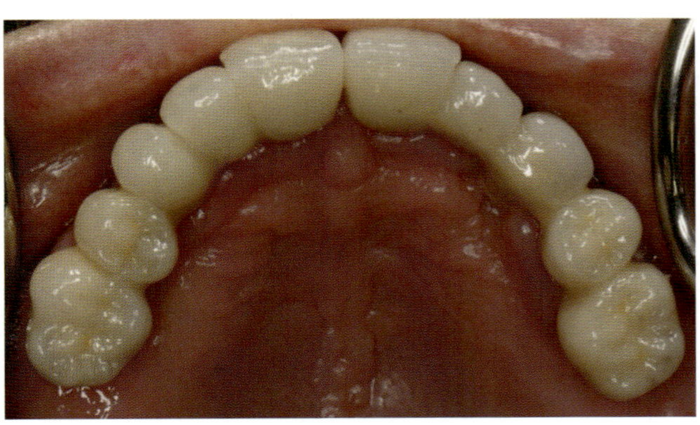

Fig 21.23 A cement-retained implant bridge on six implants in the maxilla.

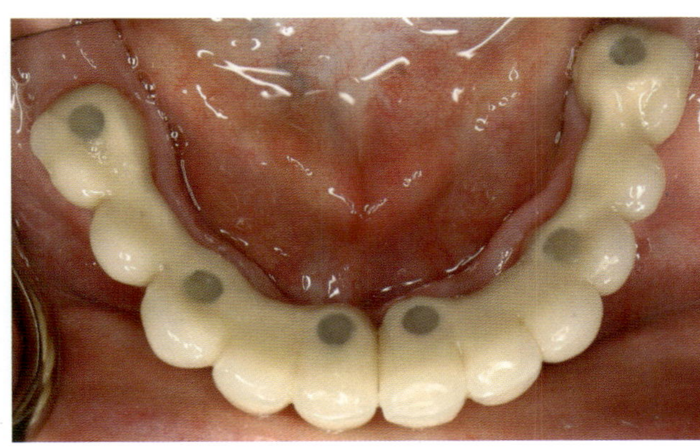

Fig 21.24 A screw-retained implant bridge on six implants in the mandible.

Implant-supported fixed prosthesis option

As a general rule, a minimum of six implants in the maxilla and four implants in the mandible are required to support a fixed bridge prosthesis. Furthermore, apart from correct positioning and angulation, various other factors should be considered, which were discussed in Chapter 16. A fixed prosthesis can be cemented (Figure 21.23) or screw retained (Figure 21.24). It places greater demands on the patient with regard to everyday cleaning and maintenance of implants, in addition to being a much costlier option.

Summary

Numerous techniques may be utilized to restore teeth using dental implants. Implant companies manufacture a vast array of abutments offering a multitude of treatment options. However, thorough presurgical planning and surgical execution is important to avoid restorative complications. The cases discussed in this chapter illustrate various clinical situations and how they can be successfully restored with dental implants.

Chapter 22

Implant failures

Implant placement has become a common procedure with predictable outcome and survival rates as high as 95% have been reported. This is true of single- or multiple-tooth replacements. Nonetheless, failures resulting in loss of implant do occur with consequential loss of intended treatment objectives, resulting in disappointment. From a patient's perspective, this involves additional treatment and associated costs.

The majority of implant failures tend to be early failures—either before a restoration is delivered or soon thereafter. Thereafter, the long-term failures are generally prosthetic phase failures or tend to occur as a result of marginal bone loss and infections.

Causes for implant failure include the following:

- Patient-related factors (underlying medical history, smoking, bone quality, and oral hygiene)
- Implant-related factors (implant surface, shape, location, etc.)
- Dentist-related factors (occlusal forces, loading protocol, ease of cleansing around the prosthesis, etc.)

This chapter briefly discusses how to monitor and maintain implant restorations. The chapter concludes with a series of clinical cases demonstrating implant failures due to various causes.

What is peri-implant disease? Describe its aetiology and discuss the recommended treatment

Peri-implant diseases usually refer to peri-implant mucositis and peri-implantitis. They represent the inflammatory lesions that develop around implants. Peri-implant mucositis is a reversible inflammation limited to the soft tissues, and if the condition is untreated, it may progress to peri-implantitis and extend into the supporting bone with loss of attachment around the implant.

The prevalence of peri-implant mucositis and peri-implantitis is high. Peri-implant mucositis occurs in approximately 80% of subjects (50% of sites) restored with implants and peri-implantitis in between 28 and 56% of subjects (12–40% of sites).

Implants should be reviewed on a regular basis. Patients should be advised to visit their dentist every 6 months to have their teeth and implants checked. Clinical probing using a light force of 0.25 N is essential for diagnosis of peri-implant diseases to identify signs of clinical inflammation in the peri-implant mucosa (i.e., bleeding on probing). Suppuration on probing is frequently associated with bone loss around an implant.

Accurate radiographs are required to help confirm a diagnosis of peri-implantitis, where loss of supporting peri-implant bone in the presence of clinical inflammation is noted.

As with periodontal disease, the aetiology of peri-implant mucositis and peri-implantitis is the bacterial biofilm. Modifying risk factors may also be involved—for example, patients with poor oral hygiene, inaccessibility for oral hygiene at implant restorations, smokers, and patients with a history of treated periodontitis who have an increased risk for peri-implantitis. High levels and proportions of Gram-negative anaerobic bacteria at sites with peri-implant mucositis and peri-implantitis have been reported.

Therefore, the treatment should be aimed at disruption or removal of bacterial biofilm and reduction in Gram-negative anaerobic species. Early treatment of peri-implant mucositis is highly desirable in order to limit the progression to peri-implantitis. The former responds well to mechanical nonsurgical therapy with concomitant improvement in oral hygiene maintenance.

On the contrary, peri-implantitis does not seem to respond equally well to mechanical nonsurgical therapy, with or without the use of adjunctive antiseptics or antibiotics. Depending on the extent and severity of bone loss, surgical access to debride the area might be necessary. Regenerative techniques with particulate bone graft materials along with a barrier membrane are performed to reconstruct the peri-implant bone defect. However, re-osseointegration of a contaminated implant surface is unpredictable and lacks scientific evidence.

Describe the various prosthetic complications and failures associated with implant restorations

Implant failures do not only relate to the actual loss of an implant fixture. One should remember that failure or complication associated with the prosthesis is also important. Therefore, at the outset, the patient should be informed about the long-term maintenance requirements, possible complications, and failures that may occur within the restoration.

The most common complications and failures include the following:

- Screw loosening
- Screw fracture
- Cementation failure
- Ceramic fracture

As described in Chapter 21, screws are used to attach the prosthetic components to the implant. Screw loosening has been reported as one of the most common and frustrating complications. Fortunately, this problem is easily resolved by re-tightening of the screw.

In contrast, screw fracture can pose a major challenge to the clinician. Although in the majority of instances, the apical part of the screw is quite loose to allow retrieval with a sharp probe, occasionally a special screw retrieval kit, specifically designed for each implant system, is required.

A cement-retained restoration is usually luted with a temporary (soft) cement. There is no pulp tissue in implants; hence, microleakage is not an issue. Use of soft cement allows easy removal of the restoration should this need arise due to screw loosening or fracture within the underlying abutment or implant. By their nature, such crowns or bridges occasionally debond and require recementation.

Ceramic fracture or delamination from the underlying metal or ceramic core is another common complication. Unlike teeth, implants are ankylosed to bone and therefore the damping or shock-absorbing effect of the periodontal ligament is lacking. Thus, any inadvertent occlusal impact can result in fracture or chipping of brittle ceramic restoration. Furthermore, if the underlying metal or zirconia substructure is not properly designed to provide optimal support for overlying ceramic, fracture or delamination may well ensue.

Removable implant prostheses are not immune to complications or failures either. In fact, research suggests that removable prostheses develop more complications and require a greater long-term maintenance in comparison to fixed prostheses in edentulous patients.

What are the common aesthetic failures when replacing teeth with dental implants?

Whereas achieving osseointegration is predictable with high long-term success and survival rates, achieving optimal aesthetic result remains a major challenge. The goal of the treatment is to provide an imperceptible restoration that matches the natural adjacent dentition.

In implant dentistry, the terms "pink" and "white" aesthetics are used. The former implies that the peri-implant tissue should be in harmony with the adjacent teeth. This includes the two papillae, facial mucosal height and contour, colour, and texture.

The white aesthetics, on the other hand, refers to the implant crown. This should be comparable to the natural tooth/teeth and includes parameters such as the size, shape, contour, texture, and colour of the restoration.

It is pertinent to reiterate that proper treatment planning and restoratively driven implant placement respecting the three dimensions of the bone and other tissues will avoid most aesthetic problems. It is also well documented that immediate placement of implants at the time of extraction results in more aesthetic failures, especially with greater mucosal recession and longer than intended clinical crowns. Insufficient labial bone thickness also results in greater recession and greyish hue of the soft tissue from underlying metal structure.

Therefore, thorough aesthetic risk assessment is recommended in order to manage each case based on individual needs. As a result, patient expectations can be accordingly managed at a very early stage.

Clinical case examples of implant failures

Case 1

LR6 has been replaced with two implants. The implants are converging and too close to each other (Figure 22.1). Usually, a single, larger-diameter implant is adequate to replace a molar. The radiograph confirms extensive bone loss (peri-implantitis) at both implants (Figure 22.2).

Case 2

On the LR5, there is evidence of excessive residual cement at the implant–abutment junction that has resulted in peri-implantitis (Figure 22.3).

Case 3

The implant replacing LL6 shows an intrabony, crater-like defect (Figure 22.4). Nearly half the bone support on this implant is lost. The crown on LL6 is overcontoured, thereby harbouring plaque at the gingival margin. Incidentally, secondary caries is also noted in the LL5.

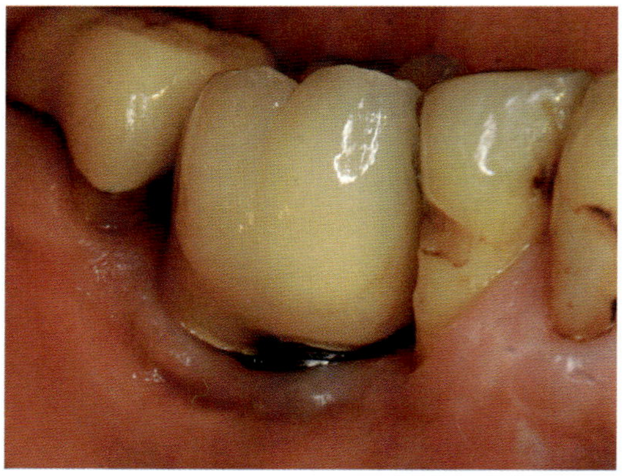

Fig 22.1 A lower molar replaced on two inappropriately placed implants.

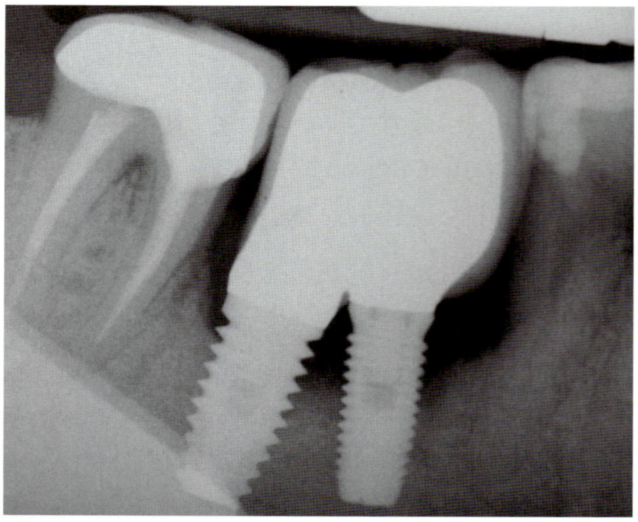

Fig 22.2 Radiograph shows that implants are converging, too close, and have lost between 25 and 50% bone support.

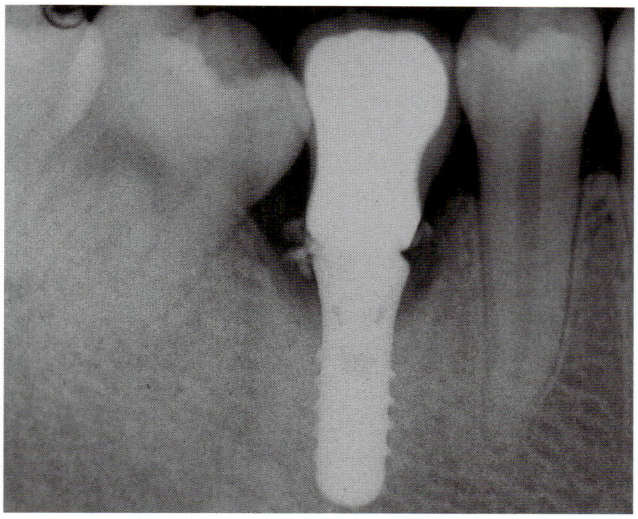

Fig 22.3 Radiograph of a lower premolar. The crown is not fully seated and excess cement residue is present, which has resulted in peri-implantitis.

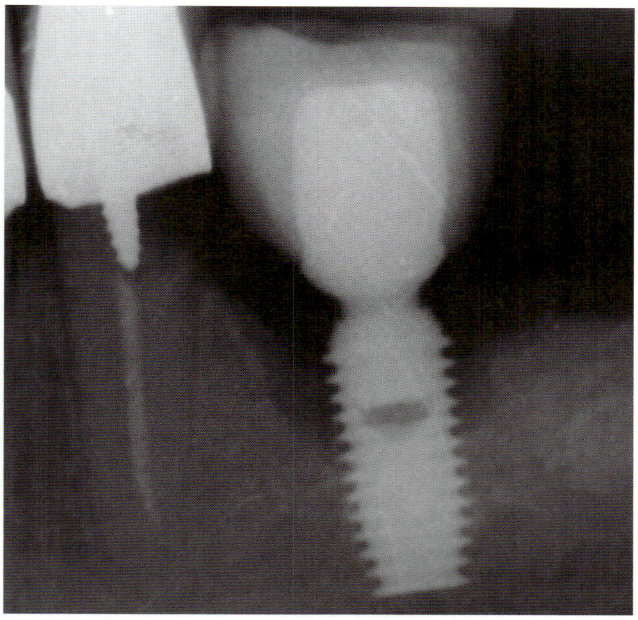

Fig 22.4 A lower molar with evidence of peri-implantitis and secondary caries in LL5.

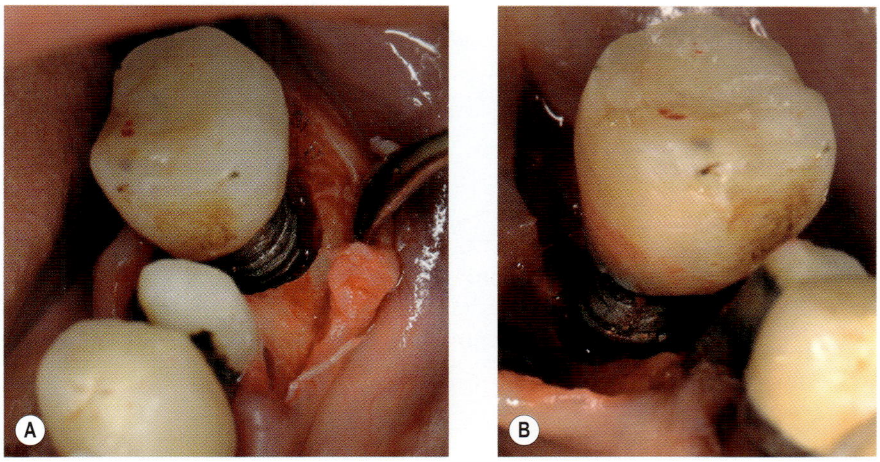

Fig 22.5 A circumferential crater-like defect with an intrabony component is noted at surgery.

Surgical exposure confirms the extensive peri-implant bone loss buccally (Figure 22.5A) and lingually (Figure 22.5B). The infected, granulation tissue was excavated and the implant thoroughly cleaned with 0.2% chlorhexidine. The defect was treated using a regenerative technique with bovine particulate bone and collagen barrier membrane (Figure 22.6). The cervical portion of the crown was recontoured to allow cleansibility.

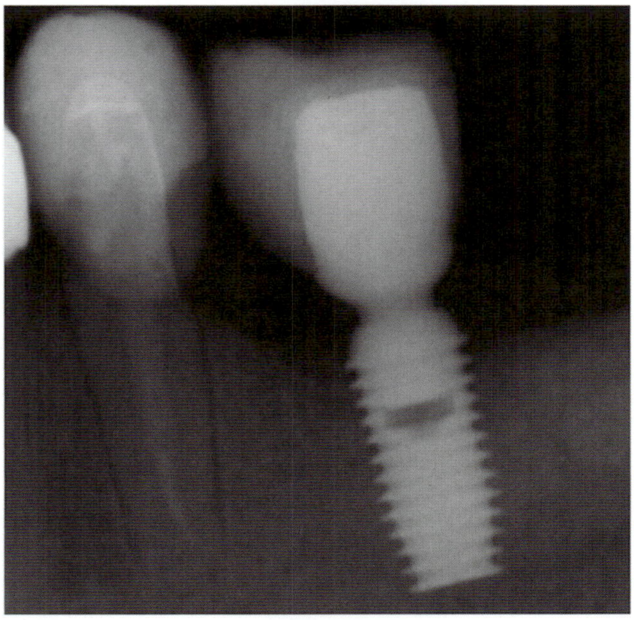

Fig 22.6 Following GBR, bone fill is noted within the intrabony component of the defect.

Case 4

There is an aesthetic failure in a patient with a three-unit anterior bridge on two implants in UR1 and UL2 (Figure 22.7). Pink-coloured ceramic has been used to correct the soft tissue deficiency and idealize the tooth size and shape. Metal of the implant collar is visible in UL2, with inflamed peri-implant mucosa and greyish hue shining from under the peri-implant soft tissues.

Case 5

A patient with congenitally missing lateral incisors lost UR1 due to trauma. The UR1 has been replaced with a dental implant. The implant crown has an approximately 2-mm recession, resulting in a longer-looking crown compared to UL1 (Figure 22.8A). This is due to the implant being deeper than necessary in apico-coronal dimension (Figure 22.8B).

Case 6

This case demonstrates a typical error by the clinician in poor positioning of the implant during its placement. The dental implant has been placed with the intention of replacing UR2. The implant shoulder (margin) is exposed with soft tissue deficiency. The implant is deep (Figure 22.9A) and too far labially placed (Figure 22.9B). The position of the implant will inevitably result in a poor aesthetic outcome.

Case 7

This case demonstrates peri-implantitis at UR1, resulting in a severely compromised aesthetic outcome. The peri-implant mucosa has receded, leaving the metal collar of the implant exposed (Figure 22.10A). The labial tissues are inflamed and swollen with deep pocketing. The radiograph reveals the extent of the peri-implant bone loss (Figure 22.10B).

Case 8

In this case, a three-unit screw-retained bridge has replaced teeth in the UL posterior region. Ceramic has fractured on the palatal aspect of the UL4 (Figure 22.11).

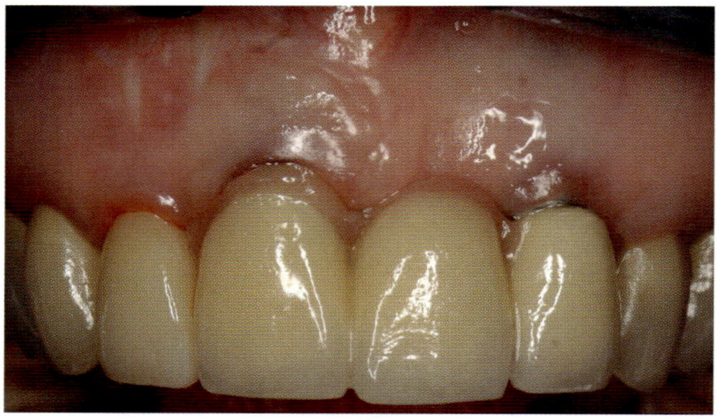

Fig 22.7 Compromised pink aesthetic outcome that has been masked with pink-coloured ceramic. Note the exposure of the implant fixture, resulting in unsightly aesthetic outcome.

Case 9

This case demonstrates an example of very poor rehabilitation with dental implants. In the anterior maxilla, the aesthetics are severely compromised (Figure 22.12A).

Implant in the LR1 and LR2 region is emerging through the embrasure space, which affects aesthetics and impairs access to cleaning (Figure 22.12B).

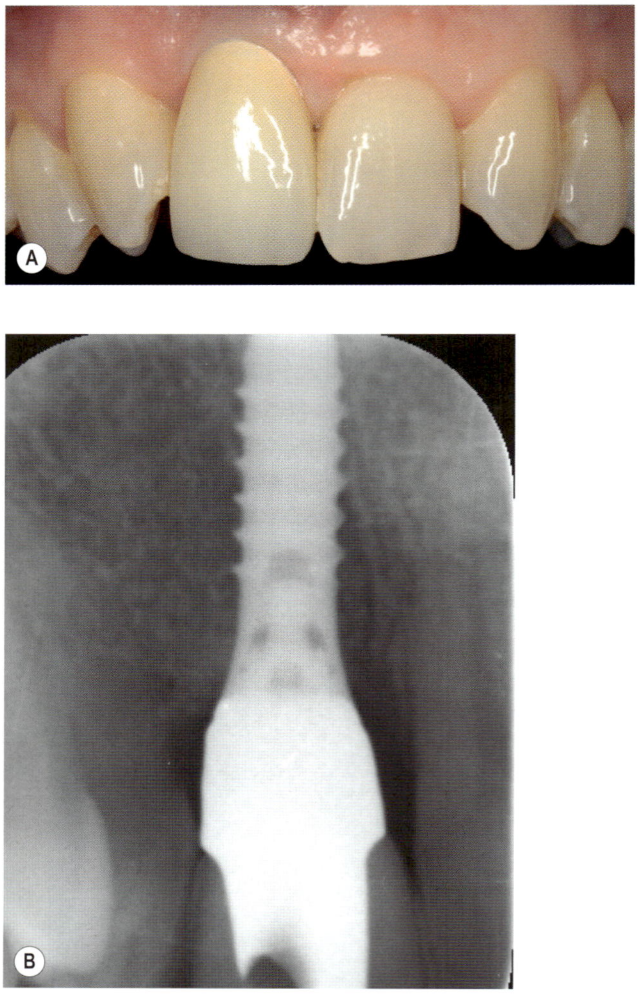

Fig 22.8 An implant that is too deep, resulting in recession and longer than intended crown.

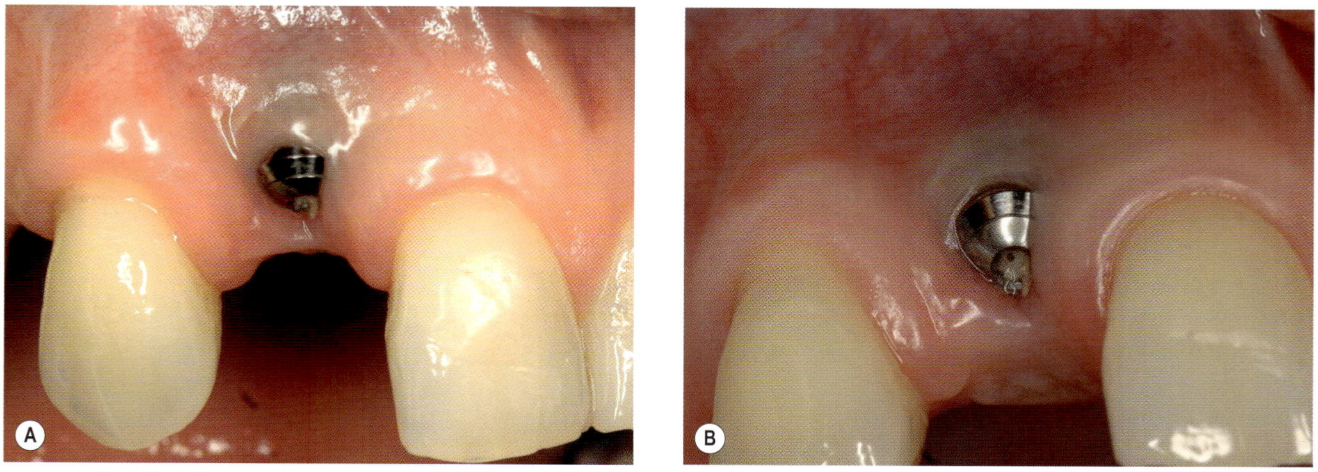

Fig 22.9 A deep and labially positioned implant will inevitably result in poor aesthetic outcome.

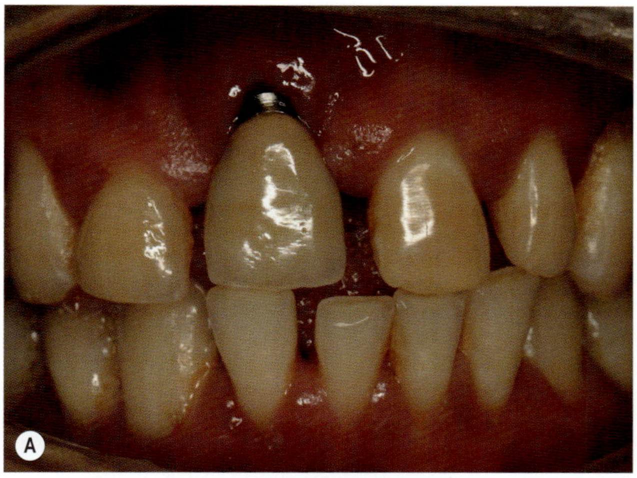

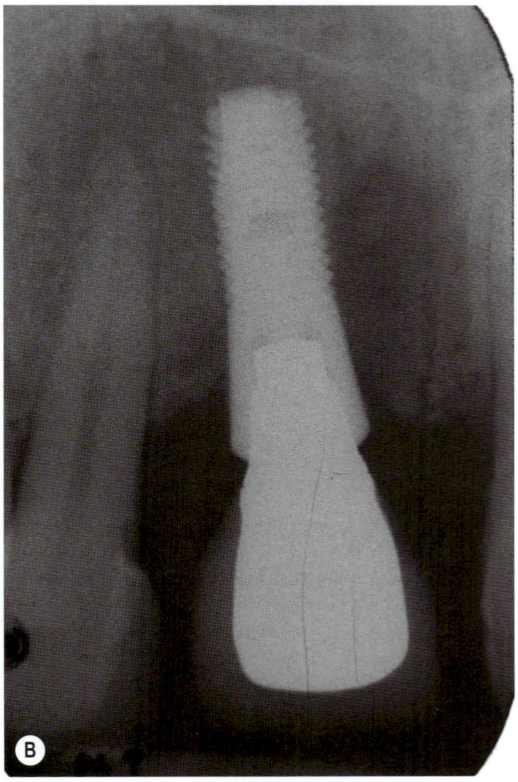

Fig 22.10 Malpositioned implant with peri-implantitis.

Most of the restorations have fractured ceramic and evidence of poor treatment outcome (Figure 22.12C). Exudation of pus is noted from LR5, confirming peri-implantitis (Figure 22.12D).

The orthopantomogram (Figure 22.13) shows a range of issues while confirming the extent of rehabilitation with implants. Complete loss of bone surrounding LR5 is noted. Peri-implantitis is also confirmed in LL3. Restoration misfit is evident in LL6.

Case 10

Maxillary arch reconstruction on dental implants in which severe peri-implant bone loss has resulted in a very unsightly outcome (Figure 22.14A). Most of the implants have lost nearly half of the bone support, resulting in exposure of rough implant surface (Figure 22.14B). A composite resin-based prosthesis has been provided. The implants in UL4 and UL5 have failed and have been removed.

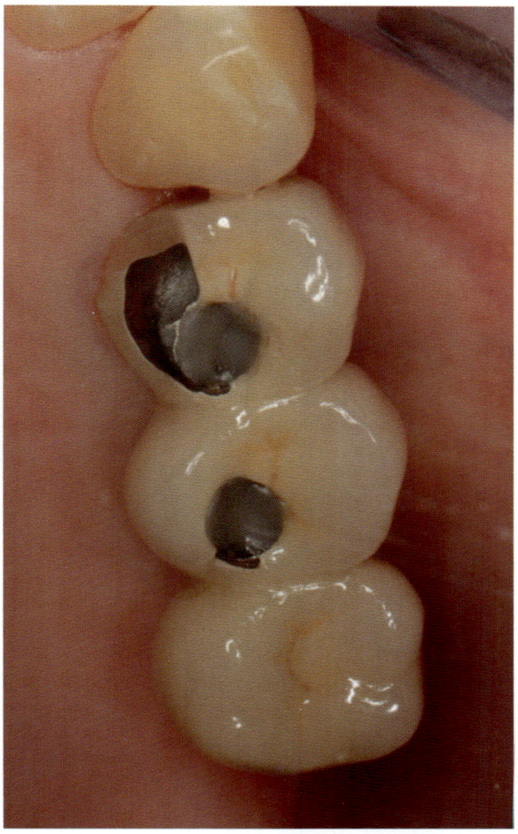

Fig 22.11 Delamination of ceramic from a three-unit implant bridge.

Case 11

A 72-year-old female patient was restored with three intraforaminal implants (Figure 22.15A) to support a mandibular overdenture. At 5-year review, initiation of peri-implantitis at the distal implant on the left side was evident (Figure 22.15B). During the next 5 years, this progressed to severe peri-implant crater-like bony defects (Figures 22.15C).

As the patient became older and frail, she lost manual dexterity to maintain oral hygiene around implants and underneath the denture, thereby increasing susceptibility to peri-implantitis (Figure 22.15D).

A fractured clip (seen in Figure 22.15D) is another common maintenance issue in implant-retained overdentures. Although these can be replaced chairside, they remain a nuisance.

Case 12

Implant-retained overdentures, and often fixed prostheses, are rehabilitated using artificial denture teeth that are used in conventional dentures. Irrespective of its mode of retention, the functional force in implant prosthesis is significantly higher compared to that in conventional dentures and is comparable to natural dentition. As a result, rapid functional wear of denture teeth is noticed, and in some cases this wear can occur within 2 or 3 years (Figure 22.16), thereby necessitating remake of prostheses. Such additional costs should be factored in and discussed with patients at the outset of treatment.

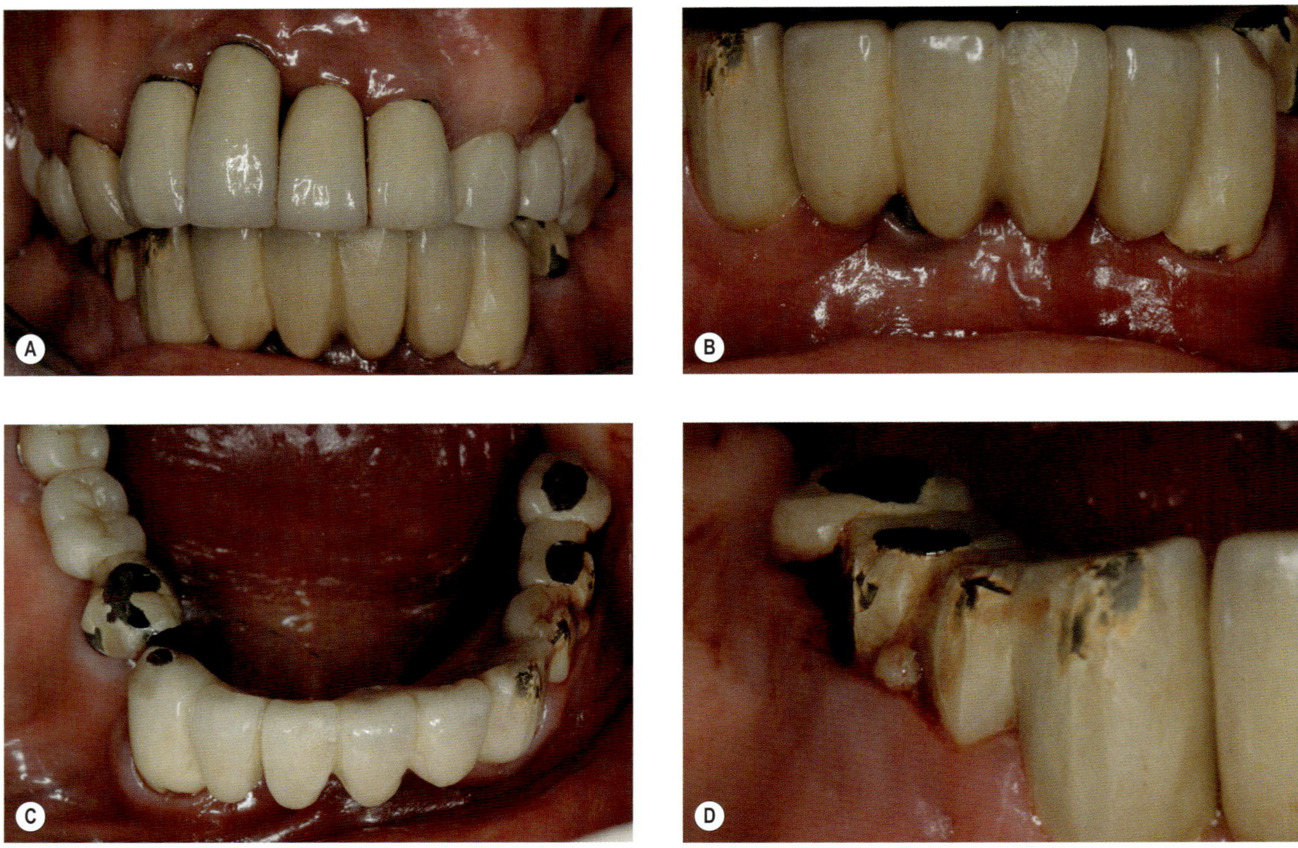

Fig 22.12 A case demonstrating poor clinical outcome. Several restorations are failing, including peri-implantitis and aesthetic failure.

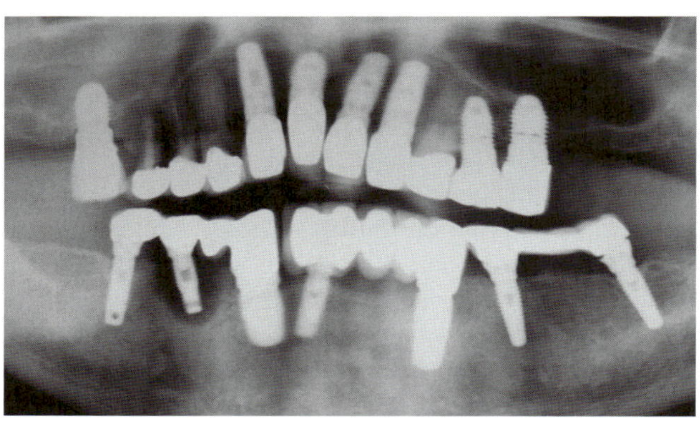

Fig 22.13 Orthopantomogram radiograph confirming a failed implant in LR5 and other implants showing peri-implantitis and misfitting prostheses.

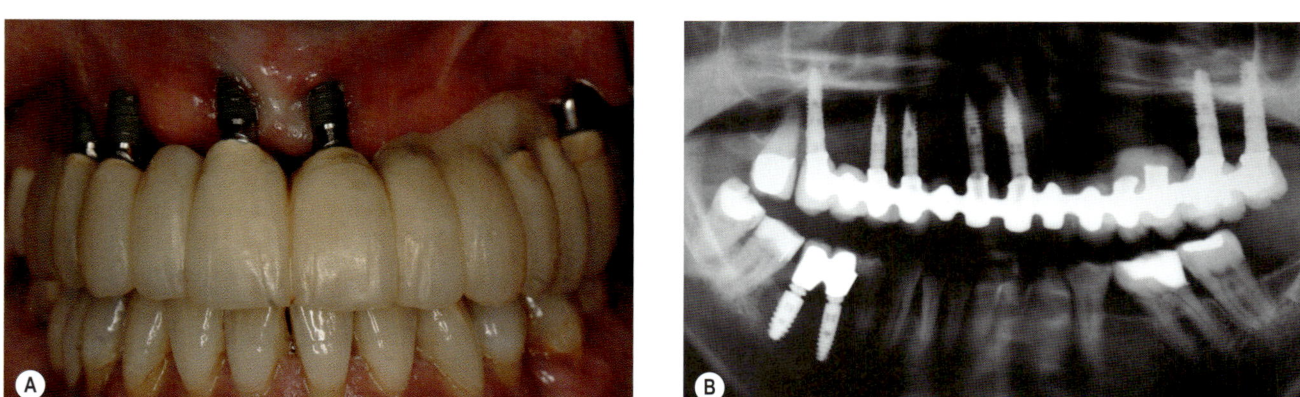

Fig 22.14 (A) A failing maxillary arch reconstruction with generalized peri-implantitis, and (B) radiograph confirms implants are already lost at UL4 and UL5 sites.

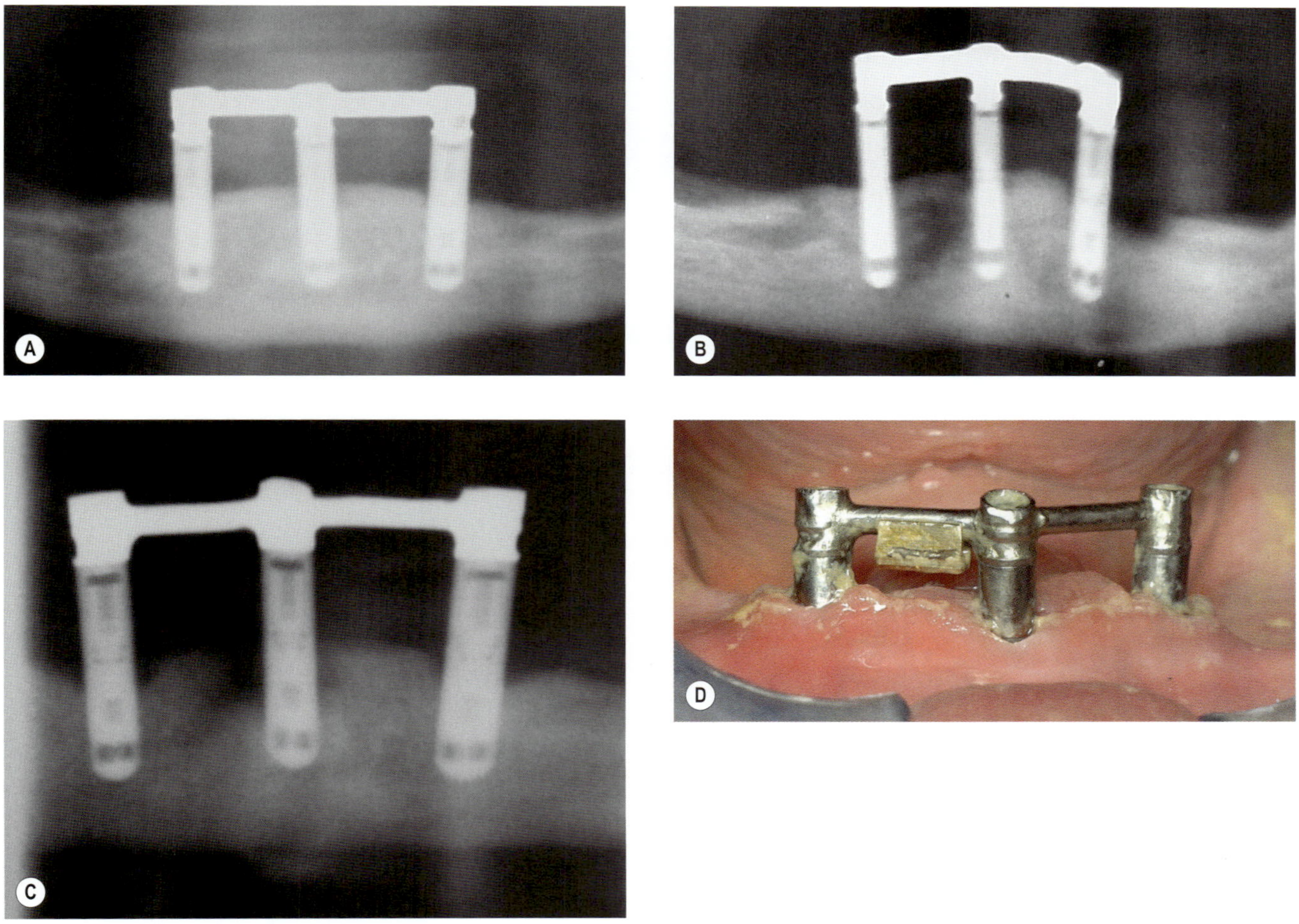

Fig 22.15 (A–C) Three radiographs taken 5 years apart showing progressive peri-implant bone loss. (D) Clinically, poor oral hygiene and inflamed peri-implant soft tissues are noted.

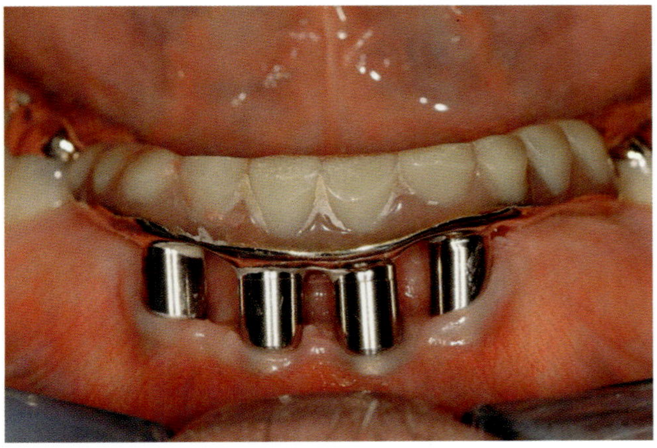

Fig 22.16 A fixed implant prosthesis with severe wear of denture teeth.

Summary

The preceding chapters focused on assessment, treatment planning, and delivery of successful implant treatment. It is a misconception that "implants are for life." The cases in this chapter demonstrate several causes of complications and failure of implants and their restorations. It is true that thorough planning will avoid most of the complications; however, it is equally true that long-term maintenance is necessary to avoid catastrophic failures. Patient compliance, excellent oral hygiene, and regular recall appointments are recommended for ensuring lasting success.

Further reading

We have provided a list of references for further reading. These include a number of standard (fully referenced) textbooks, together with a number of specific journal references and URLs that include some important primary studies together with a number of both systematic and narrative reviews of specific topics.

Additional textbooks

Buser, D., Belser, U.C., Wismeijer, D. (Eds.), 2007. ITI Treatment Guide: Volume 1. Implant Therapy in the Esthetic Zone: Single-Tooth Replacements. Quintessence, Berlin, pp. 9–24.

Cawson, R.A., Odell, E.W., 2008. Cawson's Essentials of Oral Pathology and Oral Medicine, 8th edn. Churchill Livingstone, New York.

Dawson, A., Chen, S. (Eds.), 2009. The SAC Classification in Implant Dentistry. Quintessence, Berlin.

Lindhe, J., Lang, N.P., Karring, T., 2008. Clinical Periodontology and Implant Dentistry, 5th edn. Wiley-Blackwell, New York.

Newman, M.G., Takei, H., Klokkevold, P.R., Carranza, F.A., 2011. Carranza's Clinical Periodontology, 11th edn. Elsevier, Philadelphia.

Wolf, H., Rateitschak-Pluss, E., 2005. Color Atlas of Dental Medicine: Periodontology, 3rd edn. Georg Thieme Verlag, New York.

Section 1. Periodontal assessment and diagnosis

Armitage, G.C., 1999. Development of a classification system for periodontal diseases and conditions. Ann. Periodontol. 4, 1–6.

Bergstrom, J., 2003. Tobacco smoking and risk for periodontal disease. J. Clin. Periodontol. 30, 107–113.

Bouchard, P., Boutouyrie, P., D'Aiuto, F., Deanfield, J., Deliargyris, E., Fernandez-Avilés, F., et al., 2010. European workshop in periodontal health and cardiovascular disease. Eur. Heart J. Suppl. 12 (Suppl. B), B13–B22.

British Society of Periodontology, 2011. Basic periodontal examination. http://www.bsperio.org.uk/publications/index.php.

Chambrone, L., Chambrone, D., Lima, L.A., Chambrone, L.A., 2010. Predictors of tooth loss during long-term periodontal maintenance: A systematic review of observational studies. J. Clin. Periodontol. 37, 675–684.

Garcia, R.I., Nunn, M.E., Dietrich, T., 2009. Risk calculation and periodontal outcomes. Periodontol. 2000 50, 65–77.

Haubek, D., Ennibi, O.K., Poulsen, K., Vaeth, M., Poulsen, S., Kilian, M., 2008. Risk of aggressive periodontitis in adolescent carriers of the JP2 clone of Aggregatibacter (Actinobacillus) actinomycetemcomitans in Morocco: A prospective longitudinal cohort study. Lancet 371, 237–242.

Michalowicz, B.S., Aeppli, D., Virag, J.G., Klump, D.G., Hinrichs, J.E., Segal, N.L., et al., 1991. Periodontal findings in adult twins. J. Periodontol. 62, 293–299.

National Institute for Health and Clinical Excellence, 2006. Brief interventions and referral for smoking cessation in primary care and other settings. http://guidance.nice.org.uk/PH1.

Pihlstrom, B.L., 2001. Periodontal risk assessment, diagnosis and treatment planning. Periodontol. 2000 25, 37–58.

Simpson, T.C., Needleman, I., Wild, S.H., Moles, D.R., Mills, E.J., 2010. Treatment of periodontal disease for glycaemic control in people with diabetes. Cochrane Database Syst. Rev., CD004714.

UK Department of Health, 2009. Adult dental health survey. http://www.ic.nhs.uk/statistics-and-data-collections/primary-care/dentistry.

Section 2. Periodontal treatment

Axelsson, P., Lindhe, J., 1981. Effect of controlled oral hygiene procedures on caries and periodontal disease in adults: Results after 6 years. J. Clin. Periodontol. 8, 239–248.

Axelsson, P., Nystrom, B., Lindhe, J., 2004. The long-term effect of a plaque control program on tooth mortality, caries and periodontal disease in adults: Results after 30 years of maintenance. J. Clin. Periodontol. 31, 749–757.

Cairo, F., Pagliaro, U., Nieri, M., 2008. Treatment of gingival recession with coronally advanced flap procedures: A systematic review. J. Clin. Periodontol. 35, 136–162.

Esposito, M., Grusovin, M.G., Papanikolaou, N., Coulthard, P., Worthington, H.V., 2009. Enamel matrix derivative (Emdogain(R)) for periodontal tissue regeneration in intrabony defects. Cochrane Database Syst. Rev., CD003875.

Herrera, D., Alonso, B., Leon, R., Roldan, S., Sanz, M., 2008. Antimicrobial therapy in periodontitis: The use of systemic antimicrobials against the subgingival biofilm. J. Clin. Periodontol. 35, 45–66.

Needleman, I.G., Worthington, H.V., Giedrys-Leeper, E., Tucker, R.J., 2006. Guided tissue regeneration for periodontal infra-bony defects. Cochrane Database Syst. Rev., CD001724.

Pihlstrom, B.L., McHugh, R.B., Oliphant, T.H., Ortiz-Campos, C., 1983. Comparison of surgical and nonsurgical treatment of periodontal disease: A review of current studies and additional results after 6 1/2 years. J. Clin. Periodontol. 10, 524–541.

Ramfjord, S.P., Caffesse, R.G., Morrison, E.C., Hill, R.W., Kerry, G.J., Appleberry, E.A., et al., 1987. 4 modalities of periodontal treatment compared over 5 years. J. Clin. Periodontol. 14, 445–452.

Section 3. Introduction to dental implantology

Berglundh, T., Zitzmann, N.U., Donati, M., 2011. Are peri-implantitis lesions different from periodontitis lesions? J. Clin. Periodontol. 38, 188–202.

Bornstein, M.M., Cionca, N., Mombelli, A., 2009. Systemic conditions and treatments as risks for implant therapy. Int. J. Oral Maxillofacial Implants 24 (Suppl.), 12–27.

Cavalcanti, R., Oreglia, F., Manfredonia, M.F., Gianserra, R., Esposito, M., 2011. The influence of smoking on the survival of dental implants: A 5-year pragmatic multicentre retrospective cohort study of 1727 patients. Eur. J. Oral Implantol. 4, 39–45.

Flemmig, T.F., Beikler, T., 2009. Decision making in implant dentistry: An evidence-based and decision-analysis approach. Periodontol. 2000 50, 154–172.

Jung, R.E., Pjetursson, B.E., Glauser, R., Zembic, A., Zwahlen, M., Lang, N.P., 2008. A systematic review of the 5-year survival and complication rates of implant-supported single crowns. Clin. Oral Implants Res. 19 (2), 119–130.

Martin, W., Lewis, E., Nicol, A., 2009. Local risk factors for implant therapy. Int. J. Oral Maxillofacial Implants 24 (Suppl.), 28–38.

Pjetursson, B., Lang, N., 2007. Prosthetic treatment planning on the basis of scientific evidence. J. Oral Rehabil. 35 (S1), 72–79.

Renvert, S., Polyzois, I., Claffey, N., 2011. How do implant surface characteristics influence peri-implant disease? Surface characteristics and peri-implantitis. J. Clin. Periodontol. 38, 214–222.

Zitmann, N.U., Margolin, M.D., Filippi, A., Weiger, R., Krastl, G., 2008. Patient assessment and diagnosis in implant treatment. Aust. Dent. J. 53 (1 Suppl.), S3–S10.

Index

Page numbers followed by "f" indicate figures and "t" indicate tables.

C

R